INFLAMMATORY DISEASES – A MODERN PERSPECTIVE

Edited by **Amit Nagal**

Inflammatory Diseases – A Modern Perspective
Edited by Amit Nagal

Published by InTech

Janeza Trdine 9, 51000 Rijeka, Croatia

Publishing Process Manager Marko Rebrovic

Technical Editor Teodora Smiljanic

Cover Designer InTech Design Team

Additional hard copies can be obtained from orders@intechopen.com

Inflammatory Diseases – A Modern Perspective, Edited by Amit Nagal
p. cm.
ISBN 978-953-307-444-3

For EU product safety concerns:
IN TECH d.o.o., Prolaz Marije Krucifikse Kozulić 3, 51000 Rijeka, Croatia, info@intechopen.com or visit our website at intechopen.com.

Meet the editor

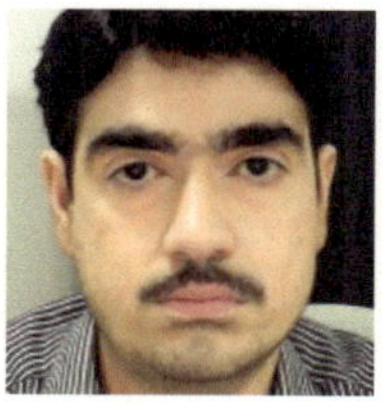

Dr. Amit Nagal is a Bioinformatics scientist in the area of rational drug design and Next- generation sequencing data analysis. He is currently working in Ocimum Biosolution, India and has several years of experience in this field. So far he had published several papers in peer reviewed journals and has presented on many international symposiums. Dr. Nagal has done his thesis on computational and molecular aspects of lens regeneration under the influence of retinoid, explaining how retinoid and their derivatives interact with Retinoid X receptor (Rxr alpha) and in line with that he developed lens regeneration tools and a database. He also worked on development of Target and lead based modern lead designing pipeline where he used a novel QSAR ranking method with help of a support vector machine algorithm to classify scaffold and their biological activity. The main aim of this project is to develop a unique platform in the area of computer aided molecule design. Currently he is working on Next-generation sequencing data analysis and he is a member of ISCB and HUGO organization.

Contents

Preface

"Inflammatory Diseases – A Modern Perspective" represents an extended and thoroughly revised collection of papers on inflammation. This book explores a wide range of topics relevant to inflammation and inflammatory diseases while its main objective is to help in understanding the molecular mechanism and a concrete review of inflammation. One of the interesting things about this book is its diversity in topics which include pharmacology, medicine, rational drug design, microbiology and biochemistry. Each topic focuses on inflammation and its related disease thus giving a unique platform which integrates all the useful information regarding inflammation.

About the Contents

Chapter 1 contains an introduction to Urinary trypsin inhibitor (UTI), a serine protease inhibitor which is found to be a good therapeutic option for endotoxin-related inflammatory disorders such as DIC, acute lung injury in targeted mice model.

Chapter 2 concerns structure based molecule design approaches and comparative docking studies of various hnps-PLA2 indole inhibitor derivatives. In this study they proved that molecule 13h could be a novel anti-inflammatory drug.

Chapter 3 formally supports a model wherein Th1 and IL-17^{+} T cells mechanistically interact and collaboratively contribute to BD skin pathogenesis. This is found to be a beneficial for further study in Behcet's disease skin lesions

Chapter 4 contains a review of the most Activate Protein C role in inflammatory disease

Chapter 5 is devoted to the formal theory of role and expression TrkA receptor in the pulmonary hypertension. This chapter well explains the importance of TrkA receptor.

Chapter 6 concerns review of cytokines, their major role in chronic inflammatory diseases and cancers and it also elucidates challenge and significance of the cytokinome profile.

Chapter 7 examines Periodontal Inflammation as Risk Factor for Pancreatic Diseases. It also explores and investigates pancreatic tissue for the potential presence of periodontopathogenic microorganisms.

Chapter 8 is entirely devoted to Polyunsaturated fatty acids. It well explains that they play critical roles in physiologic and pathophysiologic processes involving the immune system and have the ability to alter cellular responses as free fatty acids, most interest is on the properties of the array of metabolic products which they generate. These form a regulatory network which either down or up-regulates the inflammatory reaction.

Chapter 9 concerns the importance of asthma especially scientific knowledge which can help to address how and why this condition occurs and may contribute to a better understanding of the classification of each asthma patient.

Chapter 10 is discussion of the functional and structural characterization of AC0T7 in macrophages and their role in inflammation.

Chapter 11 contains interesting observations of dietary n-3 PUFA and n-3 PUFA-rich food such as salmon which plays crucial role to reduce inflammatory bowel disease.

Amit Nagal, PhD
Bioinformatics Analyst Ocimum Biosolution, Hyderabad,
India

Part 1

Urinary Trypsin Inhibitor

1

Urinary Trypsin Inhibitor, an Alternative Therapeutic Option for Inflammatory Disorders

Ken-ichiro Inoue[1] and Hirohisa Takano[2]
[1]*Department of Public Health and Molecular Toxicology, School of Pharmacy, Kitasato University, Tokyo*
[2]*Kyoto University Graduate School of Enginnering, Department of Environmental Engineering, Kyoto*
Japan

1. Introduction

Urinary trypsin inhibitor (UTI), a serine protease inhibitor, has been widely (and sometimes experiencely) used as a supportive drug for patients with inflammatory disorders such as pancreatitis, shock, and disseminated intravascular coagulation (DIC). Also, previous in vitro studies have demonstrated that serine protease inhibitors may have anti-inflammatory properties at sites of inflammation. However, the therapeutic effects of UTI in vivo remain unclarified, since commercial UTI have been developed to act against human, with the activity and selectivity toward the relevant animal UTI being less characterized. In this review, we introduce the roles of UTI mainly in experimental endotoxin (lipopolysaccharide: LPS)-related inflammatory disorders using UTI-deficient (-/-) and corresponding wild-type (WT) mice. Our experiments employing genetic approach suggest that endogenous UTI can serve protection against the systemic inflammatory response and subsequent organ injury induced by LPS, at least partly, through the inhibition of proinflammatory cytokine and chemokine expression, which provide important in vivo evidence and understanding about a protective role of UTI in inflammatory conditions. Using genetically targeted mice selectively lacking UTI, UTI has been evidenced to provide an attractive "rescue" therapeutic option for endotoxin-related inflammatory disorders such as DIC, acute lung injury, and acute liver injury.

2. General characteristics of UTI and clinical utility

UTI, also referred to as ulinastatin, HI-30, ASPI, or bikunin, is an acidic glycoprotein with a molecular weight of 30 kDa by SDS-polyacrylamide gel electrophoresis. UTI is a multivalent Kunitz-type serine protease inhibitor found in human urine and blood [1]. It is composed of 143 amino acid residues and its sequence includes two Kunitz-type domains (Fig. 1). UTI is produced by hepatocytes as a precursor in which UTI is linked to α_1-microgloblin [2, 3]. In hepatocytes, different types of UTI-containing proteins are formed by the assembly of UTI with one or two of the three evolutionarily related heavy chains (HC) 1, HC 2, and HC 3, through a chondroitin sulfate chain [4]; these proteins comprise inter-α-inhibitor (IαI) family members, including IαI, pre-α-inhibitor (PαI), inter-α-like inhibitor (IαLI), and free UTI. IαI, pαI, and IαLI are composed of HC1 + HC2 + UTI, HC3 + UTI, and HC2 + UTI, respectively [5, 6]. Its specific activity was 2,613 U/mg protein, one unit being the amount necessary to inhibit the activity of 2μg trypsin (3,200 NFU/mg, Canada Packers) by 50% [7]. During inflammation, UTI is cleaved from IαI family proteins through proteolytic cleavage by neutrophil elastase in the peripheral circulation or at the inflammatory site [8-11]. Therefore, plasma UTI has been considered to be one of the acute phase reactions and indeed, the plasma UTI level and its gene expression alter in severe inflammatory conditions [9]. Further, UTI is rapidly released into urine when infection occurs and is an excellent inflammatory marker, constituting most of the urinary anti-trypsin activity [12]. Various serine proteases such as trypsin, thrombin, chymotrypsin, kallikrein, plasmin,

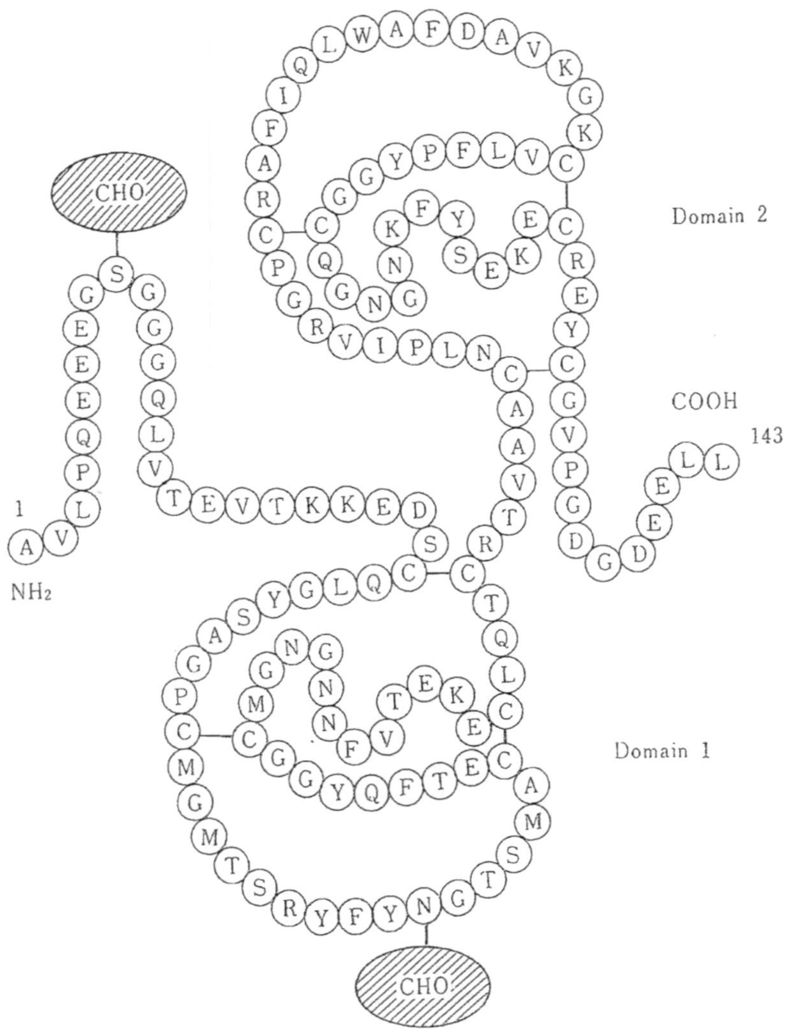

Fig. 1. Molecular structure of urinary trypsin inhibitor (UTI).

chymotrypsin, kallikrein, plasmin, elastase, cathepsin, and Factors IXa, Xa, XIa, and XIIa are inhibited by UTI [13, 14]. Furthermore, UTI can reportedly suppress urokinase-type plasminogen activator (uPA) expression through the inhibition of protein kinase C (PKC) [15, 16]. UTI appears to prevent organ injury by inhibiting the activity of these proteases [17, 18]. Based on the multivalent nature of protease inhibition, clinically, UTI is widely used, especially in Japan, to treat acute pancreatitis including post-endoscopic retrograde cholangiopancreatography pancreatitis, in which proteases are thought to play a pathophysiological role [19]; however, current understanding as for the target mechanisms/pathways remains limited.

3. Anti-inflammatory potential of UTI in *in vitro*, *in vivo*, and humans

Beyond its inhibition of inflammatory proteases mentioned above, UTI exhibits anti-inflammatory activity and suppresses the infiltration of neutrophils and release of elastase and chemical mediators from them [11, 20, 21]. Likewise, UTI reportedly inhibits the production of tumor necrosis factor (TNF)-α[22, 23] and interleukin (IL)-1 [23] in LPS-stimulated human monocytes and LPS- or neutrophil elastase-stimulated IL-8 gene expression in HL60 cells [24] or bronchial epithelial cells [25] *in vitro*. Matsuzaki et al. demonstrated that UTI inhibits LPS-induced TNF-α and subsequent IL-1β and IL-6 induction by macrophages, at least partly, through the suppression of mitogen-activated protein kinase (MAPK) signaling pathways such as ERK1/2, JNK, and p38 *in vitro* [26]. Nakatani and colleagues demonstrated that UTI inhibits neutrophil-mediated endothelial cell injury *in vitro*, suggesting that UTI can act directly/indirectly on neutrophils and suppress the production and secretion of activated elastase from them [21]. Furthermore, UTI down-regulates stimulated arachidonic acid metabolism such as thromboxane B2 production *in vitro* [27], which plays a role in the pathogenesis of sepsis [28].

A large number of *in vivo* reports have provided evidence that UTI protects against pathological traits related to septic shock induced by gram-negative bacteria: UTI reduces LPS-elicited circulatory failure such as hypotension, lactic acidosis, and hyperglycemia [29-31] through modulating TNF-α production via the inhibition of early growth response factor (Egr)-1 in monocytes and pulmonary induction of inducible nitric oxide synthase (iNOS) [29] and reduces mortality caused by sepsis [32]. Also, UTI can alleviate coagulatory disturbance accompanied by sepsis such as an increase in the serum level of fibrinogen and fibrinogen degradation products [33]. Likewise, UTI has a protective effect against ischemia-reperfusion injury in the liver [35], kidney [36], heart [37], and lung [38] *in vivo* via the actions of its radical scavenging elements [39]. As for its mechanism, UTI reduces C-X-C chemotactic molecule production during liver ischemia/reperfusion *in vivo* [40]. In humans, prepump administration (5,000 U/kg) of UTI reportedly improves cardiopulmonary bypass-induced hemodynamic instability and pulmonary dysfunction through the attenuation of IL-6 and IL-8 production/release in humans [41]. Also, UTI can inhibit coagulatory activation accompanied by severe inflammation such as tissue factor (TF) expression on monocytes *in vitro* and *in vivo* [33] as well as coagulation and fibrinolysis during surgery in humans [42].

Koizumi et al. have shown that UTI prevents experimental crescentic glomerulonephritis in rats, at least in part, by inhibiting the intraglomerular infiltration of inflammatory cells [50]. Interestingly, Tsujimura and colleagues reported a case of infectious interstitial pneumonia

associated with mixed connective tissue disease, in whom the bolus infusion of UTI improved the pathology [52]. Also, Komori et al. illustrated that UTI improves peripheral microcirculation and relieves bronchospasm associated with systemic anaphylaxis in rabbits [53].
Moreover, UTI has been shown to down-regulate the expression of the cancer metastasis-associated molecules uPA and uPA receptor (uPAR) possibly through MAPK- dependent signaling cascades *in vitro* and *in vivo* [61, 62]. In addition, UTI has anti-inflammatory effects against several forms of malignancy *in vitro* [58, 63]. These studies suggest that UTI is a candidate anti-cancer drug, although further studies are required in the future.

4. *In vivo* mouse model supporting role of UTI in physiologic and pathologic conditions

4.1 Generation of *UTI*-gene knockout mouse

To further investigate the physiobiological functions of UTI *in vivo,* we generated UTI (-/-) mice [64]. UTI (-/-) mice were produced as follows: a targeting vector was designed to disrupt the exons encoding UTI, leaving the exons encoding α1m intact. Germline transmission was observed in 3 chimeric male mice derived from 3 independent targeted ES clones. We generated mice that were homozygous for the mutant UTI gene (UTI [-/-] mice) by intercrossing the heterozygous mice. Under specific pathogen-free conditions, UTI (-/-) mice were born and developed normally. They grew to a normal body size and showed no apparent behavioral abnormalities. A histological study of various organs revealed no apparent differences between wild-type (WT) and UTI (-/-) mice. The ages at vaginal opening during postnatal development and the estrous cycle of UTI (-/-) female mice determined by the vaginal smear method were also normal [64].
Thereafter, we conducted a series of studies on the role of UTI in the inflammation related to LPS using the UTI (-/-) mice.

4.2 Protective role of UTI in systemic inflammation

In a study [65], both UTI (-/-) and wild-type (C57/BL6: WT) mice were injected intraperitoneally (i.p.) with vehicle or LPS at a dose of 1 mg/kg body weight. Evaluation of the coagulatory and fibrinolytic parameters and white blood cell (WBC) counts at 72 hours after i.p. challenge showed that fibrinogen levels were significantly greater in LPS- than in vehicle-challenged mice with the same genotypes. In the presence of LPS, however, they were also significantly higher in UTI (-/-) than in WT mice. WBC counts significantly decreased after LPS challenge in UTI (-/-) mice. In the presence of LPS, the prothrombin time was significantly shorter in UTI (-/-) than in WT mice. Furthermore, histopathological changes in the lung, kidney, and liver of both genotypes after LPS challenge revealed severe neutrophilic inflammation in UTI (-/-) lungs challenged with LPS, whereas little neutrophilic infiltration was found in LPS-treated WT mice. The overall trend was similar regarding findings in the kidney and liver.
The protein expression levels of proinflammatory molecules such as macrophage chemoattractant protein (MCP)-1 in the lungs, MCP-1 and keratinocyte-derived chemoattractant (KC) in the kidneys, and IL-1β, macrophage inflammatory protein (MIP)-2, MCP-1, and KC in the livers, were significantly greater in UTI (-/-) than in WT mice after LPS challenge. These results indicate that UTI protects against systemic inflammation induced by the intraperitoneal administration of LPS, at least partly, through the inhibition

of proinflamatory cytokine production/release [65], suggesting that UTI may be therapeutic against sepsis in humans.

4.3 Protective role of UTI in acute lung inflammation

A previous study showed that UTI improves acute lung injury *in vivo* [66]; however, no evidence has been reported using a genetic approach. In another series of studies [67, 68], therefore, UTI (-/-) and WT mice were intratracheally treated with vehicle or LPS (125μg/kg), and sacrificed 24 hours later. In both genotypes, LPS treatment induced significant increases in the numbers of total cells and neutrophils in bronchoalveolar lavage (BAL) fluid as compared with vehicle treatment, which was significantly greater in UTI (-/-) than in WT mice. Also, UTI (-/-) mice showed a significantly greater increase in the lung water content when compared to WT mice following LPS treatment. Lung specimens stained with hematoxylin and eosin 24 hours after intratracheal instillation showed that, in the presence of LPS, WT mice showed the moderate infiltration of neutrophils, whereas in UTI (-/-) mice, LPS treatment led to the marked recruitment of neutrophils and interstitial edema. LPS treatment induced a significant elevation of the protein levels of IL-1β, MIP-1α, MCP-1, and KC in lung homogenates when compared to vehicle treatment in both genotypes; however, in the presence of LPS, the expression was higher in UTI (-/-) than in WT mice. Furthermore, immunohistochemical examination showed that, in the presence of LPS, immunoreactive 8-hydroxy-2′-deoxyguanosine was detected in the lungs of both genotypes of mice, but the staining was more prominent in UTI (-/-) than in WT mice. In addition, immunoreactive nitrotyrosine was strongly detected only in UTI (-/-) mice challenged with LPS. Quantitative gene expression analyses of lung homogenates after intratracheal challenge showed that, compared to vehicle treatment, LPS treatment resulted in a significant elevation of gene expression for iNOS in both genotypes of mice; however, in the presence of LPS, the expression was higher in UTI (-/-) than in WT mice. These results indicate that UTI also protects against acute lung inflammation induced by the intratracheal administration of LPS, at least in part, via the local suppression of proinflammatory cytokines [67] and oxidative stress [68], suggesting that UTI may be a therapeutical tool for acute lung injury in humans.

4.4 Protective role of UTI in acute liver inflammation

One study has shown that plasma UTI levels increase in patients with acute hepatitis and markedly decrease in those with fulminant hepatitis, suggesting that the plasma UTI level is closely linked to the severity of liver damage [69]. Further, the plasma UTI level is reportedly correlated with the degree of liver damage in patients with chronic liver diseases such as liver cirrhosis and hepatocellular carcinoma [70]. In a liver inflammation and coagulatory disturbance model induced by LPS (3μg/kg) and D-galactosamine (800 mg/kg: LPS/D-GalN), LPS/D-GalN treatment caused severe liver injury characterized by neutrophilic inflammation, hemorrhagic change, necrosis, and apoptosis, which was more prominent in UTI (-/-) than in WT mice [71]. In both genotypes of mice, interestingly, LPS/D-GalN challenge caused elevations of aspartate amino-transferase and alanine amino-transferase, prolongation of the prothrombin and activated partial thromboplastin time, and decreases in fibrinogen and platelet counts, as compared with vehicle challenge. These changes, however, were significantly greater in UTI (-/-) than in WT mice. Circulatory levels of TNF-α and interferon (IFN)-γ were also greater in UTI (-/-) than in WT mice after LPS/D-GalN challenge. These results suggest that UTI protects against severe liver injury and subsequent coagulatory disturbance induced by LPS/D-GalN, which was mediated, at least partly, through the suppression of TNF-α production along with its anti-protease activity [71]. Furthermore, after LPS/D-GalN challenge, protein levels of IL-1β, TNF-α, IFN-γ, MIP-1α, and MCP-1 in the lung homogenates were elevated in both genotypes, but to a greater extent in UTI (-/-) than in WT mice. The IFN-γ level was also significantly greater in LPS/D-GalN-challenged UTI (-/-) than in other mice. These results indicate that UTI protects against the local inflammatory response accompanied by severe liver injury, which supports its anti-inflammatory properties *in vivo* [72], implicating a therapeutic potential of UTI in fulminant hepatitis in humans. In this regard, Nobuoka and colleagues have recently implicated UTI in normal liver regeneration using UTI (-/-) mice via the regulation of systemic (serum) levels of cytokines such as IL-6 and IL-10 and chemokines such as MCP-1 and MIP-1α [73].

5. Concluding remarks

As described above, UTI protects against endotoxin-related inflammatory diseases' pathology and subsequent organ damage induced by LPS in mice, at least partly, via the regulation of neutrophil-derived proteases such as elastase, proinflammatory cytokines and chemokines such as IL-1β, MIP-1α, MCP-1, and KC and oxidative stress (Fig. 2). Our

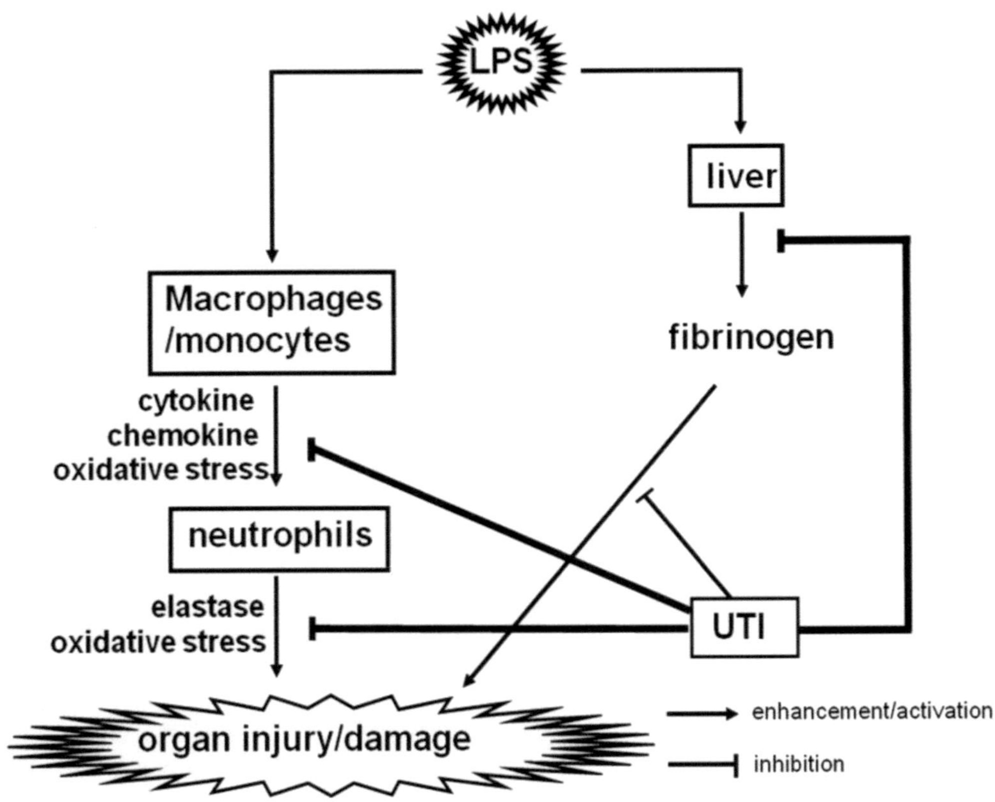

Fig. 2. Schematic representation of the protective role of UTI against endotoxin-related inflammation in mice. Our data suggest that UTI protects against: 1) endothelial activation/damage, 2) proinflammatory cytokine and chemokine production/release, 3) fibrinogen synthesis, 4) neutrophil recruitment into organs, and/or 5) organ injury.

consecutive *in vivo* results provide direct and novel molecular evidence for the "rescue" therapeutic potential of UTI against endotoxin-related inflammatory diseases such as DIC, acute lung injury, and acute liver injury.

6. Acknowledgement

This study was financially supported in part by Mochida Pharmaceutical Co., Ltd.

7. References

[1] Jonsson-Berling BM, Ohlsson K, Rosengren M. Radioimmunological quantitation of the urinary trypsin inhibitor in normal blood and urine. Biol Chem Hoppe Seyler 1989; 370:1157-61.

[2] Salier JP, Rouet P, Raguenez G, Daveau M. The inter-alpha-inhibitor family: from structure to regulation. Biochem J 1996; 315:1-9.

[3] Sjoberg EM, Fries E. Biosynthesis of bikunin (urinary trypsin inhibitor) in rat hepatocytes. Arch Biochem Biophys 1992; 295:217-22.

[4] Thogersen IB, Enghild JJ. Biosynthesis of bikunin proteins in the human carcinoma cell line HepG2 and in primary human hepatocytes. Polypeptide assembly by glycosaminoglycan. J Biol Chem 1995; 270:18700-9.

[5] Heron A, Bourguignon J, Calle A, Borghi H, Sesboue R, Diarra-Mehrpour M, Martin JP. Post-translational processing of the inter-alpha-trypsin inhibitor in the human hepatoma HepG2 cell line. Biochem J 1994; 302:573-80.

[6] Heron A, Bourguignon J, Diarra-Mehrpour M, Dautreaux B, Martin JP, Sesboue R. Involvement of the three inter-alpha-trypsin inhibitor (ITI) heavy chains in each member of the serum ITI family. FEBS Lett 1995; 374:195-8.

[7] Ohnishi H, Suzuki K, Hiho T, Ito C, Yamaguchi K. Protective effects of urinary trypsin inhibitor in experimental shock. Japan J Pharmacol 1985; 39: 137-44.

[8] Albani D, Balduyck M, Mizon C, Mizon J. Inter-alpha-inhibitor as marker for neutrophil proteinase activity: an in vitro investigation. J Lab Clin Med 1997; 130:339-47.

[9] Balduyck M, Albani D, Jourdain M, Mizon C, Tournoys A, Drobecq H, Fourrier F, Mizon J. Inflammation-induced systemic proteolysis of inter-alpha-inhibitor in plasma from patients with sepsis. J Lab Clin Med 2000; 135:188-98.

[10] Mizon C, Piva F, Queyrel V, Balduyck M, Hachulla E, Mizon J. Urinary bikunin determination provides insight into proteinase/proteinase inhibitor imbalance in patients with inflammatory diseases. Clin Chem Lab Med 2002; 40:579-86.

[11] Hirose J, Ozawa T, Miura T, et al. Human neutrophil elastase degrades inter-alpha-trypsin inhibitor to liberate urinary trypsin inhibitor related proteins. Biol Pharm Bull 1998; 21:651-6.

[12] Balduyck M, Mizon J. [Inter-alpha-trypsin inhibitor and its plasma and urine derivatives]. Ann Biol Clin (Paris) 1991; 49:273-81.

[13] Nishiyama T, Aibiki M, Hanaoka K. The effect of ulinastatin, a human protease inhibitor, on the transfusion-induced increase of plasma polymorphonuclear granulocyte elastase. Anesth Analg 1996; 82:108-12.

[14] Pugia MJ, Valdes R, Jr., Jortani SA. Bikunin (urinary trypsin inhibitor): structure, biological relevance, and measurement. Adv Clin Chem 2007; 44:223-45.

[15] Kobayashi H, Suzuki M, Tanaka Y, Hirashima Y, Terao T. Suppression of urokinase expression and invasiveness by urinary trypsin inhibitor is mediated through inhibition of protein kinase C- and MEK/ERK/c-Jun-dependent signaling pathways. J Biol Chem 2001; 276:2015-22.

[16] Kobayashi H, Gotoh J, Terao T. Urinary trypsin inhibitor efficiently inhibits urokinase production in tumor necrosis factor-stimulated cells. Eur J Cell Biol 1996; 71:380-6.

[17] Ohnishi H, Kosuzume H, Ashida Y, Kato K, Honjo I. Effects of urinary trypsin inhibitor on pancreatic enzymes and experimental acute pancreatitis. Dig Dis Sci 1984; 29:26-32.

[18] Okabe H, Irita K, Kurosawa K, Tagawa K, Koga A, Yamakawa M, Yoshitake J, Takahashi S. Increase in the plasma concentration of reduced glutathione observed in rats with liver damage induced by lipopolysaccharide/D-galactosamine: effects of ulinastatin, a urinary trypsin inhibitor. Circ Shock 1993; 41:268-72.

[19] Tsujino T, Komatsu Y, Isayama H, et al. Ulinastatin for pancreatitis after endoscopic retrograde cholangiopancreatography: a randomized, controlled trial. Clin Gastroenterol Hepatol 2005; 3:376-83.

[20] Endo S, Inada K, Yamashita H, et al. The inhibitory actions of protease inhibitors on the production of polymorphonuclear leukocyte elastase and interleukin 8. Res Commun Chem Pathol Pharmacol 1993; 82:27-34.

[21] Nakatani K, Takeshita S, Tsujimoto H, Kawamura Y, Sekine I. Inhibitory effect of serine protease inhibitors on neutrophil-mediated endothelial cell injury. J Leukoc Biol 2001; 69:241-7.

[22] Aosasa S, Ono S, Mochizuki H, Tsujimoto H, Ueno C, Matsumoto A. Mechanism of the inhibitory effect of protease inhibitor on tumor necrosis factor alpha production of monocytes. Shock 2001; 15:101-5.

[23] Endo S, Inada K, Taki K, Hoshi S, Yoshida M. Inhibitory effects of ulinastatin on the production of cytokines: implications for the prevention of septicemic shock. Clin Ther 1990; 12:323-6.

[24] Maehara K, Kanayama N, Halim A, el Maradny E, Oda T, Fujita M, Terao T. Down-regulation of interleukin-8 gene expression in HL60 cell line by human Kunitz-type trypsin inhibitor. Biochem Biophys Res Commun 1995; 206:927-34.

[25] Nakamura H, Abe S, Shibata Y, et al. Inhibition of neutrophil elastase-induced interleukin-8 gene expression by urinary trypsin inhibitor in human bronchial epithelial cells. Int Arch Allergy Immunol 1997; 112:157-62.

[26] Matsuzaki H, Kobayashi H, Yagyu T, et al. Bikunin inhibits lipopolysaccharide-induced tumor necrosis factor alpha induction in macrophages. Clin Diagn Lab Immunol 2004; 11:1140-7.

[27] Aibiki M, Cook JA. Ulinastatin, a human trypsin inhibitor, inhibits endotoxin-induced thromboxane B2 production in human monocytes. Crit Care Med 1997; 25:430-4.

[28] Cook JA, Geisel J, Temple GE, et al. Endotoxin activation of eicosanoid production by macrophages. In: Pathophysiology of Shock, Sepsis and Organ Failure. Schlag F, Redl H (Eds). Heidelberg, Germany, Springer-Verlag, 1993, pp 518-30.

[29] Molor-Erdene P, Okajima K, Isobe H, Uchiba M, Harada N, Okabe H. Urinary trypsin inhibitor reduces LPS-induced hypotension by suppressing tumor necrosis factor-alpha production through inhibition of Egr-1 expression. Am J Physiol Heart Circ Physiol 2005; 288:H1265-71.

[30] Okano S, Tagawa M, Urakawa N, Ogawa R. A therapeutic effect of ulinastatin on endotoxin-induced shock in dogs--comparison with methylprednisolone. J Vet Med Sci 1994; 56:645-9.

[31] Tani T, Aoki H, Yoshioka T, Lin KJ, Kodama M. Treatment of septic shock with a protease inhibitor in a canine model: a prospective, randomized, controlled trial. Crit Care Med 1993; 21:925-30.

[32] Wakahara K, Kobayashi H, Yagyu T, et al. Bikunin suppresses lipopolysaccharide-induced lethality through down-regulation of tumor necrosis factor- alpha and interleukin-1 beta in macrophages. J Infect Dis 2005; 191:930-8.

[33] Molor-Erdene P, Okajima K, Isobe H, Uchiba M, Harada N, Shimozawa N, Okabe H. Inhibition of lipopolysaccharide-induced tissue factor expression in monocytes by urinary trypsin inhibitor in vitro and in vivo. Thromb Haemost 2005; 94:136-45.

[34] Masuda T, Sato K, Noda C, et al. Protective effect of urinary trypsin inhibitor on myocardial mitochondria during hemorrhagic shock and reperfusion. Crit Care Med 2003; 31:1987-92.

[35] Aihara T, Shiraishi M, Hiroyasu S, Hatsuse K, Mochizuki H, Seki S, Hiraide H, Muto Y. Ulinastatin, a protease inhibitor, attenuates hepatic ischemia/reperfusion injury by downregulating TNF-alpha in the liver. Transplant Proc 1998; 30:3732-4.

[36] Nakahama H, Obata K, Sugita M. Ulinastatin ameliorates acute ischemic renal injury in rats. Ren Fail 1996; 18:893-8.

[37] Cao ZL, Okazaki Y, Naito K, Ueno T, Natsuaki M, Itoh T. Ulinastatin attenuates reperfusion injury in the isolated blood-perfused rabbit heart. Ann Thorac Surg 2000; 69:1121-6.

[38] Binns OA, DeLima NF, Buchanan SA, *et al.* Neutrophil endopeptidase inhibitor improves pulmonary function during reperfusion after eighteen-hour preservation. J Thorac Cardiovasc Surg 1996; 112:607-13.

[39] Okuhama Y, Shiraishi M, Higa T, Tomori H, Taira K, Mamadi T, Muto Y. Protective effects of ulinastatin against ischemia-reperfusion injury. J Surg Res 1999; 82:34-42.

[40] Yamaguchi Y, Ohshiro H, Nagao Y, et al. Urinary trypsin inhibitor reduces C-X-C chemokine production in rat liver ischemia/reperfusion. J Surg Res 2000; 94:107-15.

[41] Nakanishi K, Takeda S, Sakamoto A, Kitamura A. Effects of ulinastatin treatment on the cardiopulmonary bypass-induced hemodynamic instability and pulmonary dysfunction. Crit Care Med 2006; 34:1351-7.

[42] Nishiyama T, Yokoyama T, Yamashita K. Effects of a protease inhibitor, ulinastatin, on coagulation and fibrinolysis in abdominal surgery. J Anesth 2006; 20:179-82.

[43] Kurosawa S, Kanaya N, Fujimura N, Nakayama M, Edanaga M, Mizuno E, Park KW, Namiki A. Effects of ulinastatin on pulmonary artery pressure during abdominal aortic aneurysmectomy. J Clin Anesth 2006; 18:18-23.

[44] Yano T, Anraku S, Nakayama R, Ushijima K. Neuroprotective effect of urinary trypsin inhibitor against focal cerebral ischemia-reperfusion injury in rats. Anesthesiology 2003; 98:465-73.
[45] Umeki S, Tsukiyama K, Okimoto N, Soejima R. Urinastatin (Kunitz-type proteinase inhibitor) reducing cisplatin nephrotoxicity. Am J Med Sci 1989; 298:221-6.
[46] Ishigami M, Eguchi M, Yabuki S. Beneficial effects of the urinary trypsin inhibitor urinastatin on renal insults induced by gentamicin and mercuric chloride (HgCl2) poisoning. Nephron 1991; 58:300-5.
[47] Kobayashi H, Ohi H, Terao T. Prevention by urinastatin of cis-diamminedichloroplatinum-induced nephrotoxicity in rabbits: comparison of urinary enzyme excretions and morphological alterations by electron microscopy. Asia Oceania J Obstet Gynaecol 1991; 17:277-88.
[48] Yamasaki F, Ishibashi M, Nakakuki M, Watanabe M, Shinkawa T, Mizota M. Protective action of ulinastatin against cisplatin nephrotoxicity in mice and its effect on the lysosomal fragility. Nephron 1996; 74:158-67.
[49] Ishibashi M, Yamasaki F, Nakakuki M, Shinkawa T, Mizota M. Cytoprotective effect of ulinastatin on LLC-PK1 cells treated with antimycin A, gentamicin, and cisplatin. Nephron 1997; 76:300-6.
[50] Koizumi R, Kanai H, Maezawa A, Kanda T, Nojima Y, Naruse T. Therapeutic effects of ulinastatin on experimental crescentic glomerulonephritis in rats. Nephron 2000; 84:347-53.
[51] Huang Y, Xie K, Zhang J, Dang Y, Qiong Z. Prospective clinical and experimental studies on the cardioprotective effect of ulinastatin following severe burns. Burns 2008; 34:674-80.
[52] Tsujimura S, Saito K, Nakayamada S, Tanaka Y. Human urinary trypsin inhibitor bolus infusion improved severe interstitial pneumonia in mixed connective tissue disease. Mod Rheumatol 2005; 15:374-80.
[53] Komori M, Takada K, Tomizawa Y, Uezono S, Ozaki M. Urinary trypsin inhibitor improves peripheral microcirculation and bronchospasm associated with systemic anaphylaxis in rabbits in vivo. Shock 2003; 20:189-94.
[54] Inamo Y, Okubo T, Wada M, *et al.* Intravenous ulinastatin therapy for Stevens-Johnson syndrome and toxic epidermal necrolysis in pediatric patients. Three case reports. Int Arch Allergy Immunol 2002; 127:89-94.
[55] Harashima S, Tsukamoto H, Nishizaka H, Otsuka J, Hiriuchi T. Successful treatment of invasive pulmonary aspergillosis by transbronchial injection of urinary trypsin inhibitor and amphotericin B. Acta Haematol 2003; 109:156-7.
[56] Sato A, Kuwabara Y, Shinoda N, Kimura M, Ishiguro H, Fujii Y. Use of low dose dopamine, gabexate mesilate and ulinastatin reduces the water balance and pulmonary complication in thoracic esophagectomy patients. Dis Esophagus 2005; 18:151-4.
[57] Kobayashi H, Suzuki M, Tanaka Y, Kanayama N, Terao T. A Kunitz-type protease inhibitor, bikunin, inhibits ovarian cancer cell invasion by blocking the calcium-dependent transforming growth factor-beta 1 signaling cascade. J Biol Chem 2003; 278:7790-9.

[58] Kobayashi H, Yagyu T, Inagaki K, Kondo T, Suzuki M, Kanayama N, Terao T. Therapeutic efficacy of once-daily oral administration of a Kunitz-type protease inhibitor, bikunin, in a mouse model and in human cancer. Cancer 2004; 100:869-77.

[59] Suzuki M, Kobayashi H, Tanaka Y, et al. Suppression of invasion and peritoneal carcinomatosis of ovarian cancer cell line by overexpression of bikunin. Int J Cancer 2003; 104:289-302.

[60] Yoshioka I, Tsuchiya Y, Aozuka Y, Onishi Y, Sakurai H, Koizumi K, Tsukada K, Saiki I. Urinary trypsin inhibitor suppresses surgical stress-facilitated lung metastasis of murine colon 26-L5 carcinoma cells. Anticancer Res 2005; 25:815-20.

[61] Kobayashi H, Suzuki M, Kanayama N, Nishida T, Takigawa M, Terao T. Suppression of urokinase receptor expression by bikunin is associated with inhibition of upstream targets of extracellular signal-regulated kinase-dependent cascade. Eur J Biochem 2002; 269:3945-57.

[62] Kobayashi H, Suzuki M, Hirashima Y, Terao T. The protease inhibitor bikunin, a novel anti-metastatic agent. Biol Chem 2003; 384:749-54.

[63] Kobayashi H. Suppression of urokinase expression and tumor metastasis by bikunin overexpression [mini-review]. Hum Cell 2001; 14:233-6.

[64] Sato H, Kajikawa S, Kuroda S, et al. Impaired fertility in female mice lacking urinary trypsin inhibitor. Biochem Biophys Res Commun 2001; 281:1154-60.

[65] Inoue K, Takano H, Shimada A, Yanagisawa R, Sakurai M, Yoshino S, Sato H, Yoshikawa T. Urinary trypsin inhibitor protects against systemic inflammation induced by lipopolysaccharide. Mol Pharmacol 2005; 67:673-80.

[66] Ito K, Mizutani A, Kira S, Mori M, Iwasaka H, Noguchi T. Effect of Ulinastatin, a human urinary trypsin inhibitor, on the oleic acid-induced acute lung injury in rats via the inhibition of activated leukocytes. Injury 2005; 36:387-94.

[67] Inoue K, Takano H, Yanagisawa R, Sakurai M, Shimada A, Yoshino S, Sato H, Yoshikawa T. Protective role of urinary trypsin inhibitor in acute lung injury induced by lipopolysaccharide. Exp Biol Med (Maywood) 2005; 230:281-7.

[68] Inoue K, Takano H, Yanagisawa R, Sakurai M, Shimada A, Sato H, Kato Y, Yoshikawa T. Antioxidative role of urinary trypsin inhibitor in acute lung injury induced by lipopolysaccharide. Int J Mol Med 2005; 16:1029-33.

[69] Lin SD, Endo R, Sato A, Takikawa Y, Shirakawa K, Suzuki K. Plasma and urine levels of urinary trypsin inhibitor in patients with acute and fulminant hepatitis. J Gastroenterol Hepatol 2002; 17:140-7.

[70] Lin SD, Endo R, Kuroda H, Kondo K, Miura Y, Takikawa Y, Kato A, Suzuki K. Plasma and urine levels of urinary trypsin inhibitor in patients with chronic liver diseases and hepatocellular carcinoma. J Gastroenterol Hepatol 2004; 19:327-32.

[71] Takano H, Inoue K, Shimada A, Sato H, Yanagisawa R, Yoshikawa T. Urinary trypsin inhibitor protects against liver injury and coagulation pathway dysregulation induced by lipopolysaccharide/D-galactosamine in mice. Lab Invest 2009; 89:833-9.

[72] Inoue KI, Takano H, Sato H, Yanagisawa R, Yoshikawa T. Protective role of urinary trypsin inhibitor in lung expression of proinflammatory cytokines accompanied by lethal liver injury in mice. Immunopharmacol Immunotoxicol 2009:1-5.
[73] Nobuoka T, Mizuguchi T, Oshima H, *et al.* Impaired liver regeneration with humoral and genetic disturbances in urinary trypsin inhibitor-deficient mice. Liver Int 2009; 29:979-87.

Part 2

Design of hn-SPLA2 Inhibitors: A Structure Based Molecule Design Approach

2

Design of Human Non-Pancreatic Secretary Phospholipase A2 (hnps-PLA2) Inhibitors: A Structure Based Molecule Design Approach

Amit Nagal
Advanced Bioinformatics Center
Birla Institute of Scientific Research,
Statue Circle, Jaipur
India

1. Introduction

Phospholipase A2 (PLA2) catalyzes the hydrolysis of the SN-2 acyl ester linkage of phospholipids and producing fatty acids and lysophospholipids. Their activity is one of the rate-limiting steps in the formation of arachidonic acid and in the synthesis of leukotrienes and prostaglandins. These prostaglandins have vital role in carcinogenesis. In the present study structure based drug design approach has applied to the hnps-PLA2 inhibitors. It can be concluded that indole-3-acetamide derivative molecule 13 h was showing better interaction with the active site of hnps-PLA2. The comparative in silico ADME studies proved that 13h molecule could be a potential anticancer drug. Phospholipase is an enzyme that converts phospholipids into fatty acid and other lipophillic-substances. There are four major classes of Phospholipase, termed A, B, C and D. These classes are distinguished by the catalyzing type of reactions. Phospholipase A has two subtypes: Phospholipase A1 which cleaves the SN-1 acyl chain and Phospholipase A2 which cleaves the SN-2 acyl chain.

2. Material and method

Ligand fit (Discovery studio 2.1) software was used for molecular docking studies (Venkatachalam, C.M. et al. 2003). It is based on a cavity detection algorithm and Monte Carlo conformational search algorithm for generating ligand poses consistent with the active site shape. The crystal structure of hnps-PLA2 (1DB4) complex with potent indole inhibitor was determined and used in structure based drug design (Schevitz RW et al 1995). The PDB structure 1DB4 was chosen for our study has 2.20 A° resolution and has RMSD value below 2 A°.

2.1 Ligand and receptor preparation

The hnps-PLA2 inhibitors, 74 indole-3-acetic acid derivatives (Robert D. Dillard et al 1996) were sketched. The structure of all molecules used in the present study was designed on the

basis of the reported scaffold and the substituent table from NCBI pubchem. The Generic drugs with diverse scaffolds were downloaded from pubchem library. The Hydrogen Bonds were added and CHARMm force field was applied to all molecules.
The crystal structure of hnps-PLA2 protein (1DB4) was downloaded from the PDB. After applying CHARMm force field macro molecule hnps-PLA2 was assigned as receptor. The receptor cavity was searched using flood filling algorithm and partition site was adjusted for the better fitments of molecule in the partition site of receptor. The comparative docking studies for all 100 molecules were performed. The determination of the ligand binding affinity was calculated using Ligscore1, Ligscore2 and Dock score were used to estimate the ligand-binding energies.In the present study ADME Tox software was used to study the toxicity of hnps-PLA2 inhibitors.We have used top ten ranked dock molecule of hnps-PLA2 for the present study.The Hydrogen Bonds were added and CHARMm force field was applied to all molecules and the ADME properties were calculated.

3. Result and analysis

In the present study we have taken generic drugs with diverse scaffolds and indole inhibitors of hnps- PLA2 which were biologically tested and synthesized (Robert D. Dillard et al 1996). The structure based studies of the molecules described above were carried out using Discovery Studio. The RMSD value between the top ten ranked (based on docked energy) reference molecules and hnp-SPLA2 was reported around 2A°.
Table 1 had shown the different score values of top ranked ligands against hnsp-SPLA2 receptor. The score values include Ligscore1 and Ligscore 2 which is based on protein-ligand affinity energy (Krammer et al 2005). It has been observed that Ligscore1 (6.16), Ligscore2 (7.06) were found highest for the 13 h molecule in comparison with the other 100 molecules. During the study it has been observed that molecule 13 h which was found highest docked energy score 80.47 has high inhibitory concentration (IC50 .03 $_{uM}$) which proved that the drugs found most effective in prior experimental studies was also giving high dock scores.
It has been reported that indole inhibitors when substituted with additional alkyl group at different positions of indole the efficacy of the compound had increased towards hnps-PLA2 (Lin et al 2003). In the present study the molecules having indole ring proved more efficient when substituting with other additional groups on indole ring. In comparison with the binding affinity of the other molecules it has been observed that indole-3- derivatives were found most effective scaffold. The top 7 Ranked docked molecules had indole ring and a additional acid side chain on the fifth position with acid group (13h (80.47 J/mol), 41 (71.59 J/mol), 2n (70.59 J/mol), 71 (70.48 J/mol), 7i (68.14 J/mol), 16b (67.71 J/mol), 60a (67.71 J/mol)) It has been observed that indole-3-acetamides series molecule possessed potency and selectivity as inhibitors of hnps-PLA2 (Robert D. Dillard et al 1996). It was observed that the top 6 docked molecules (molecule 13h (80.47 J/mol), 41 (71.59 J/mol), 71 (70.48 J/mol), 7i (68.14 J/mol), 16b (67.71 J/mol), 60a (67.71 J/mol)) had 3-acetamide side chain at Indole ring. The molecule 13 h had oxy propyl phosphonic acid group on fifth position which had shown strong hydrogen bonding formation with the active site residue histidine of hnp-SPLA2 receptor.(Fig 1).

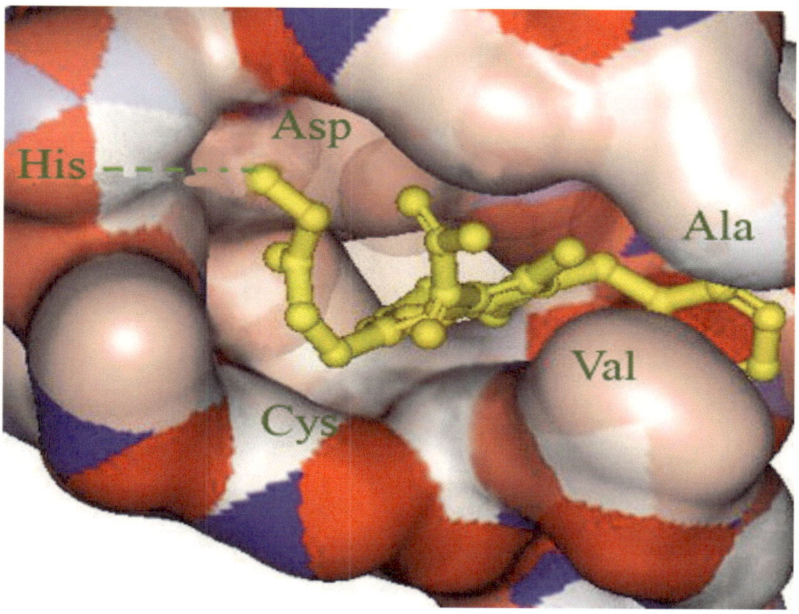

Fig. 1. Molecule 13h showing hydrogen bonding with histidine

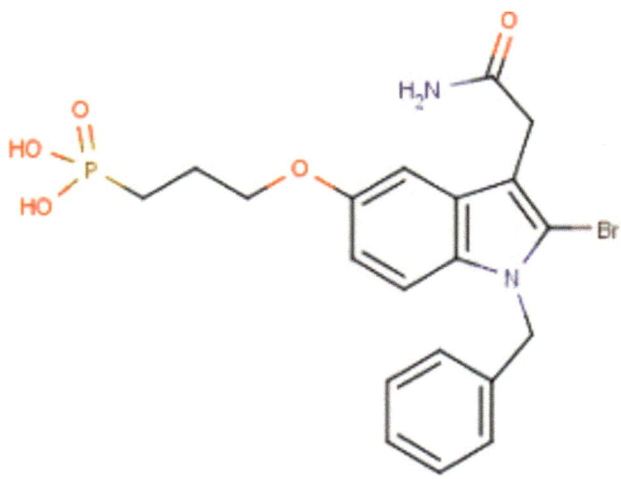

Fig. 2. Molecule 13h

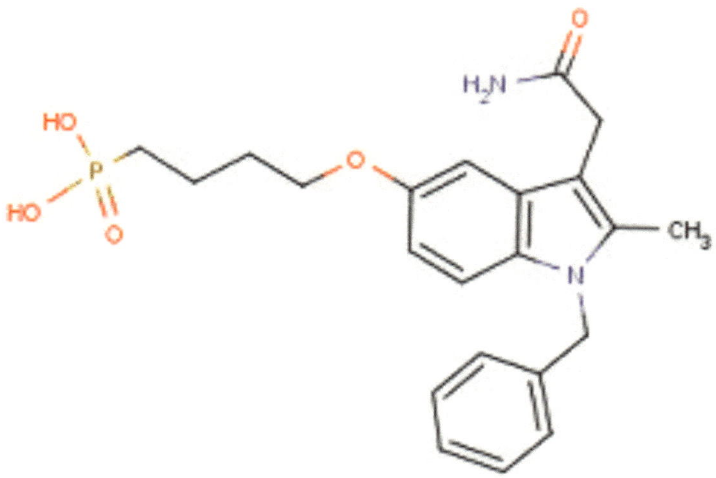

Fig. 3. Molecule 41 showing similarties with mol 13h

The structural similarity of two top ranked dock score molecules suggested that both had 3-indole acetamide ring as basic scaffold and phosphonic acid group which was attached to fifth position of indole and a benzyl ring which was attached to first position of indole.(Fig 2,3)

The top ten ranked dock molecules were chosen for ADME analysis. The ADME properties of 13h were found very satisfactory. The aqueous solubility value was found within optimal range-(4.028) whereas the molecule indomethcin (3.24), indoprofen (3.54) was found not good solubility value. The molecule 16b, 7i, 71, 60a had poor (3) intestinal absorption level whereas molecule 13 h had very good (0) intestinal absorption level. The Plasma protein binding was found more than 90% for molecule 13 h but it was reported more than 95% for the molecule 41 and 2n. The Blood Brain Penetration Level for molecule 13h was found to be extremely low (4) level and the cytochrome P450 enzyme (1) level was not found to be inhibited by molecule 13 h. Thus comparing with the other molecules ADME properties 13 h had a good therapeutic index.

Name	LigScore1	LigScore2	DOCK_SCORE
13h	6.16	7.06	80.47
Bendazac	2.79	2.97	71.766
41	6	6.62	71.496
2n	3.33	2.89	70.596
71	5.64	6.39	70.48
7i	6.14	6.27	68.147
16b	4.27	5.19	67.71
60a	4.88	6.63	67.487
Indometacin	3.54	4.26	66.921
Indoprofen	2.86	2.85	66.375
13f	5.81	6.9	65.9
4n	4.76	5.46	65.728
7o	5.47	5.84	65.64
7r	5.32	6.4	65.526

Table 1. Sketched molecules with Best dock score

4. Conclusion

In the present study it can be concluded that Indole derivative molecule 13 h is proved to better molecule in terms of experimental studies, molecular interaction with hnp-SPLA2 receptor and computational ADME studies. So the present study proved that hnps-PLA2 based inhibitor molecule 13 h (Fig 4) could be a better substitute for NSAID (Non-steroid anti inflammatory drug).

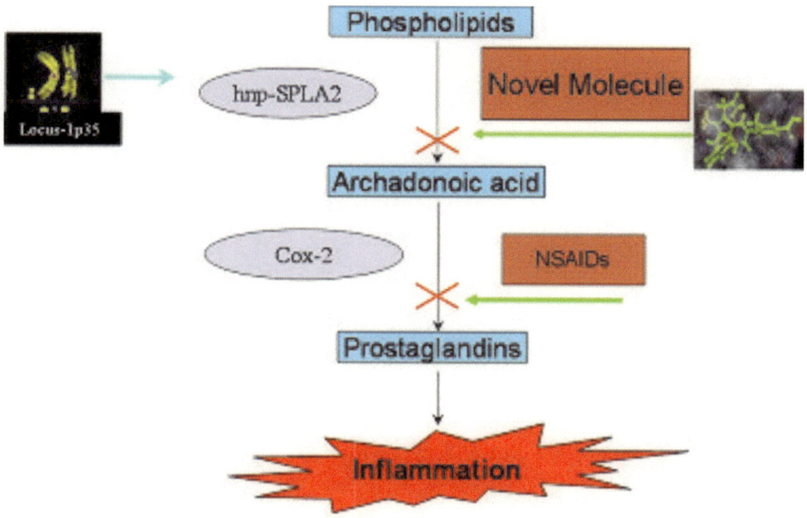

Fig. 4. Showing alternate pathway for inflammation

5. References

Robert D. Dillard & Nicholas. (1996). Indole Inhibitors of Human Nonpancreatic Secretory Phospholipase A2. Indole-3-acetamides with Additional Functionality. *J. Med. Chem, Vol 39,* pp. *5137–5158.*

Robert D. Dillard & Nicholas. (1996). Indole Inhibitors of Human Nonpancreatic Secretory Phospholipase A2. Indole-3-acetamides. *J. Med. Chem, Vol.*39, pp. 5119–5136.

Lars Linderoth & Thomas L. (2008). Molecular Basis of Phospholipase A_2 Activity toward Phospholipids with *sn*-1 Substitutions. *Biophys J.* Vol 94, pp. 14–26

Venkatachalam CM & Jiang.(2003) LigandFit: A Novel Method for the Shape-Directed Rapid Docking of Ligands to Protein Active Sites.*J Mol Graph Modell*, Vol 21, pp. 289-307.

Krammer A & Kirchhoff PD. (2005) LigScore: a novel scoring function for predicting binding affinities. *J Mol Graph Model,* Vol 23, pp. 395-407.

Schevitz RW & Bach NJ. (1995). Structure-based design of the first potent and selective inhibitor of human non-pancreatic secretory phospholipase A2. *Nat Struct Biol.,* Vol 2, pp .458-65.

Part 3

Bachcet's Disease

3

Th17 Trafficking Cells in Behcet's Disease Skin Lesions

Hamzaoui Kamel, Bouali Eya
and Houman Habib
Tunis El Manar University; Homeostasis and Cell Dysfunction Unit Research Medicine Faculty of Tunis, La Rabta Hospital, Internal Medicine Department; unit research on Behcet's didease
Tunisia

1. Introduction

Behçet's disease (BD) is a vasculitis characterized by oral, genital ulcers and uveitis with varying other manifestations associated with vascular inflammation. Additional target organ, including vascular, neurological, and gastrointestinal manifestations, were added to the disease spectrum [Yazici et al., 2003]. The etiology of BD is considered to be a complex systemic vasculitis, caused by T-helper-1 (Th1) cytokine skewed neutrophilic and lymphohistiocytic inflammation [Suzuki et al., 2006; Kulaber et al., 2007; Koarada et al., 2004; Keller et al., 2005].

The pathogenesis of BD is still unclear, but immune dysfunction, viral and bacterial agents, such as Staphylococcus spp. and herpes simplex virus, have been postulated [Onder et al., 2001]. Cytokines play crucial roles in the inflammatory responses in BD [Hamzaoui et al., 2002; Direskeneli et al., 2003]. BD as many autoimmune diseases are considered to be T cell-regulated diseases, further classified as Th1-mediated diseases, with Th1-like diseases featuring a high production of IFN-γ. However, this classification fails to explain the involvement of inflammatory cells as seen in many autoimmune/inflammatory diseases. A unifying feature of the inflammation observed in BD is the nonspecific hyperreactivity of tissue to minor trauma, termed the skin pathergy reaction (SPR), which remains the most diagnostically relevant lesion in BD patients, where an exaggerated inflammatory response develops in the skin of BD patients that is characterized by dermal infiltration of activated dentritic cells (DCs) and the presence of a Th1-type immunological cascade [Melikoglu et al., 2006]. The immunohistochemistry of patients with sterile, pustular skin eruptions in the context of a systemic autoinflammatory disease revealed a substantially denser, lymphocyte rich cell infiltrate (mainly $CD4^+$ and some $CD8^+$ T cells than in normal skin). The majority of T cells detected were immigrating, inflammatory T cells, as they expressed CCR6, the receptor for CCL20 (MIP-3α) [Keller et al., 2005].

Studies show that $CD4^+$ IL-17^+ and $CD8^+$ IL-17^+ T cells (Th17) play an active role in inflammation and autoimmune diseases in murine systems [Komiyama et al., 2006; Bettelli et al., 2007; Kryczek et al. 2007], and have never been studied in skin lesions from BD patients. The question addressed in this study is why Th1 and Th17 cells often colocalized in pathological environments and what is the mechanism and pathological relevance of this colocalization. We studied skin lesions from BD patients. Previous studies implicated Th1 cells promoting cytokine in skin lesions from BD patients [Melikoglu et al., 2006].

In the current investigation, we explored the phenotype and function of IL-17-secreting T cells in BD and healthy skin, and the factors supporting their trafficking to and induction in lesional skin. Specifically, we show that IFN-γ is demonstrated as a potent promoter of IL-17^{+} T cell trafficking, induction, and function. Our observations support a model wherein Th1 and IL-17^{+} T cells mechanistically interact and collaboratively contribute to BD skin pathogenesis.

2. Materials and methods

2.1 Patients skin testing, and tissue samples

The study was approved by the Ethical Committee of our University. A total of 12 patients with active BD (3 females, 9 males) fulfilling the International Study Group Criteria for BD [ISG. 1990] were enrolled into this study. BD patients were aged: 39 years (range 26-47 years) and the mean disease duration were 76 months (range 10-132 months). Disease activity was evaluated according to published criteria [Lawton & Bhakta, 2004]. Of 12 patients, all had oral ulcerations, 8 had genital ulcers, 6 had erythema nodosum, 10 had papulopustular lesions, 8 had arthritis, 7 had uveitis, 6 had deep venous thrombosis, and 11 had a positive skin pathergy reaction (SPR). Consistent with previous published reports, there were no demographic or clinical differences discernible between BD patients with a positive or negative SPR in our study [Krause et al., 2000].

The skin lesions were scored [Diri et al., 2001]: 0 = no lesions; 1 = 1-5 lesions; 2 = 6-10 lesions; 3 = 11-15 lesions; 4 = 16-20 lesions; and 5 = more than 20 lesions. Table I describes BD patients with skin lesions. Patients were treated with steroids and colchicines. Seven donors of healthy human skin were included in this study. Punch-biopsy specimens (4 mm) were obtained from affected skin (pustular eruption) and were divided in two equal parts, one for T cell elution and one for RT-PCR analysis. All skin biopsy samples were obtained with a circular dermal punch after injection of 1% lidocaine solution into the hypodermis. Biopsy samples were snap frozen directly in liquid nitrogen for mRNA extraction and RT-PCR analysis.

2.2 Immune cell isolation

Single cell suspensions were prepared from PBMC and skin tissue samples. Skin biopsy samples were incubated in 50 U/ml dispase (BD Biosciences) at 37°C for 90 min. The skin portions were then cut into 1-mm pieces and digested in collagenase for 2 h at room temperature. Single cell suspensions of epidermal portions were generated by incubation in Cell Dissociation buffer (Invitrogen) at 37°C for 2 h. Skin explant cultures of T cells from skin biopsies were prepared as described by Clark et al. [Clark et al., 2006].

Immune cells including T cells and CD14^{+} or CD11c^{+} myeloid APCs were enriched using paramagnetic beads (StemCell Technologies) and sorted from stained single cell suspensions using a high-speed cell sorter (FACSAria; BD Immunocytometry Systems) as described by Curiel et al [Curiel et al., 2003]. Cell purity was >98% as confirmed by flow cytometry (LSR II; BD Immunocytometry Systems). CD14^{+} or CD11c^{+} myeloidAPCs were used to stimulate T cells as indicated.

2.3 APC activation and cytokine production

Fresh peripheral blood $CD11c^+$ APCs (0.5×10^6/ml) were incubated for 72 h with or without recombinant human IFN-γ (200 ng/ml; R&D Systems). These cells were washed and used for T cell stimulation or activated for 12 h with LPS (1 μg/ml; Sigma-Aldrich) or incubated 3 days (1×10^6 cells/ml) in the presence of LPS to detect cytokine levels in supernatants. All Abs were from R&D Systems.

2.4 T cell culture system

Myeloid APCs were cocultured with peripheral blood T cells in ratios from 1:3 to 1:10 (0.5×10^6 T cells/ml) for 4 days in the presence of anti-CD3 (2.5 - 5 μg/ml) and anti-CD28 (1.2 - 2.5 μg/ml) mAbs (BD Biosciences). Different cytokines and neutralizing antibodies (Abs) or their combinations including IL-1α (2.5 ng/ml), IL-1β (2.5 ng/ml), IL-23 (10 ng/ml), anti-IL-4 (1 μg/ml), anti-IFN- γ (2 μg/ml), anti-IL-1 (1 μg/ml anti-IL-1R plus 1 μg/ml anti-IL-1 α) were used as indicated (all from R&D Systems). Cells were subjected to flow cytometric phenotyping, intracellular cytokine staining, and transcript detection by real-time PCR. Culture supernatants were collected for detection of IL-17 by ELISA (R&D Systems). For flow cytometry analysis, cells were first stained extracellularly with specific monoclonal antibodies (Abs), then fixed and permeabilized with Perm/Fix solution (eBioscience), and finally stained intracellularly with specific Abs against the indicated cytokines (BD Biosciences). Samples were acquired on a LSR II (BD Biosciences) and data were analyzed with DIVA software (BD Biosciences).

2.5 Migration assays

Migration assays were performed in a Transwell system with a polycarbonate membrane of 6.5 mm diameter with a 3-μm pore size as described by Curiel et al. [Curiel et al., 2004]. Purified T cell subsets were added to the upper chamber, and CCL20 (5 ng/ml; R&D Systems) was added to the lower chamber. After 4 h of incubation at 37°C, the phenotype and number of T cells in the upper and lower chambers was determined by FACS.

2.6 Quantification of gene expression

Quantitative real-time PCR was performed on control and lesional skin samples from 12 BD patients and 7 normal healthy controls as we have recently reported [Hamzaoui et al., 2008]. Quantification of gene expression in the cultured myeloid APCs was performed as described by Kryczek et al [Kryczek et al., 2007]. The gene transcripts were quantified in a MasterCycler RealPlex system (Eppendorf Scientific) and expressed as mRNA quantities normalized to GAPDH levels.

2.7 Immunohistochemistry

Skin biopsy samples were stained with anti-CD4 or anti-CD8 Ab as described [Hamzaoui et al., 2008]. The staining was detected using the one-step avidin-biotin complex technique (BD Pharmingen).

2.8 Statistical calculations

The Wilcoxon rank-sum test was used to determine pairwise differences and the X^2 test used to determine differences between groups. A value for $p < 0.05$ was considered as significant. Differences in phenotype of T cell subsets were tested with the paired Student's t test.

Correlation was tested by Spearman's test. All statistical analysis was done on Statistical software (StatSoft).

3. Results

3.1 IL-17$^+$ T cells are increased in BD skin lesions

We investigated the distribution of CD4$^+$ and CD8$^+$ IL-17$^+$ T cells in BD-skin lesions and in healthy donors [Figure 1A and Figure 1B]. High levels of CD3$^+$ IL-17$^+$ T cells were observed in active BD compared to healthy control skin. The highest percentage of CD4$^+$ and CD8$^+$ IL-17$^+$ T cells were observed in BD-skin lesions. Notably, we observed an increased number of CD8$^+$ IL-17$^+$ T cells in BD-skin [Figure 1B]. We further analyzed the expression of IFN-γ and IL-17 per single cell level. Interestingly, 40–60% IL-17$^+$ T cells coexpressed IFN-γ in the BD-skin [Figure 1C].

The data demonstrate the prevalence, phenotype, and distribution of IL-17$^+$ T cells in patients with BD, and indicate that BD-skin lesions is an environment containing abundant IL-17$^+$ T cells including Th17 cells and CD8$^+$ IL-17$^+$ T cells.

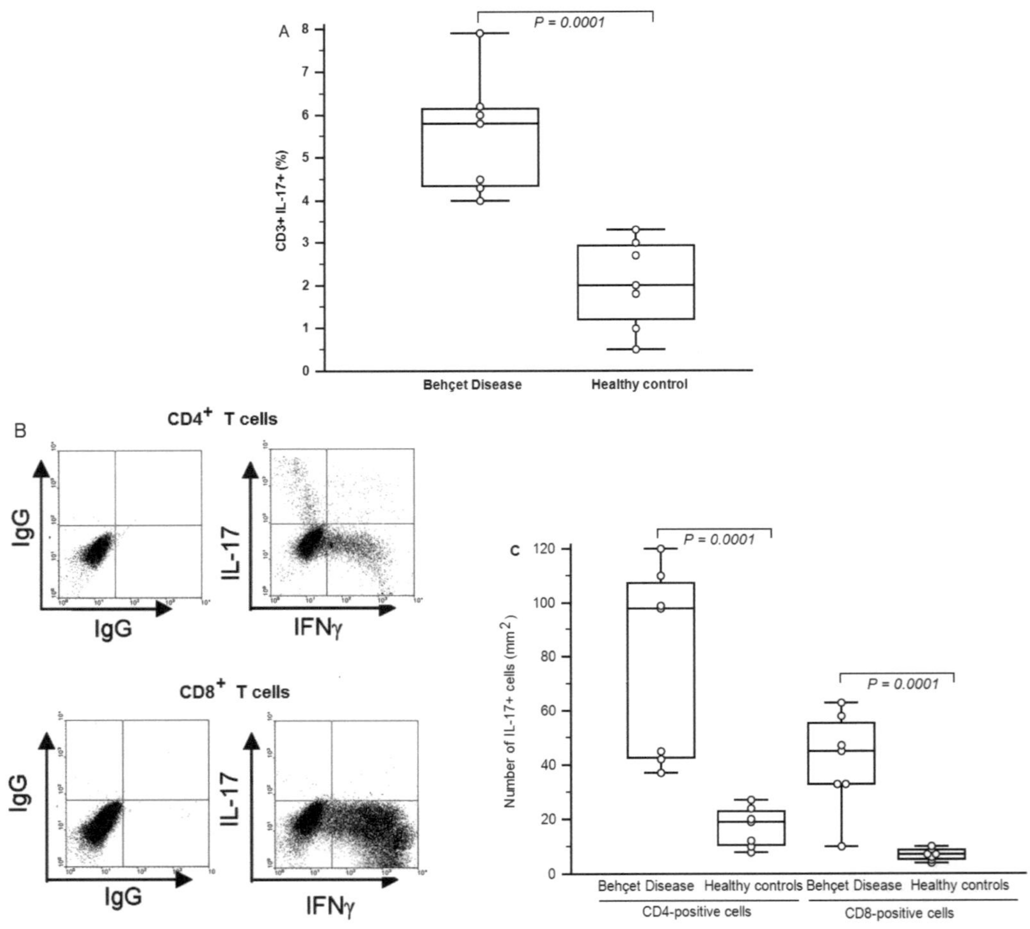

Fig. 1. IL-17$^+$ T cells in BD skin lesions.

Skin biopsy from healthy donors and patients with Behcet's disease (BD) were stained with specific antibodies as described in Materials and Methods. IL-17⁺ T cells were analyzed with FACS. (A): Results show mean percentage of $IL\text{-}17^+$ T cells in T cells. Error bar indicates SD. Representative dot plots are shown. Total number of $IL\text{-}17^+$ T cells in the skin. Total number of $IL\text{-}17^+$ T cells was calculated by multiplying the percentage of $IL\text{-}17^+$ T cells by the absolute number of T cells/mm^2 of skin, as determined previously [51]. Results shown are mean number ± SD, for n = 12 BD patients and 7 healthy donors. (B): Coexpression of IL-17 and IFN-γ on $IL\text{-}17^+$ T cells. Single cell suspensions were made from skin tissues in healthy donors and patients with BD. The expression of IFN-γ and IL-17 were analyzed by intracellular cytokine staining gated on $CD3^+$ T cells. (C): Total numbers of $CD4^+$ and $CD8^+$ $IL\text{-}17^+$ T cell subsets are shown as mean number ± SD.

3.2 IFN-γ+ T cells in patients with BD

As BD was related as Th1 disease, we examined the distribution of $CD4^+$, $CD8^+$, and IFN-γ+ T cells in BD-skin lesion. Consistent with previous reports [9], we observed a large number of $CD4^+$ and $CD8^+$ T cells in BD skin lesion [9; 20]. The distribution of $CD4^+$ and $CD8^+$ IFN-γ+ T cells is similar for T cells expressing IFN-γ and IL-17 in BD-skin. High levels of IFN-γ+ T cells [BD: 180.08 ± 62.46 cells/ mm2; HC: 25.71 ± 14.05 cells/ mm2; P = 0.0001][Figure 2A] and IFN-γ transcripts [BD: 27.75 ± 6.98 relative IFNγ mRNA expression (10-3); HC: 4.5 ± 1.87 relative IFNγ mRNA expression (10-3); P = 0.0001] [Figure 2B] were also detected in BD skin lesions compared to healthy controls.

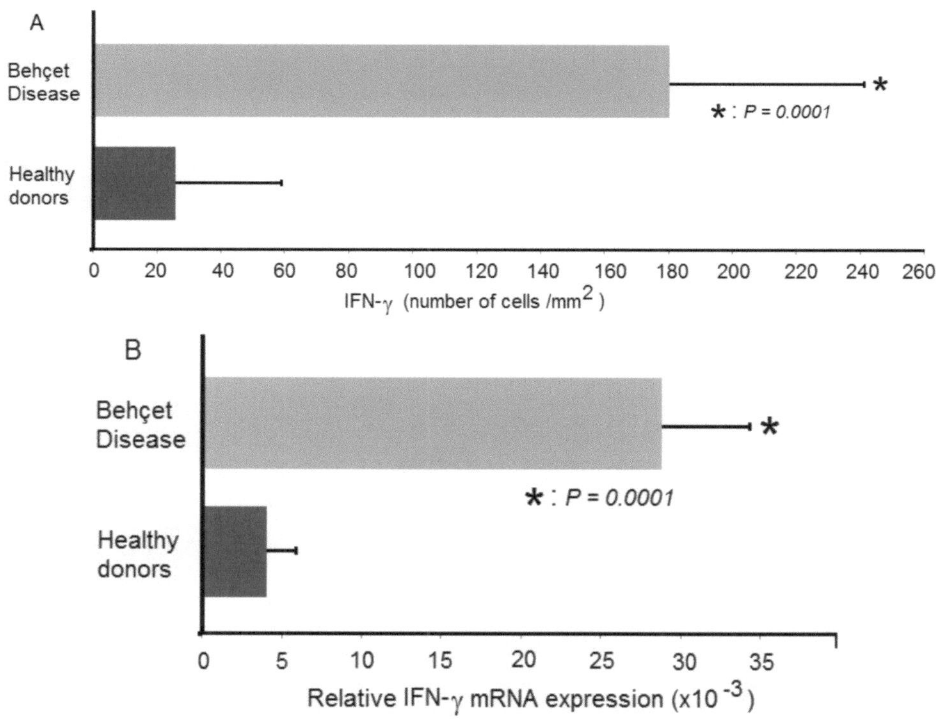

Fig. 2. IFN-γ^+ T cells in BD skin lesions. [A] and [B]: IFN-γ^+ T cells in BD lesions.

$CD45^+CD3^+$ T cells were analyzed by FACS in cell suspensions obtained from healthy skin and BD skin lesions. [A]: IFN-γ^+ T cells were analyzed by FACS and quantified in the skin. Results shown are the mean number of cells/mm^2 of skin ± SD for $n = 5$ healthy donors. [B]: Expression of IFN-γ in skin from healthy donors and patients with BD. IFN-γ was quantified by real-time PCR. Results shown are mean value of relative expression ± SD for 12 BD patients and 7 healthy donors.

3.3 Myeloid APCs induce IL-17$^+$ T cells

We sorted both $CD14^+$ and $CD11c^+$ myeloid APCs from peripheral blood and skin lesions from BD patients and healthy donors [Figure 3A]. CD14+ and CD11c+ myeloid APCs induced similar levels of Th17 cells [Figure 3B]. Then we investigated the potential role for myeloid APCs in inducing IL-17^+ T cells [Figure 3C]. Interestingly, APCs from BD peripheral blood and skin lesions were significantly more efficient than those from healthy donors in inducing IL-17 production [Figure 3C]. Myeloid APCs induced both $CD4^+$ and $CD8^+$ IL-17^+ T cells [Figure 3D]. We performed similar experiments with responder T cells from normal donors and BD patients. Our data indicate that BD myeloid APCs potently induce IL-17^+ T cells, and may thereby stimulate and maintain the IL-17^+ T cell pool in BD patients.

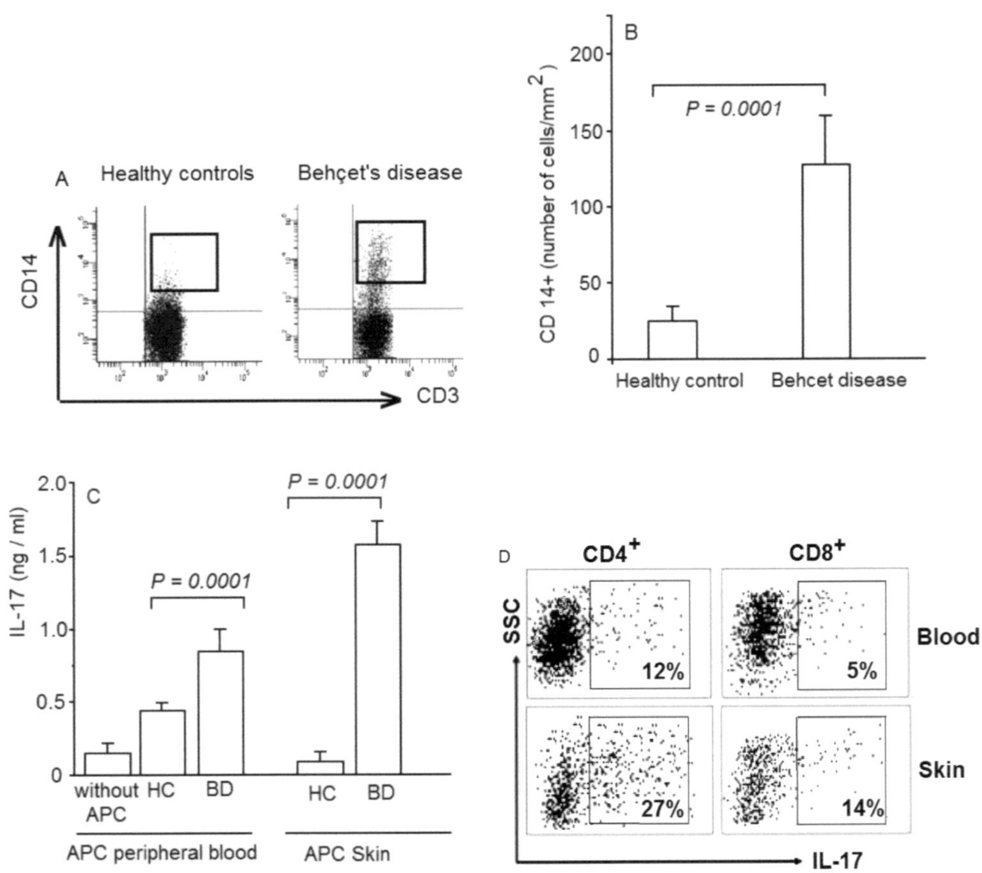

Fig. 3. Behçet's disease (BD) myeloid APCs stimulate IL-17^+ T cell expansion.

Myeloid APCs (CD45+CD14+) were analyzed by FACS in cell suspensions obtained from healthy skin and BD skin lesions. [A]: One representative dot plot of CD14+ leukocytes from the skin of a healthy donor and a patient with BD. Total number of CD3+ or CD14+ cells is indicated. [B]: Myeloid APCs were analyzed by FACS and quantified in the skin. Results shown are mean number of cells/mm^2 of skin ± SD for 5 BD patients and 4 healthy controls. [C and D]: BD myeloid APCs induce IL-17+ T cells. Normal peripheral blood T cells were stimulated for 5 days with myeloid APCs derived from skin and blood of healthy donors or patients with BD in the presence of anti-CD3 and anti-CD28. [C]: IL-17 was detected in the culture supernatants. Results shown are mean ± SD, for the same number of BD patients and controls.

3.4 IFN-γ induces myeloid APCs to stimulate IL-17+ T cells

We next studied why BD myeloid APCs are potent inducers of IL-17+ T cells. The contribution of IFN-γ was investigated, as IFN-γ is increased in serum of BD patients [Hamzaoui et al., 2007]. IFN−γ+ T cells are enriched in BD skin lesions as reported in Figure 2 and all studies implicated IFN-γ (Th1 cells) in BD pathogenesis. To test the hypothesis that IFN-γ may program myeloid APCs to stimulate IL-17+ T cells, CD11+ cells from the blood of donors were conditioned with IFN-γ and tested for their capacity to induce IL-17+ T cells. IFN−γ profoundly increased the capacity of CD11c+ cells to elicit IL-17+ T cells [Figure 4A, B, and C]. We also conditioned peripheral blood myeloid APCs from BD patients with exogenous IFN-γ, and observed that IFN-γ was able to further enhance the ability of healthy controls and BD myeloid APCs to induce IL-17-secreting T cells [Figure 4]. The data suggest that IFN-γ released by BD T cells may condition myeloid APCs to induce IL-17+ T cells.

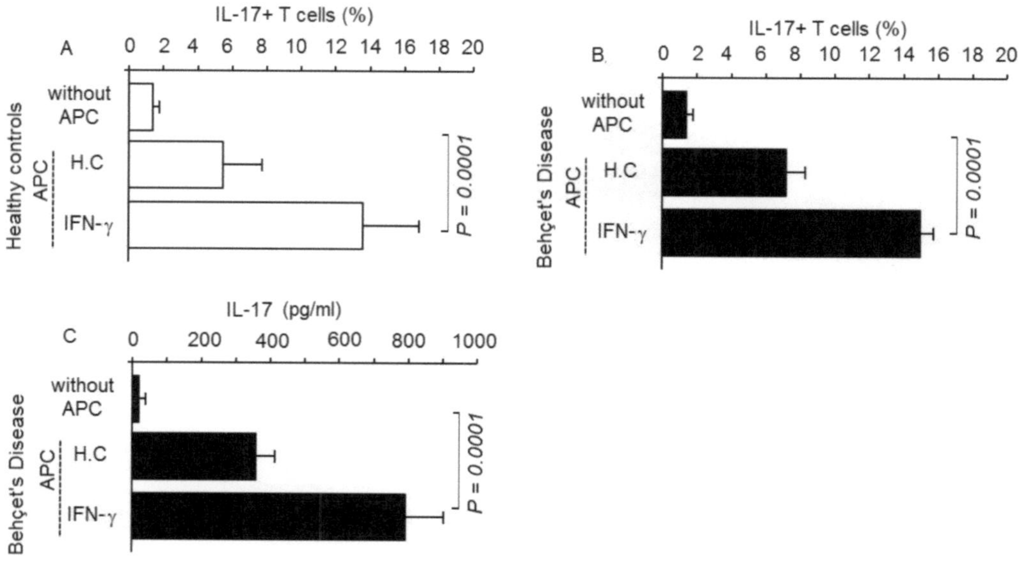

Fig. 4. IFN-γ induces BD- APCs to stimulate IL-17+ T cells.

Healthy control (A) or BD patients (B) blood-derived ex vivo CD11c+ cells were conditioned for 72 h with or without IFN-γ, and then cultured with normal T cells for 5 days in the presence of anti-CD3 and anti-CD28. [A]: IL-17^{+} T cells were detected by FACS. Results shown are mean percentage ± SD of IL-17^{+} T cells in T cells. (C): IL-17 was measured in the supernatants by ELISA. Results shown are mean percentage ± SD of IL-17. Five patients with BD and 4 healthy controls were investigated.

3.5 CCR6+ IL-17^{+} T cells and CCL20 in Behçet's disease

We examined how IL-17^{+} T cells traffic to the BD skin environment. We found that $CD4^{+}$ and $CD8^{+}$ IL-17^{+} T cells derived from BD skin lesions highly expressed CCR6 [Figure 5A and B]. We therefore asked whether IL-17^{+} T cells could migrate toward CCL20, the ligand for CCR6. We observed that T cells efficiently migrated in response to CCL20, and that the migrating cells were enriched for IL-17^{+} T cells (from 0.2% IL-17– cells in the upper chamber to 18% IL-17^{+} T cells in the lower chamber) [Figure 5C]. We further tested the role of IFN-γ in CCL20 production. We observed that IFN–γ stimulated CCL20 production from $CD11c^{+}$ APCs [Figure 5D]. High levels of CCL20 mRNA were detected in lesional BD skin [Figure 5E]. The data suggest that IFN-γ derived from BD T cells induces CCL20 and promotes homing of IL-17^{+} T cells to the BD environment. In addition to CCR6, we observed that BD- IL-17^{+} T cells highly expressed CD103 as compared with IL-17– T cells [Figure 5F]. CD103 may play a specific role in IL-17^{+} T cell trafficking.

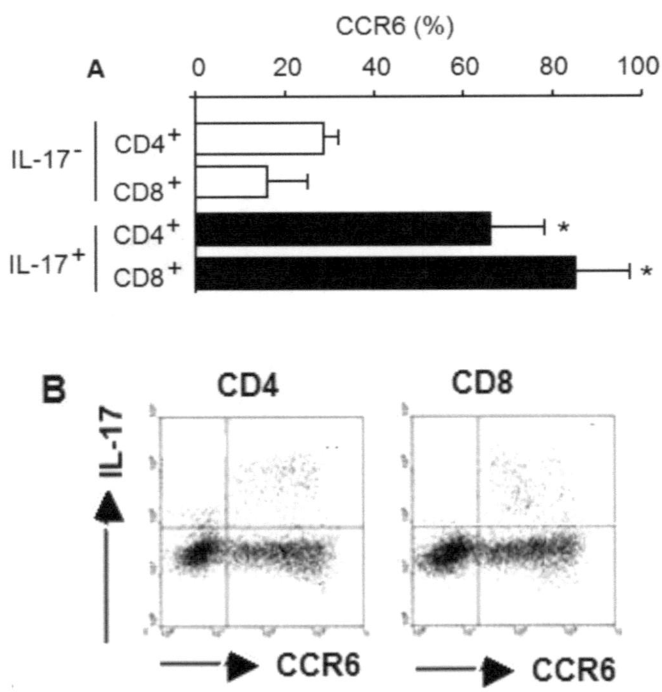

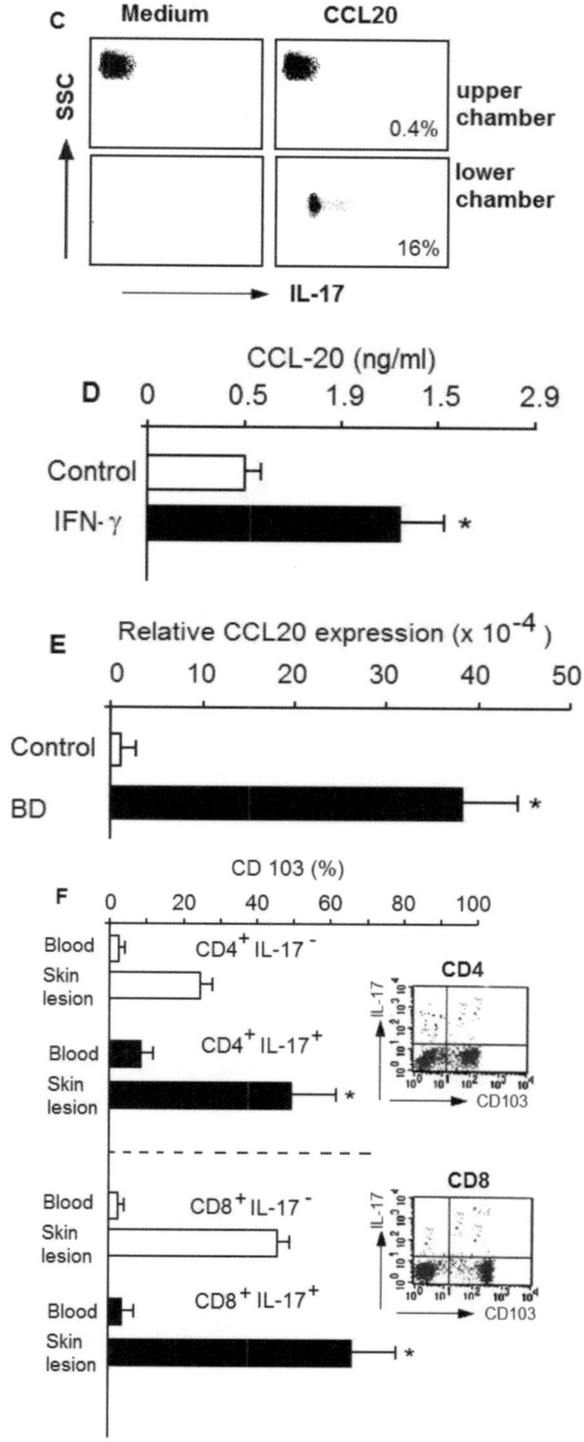

Fig. 5. CCR6+ IL-17+ T cells and CCL20 in the BD environment.

[A,B]: BD-IL-17⁺ T cells highly express CCR6. Expression of CCR6 was determined by FACS on IL-17⁺ and IL-17–T cells in BD skin. Results shown are mean of CCR6+ T cells in IL-17⁺ T cells or IL-17– T cells ± SD for 5 healthy donors and 6 BD patients. (*): $P < 0.05$ compared with IL-17– T cells. [C]: IL-17⁺ T cells migrate in response to CCL20. Migration assay was performed as described in Materials and Methods. The migrated T cells were subjected to intracellular staining for IL-17. The percentage of IL-17⁺ T cells in the upper and lower chambers is shown. [D]: IFN-γ induces CCL20 production. Blood CD11c+ cells were stimulated for 3 days with or without IFN- γ. CCL20 was detected by ELISA in the supernatants. Results shown are mean value ± SD for 8 healthy controls. (*): $P < 0.05$ compared with control. [E]: High expression of CCL20 in BD skin. CCL20 transcript was quantified by real-time PCR. Results shown are mean value of relative 1 expression ± SD for 5 healthy donors. (*): $P = 0.004$ compared with healthy skin control. [F]: High expression of CD103 on BD IL-17⁺ T cells. CD103 expression was determined by FACS on IL-17⁺ and IL-17– T cell subsets. Results shown are mean ± SD of CD103⁺ T cells in each T cell subset, for 5 healthy donors. (*): $P < 0.05$ compared with IL-17– T cells. One representative dot plot of BD CD103⁺ IL-17⁺ T cells is shown gated each on CD4⁺ and CD8⁺ T cells.

3.6 Functional characterization of $CD8^+IL\text{-}17^+$ and $CD4^+IL\text{-}17^+$ cells from BD-skin lesions

The ability of $CD8^+IL\text{-}17^+$ and $CD4^+IL\text{-}17^+$ cells-producing T cells derived from BD-skin lesions to proliferate in response to TCR-mediated stimulation was also assessed. For this purpose, CCR6-sorted and expanded cells were challenged with anti-CD3/CD28 mAb. A well-characterized Th17 line was used as a control. The response of the Th17 cells from the BD-skin lesions was significantly increased to those of the $CD8^+IL\text{-}17^+$ and $CD4^+IL\text{-}17^+$ T cells derived from healthy controls [Figure 6].

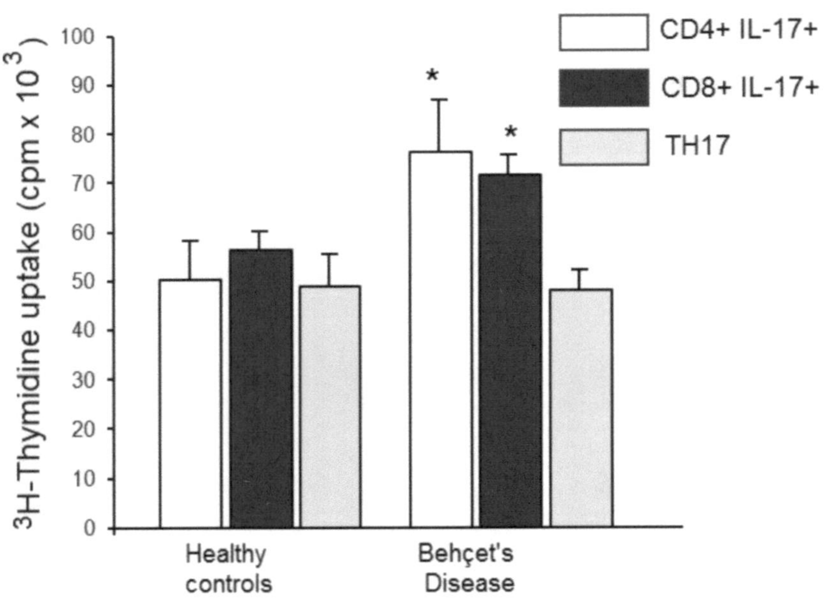

Fig. 6. Proliferative response of BD-skin-derived $CD8^+IL\text{-}17^+$ and $CD4^+IL\text{-}17^+$ T cells and a Th17 cell line.

Proliferative responses of CD8+IL-17+ and CD4+IL-17+ T cells from BD patients were more important than in healthy controls. Columns represent mean ± SD values (n=8) of proliferative response and asterisks, statistical significance [*]: $P < 0.05$.

4. Discussion

In this report we have investigated the phenotype and function of IL-17+ T cells in skin healthy controls and BD patients with skin lesions. We show that CD3+ T cells expressing IL-17 were increased in BD-skin lesions compared to skin biopsies from healthy controls. CD3+ IL-17+ T cells (Th17) are postulated to play a role in inflammatory/autoimmune pathogenesis [Wilson et al., 2007; Zaba et al., 2007; Murphy et al., 2003; Aggarwal et al., 2003]. Recent data from Melikoglu et al [Melikoglu et al., 2006] reported increased cytokines (IFN-γ, IL-12 p40, IL-15), chemokines (MIP3-α, IP-10, Mig, and iTac), and adhesion molecules (ICAM-1, VCAM-1) in the skin of BD patients with SPR+ but not in the skin of normal controls. These results suggested that BD patients experience marked cellular influx into the injury site, leading to an exaggerated lymphoid Th1-type response. Our results agree the inflammatory state in skin BD patient; our present results added a Th17-type response. We show that both CD4+ and CD8+ T cells express IL-17 in BD-skin lesions. We observed high levels of CD8+ IL-17+ T cells in the BD skin lesions. CD8+ IL-17+ T cells are ideally positioned to respond to potential keratinocyte autoantigens on HLA class I molecules. CD8+ IL-17+ T cells have been genetically implicated in skin lesions from autoimmune/inflammatory diseases [Nair et al., 206]. Our observations support the hypothesis that CD8+ IL-17+ T cells are critical mediators of the persistently altered epidermal growth and differentiation and the local inflammation that is characteristic of BD skin lesions. CD8+ IL-17+ T cells were observed in cancers [12] and in psoriasis [Kryczek et al., 2008]. Our data provide the first evidence that CD8+ IL-17+ T cells are important in BD as observed in autoimmune/inflammatory diseases [Wilson et al., 2007]. The presence of CD8+ T cells is necessary for the epidermal hyperproliferative response [Conrad et al., 2007]. We characterized the phenotype of skin BD lesions IL-17+ T cells: CD103+CCR6+ IL-17+ T cells are effector T cells often found in environments with chronic inflammation [Gudjonsson et al. 2004; Krolls et al., 2006]. IL-17+ T cells highly express CD103, which may facilitate trafficking of IL-17+ cells into inflammatory tissues [Conrad et al., 2007; Pauls et al., 2001]. We confirm that BD skin is an environment enriched with CCL20, and show that CCL20 is triggered by IFN-γ in myeloid APCs. We reported that BD Th1 cells are one of the major sources of IFN-γ, as reported recently [Hamzaoui et al., 2007], and that IL-17+ T cells efficiently migrate toward a CCL20-enriched BD environment via CCR6. Our data lead us to propose a first mode of potential interaction between Th1 and IL-17+ T cells in BD: IFN-γ derived from Th1 cells promotes trafficking of IL-17+ T cells to the environment BD lesions through the induction and maintenance of local CCL20 production.

Regarding the contribution of epidermal CD8+IL-17+ cells to the pathogenesis of BD skin lesions, we have proved that CD4+IL-17+ and CD8+IL-17+ proliferate and secrete cytokines efficiently in response to CD3/TCR-mediated stimulation and to certain mediators. In Behcet's disease, high mRNA levels of IL-8, IFN-γ, IL-12, IL-10, and MCP-1were found in lesional skin and pathergy sites [Melikoglu et al., 2006].

CD4+CD25+ regulatory T (Treg) cells were found increased in the peripheral circulation of BD patients [Hamzaoui, 2007]. Treg cells and interleukin 17 (IL-17)-producing T helper cells (TH17) carry out opposite functions, the former maintaining self-tolerance and the latter being involved in inflammation and autoimmunity [Deknuydt et al., 2009]. Several recent studies have indicated the existence of a close interplay between Treg and Th17 cells in regulating some autoimmune diseases. Whereas murine Treg cells suppress both Th1 and Th2 cells, in BD patients they enhance IL-17 secretion, likely through production of TGF-β [Mangan et al., 2006; Veldhoen et al., 2006]. Interplay between Treg cells and $CD4^+$ $IL\text{-}17^+$ cells have to be investigated in BD patients [Hamzaoui et al., 2011a; 2011b]. Memory Treg actually showed a more pronounced proficiency to give rise to Th17 cells than conventional memory $CD4^+$ T cells, suggesting that they may be at least partially committed towards the T_H17 differentiation pathway. This is consistent with the fact that memory Treg populations contain high proportions of cells expressing CCR6, the receptor of macrophage inflammatory protein3α (MIP-3α/CCL20) that has been shown to characterize the T_H17 lineage [Acosta-Rodriguez et al., 2007; Tosello et al., 2008].

The findings reported in the present study have several implications. First, one can imagine a scenario in which, during skin BD inflammation, Treg cells stimulated by APC activated by microbial products participate to innate immunity and transiently down-regulate suppressor functions, to allow the development of adaptive immunity. In a second scenario, sustained induction of Treg into Th17 cells *in vivo* will likely occur under defined permissive conditions, such as those that have been reported to lead to autoimmune/inflammatory reactions including chronic inflammation in the presence of interleukin (IL)-1 and IL-2. IL-1 was highly expressed in BD [Bilginer et al., 2010; Kôtter et al., 2005].

There are <1% $CD4^+$ and <0.5% $CD8^+$ $IL\text{-}17^+$ T cells in peripheral blood of healthy humans [Kryczek et al., 2007]. Peripheral blood of active BD patients exhibited high levels of Th17 cells in their peripheral circulation [Hamzaoui et al., 2002; Direskeneli et al.; 2003; Hamzaoui et al., 2011] and in cerebrospinal fluid [Hamzaoui et al., 2011]. High levels of Th17, $CD4^+$ $IL\text{-}17^+$ and $CD8^+$ $IL\text{-}17^+$ T cells are observed in BD inflammatory skin. How does this induction occur? In addition to migration from peripheral blood, $IL\text{-}17^+$ T cells may be induced within the BD lesions environment. It has been reported that myeloid cell-derived genes contribute to pathogenic manifestations in inflammatory diseases [Haider et al., 2008; Szegedi et al., 2003]. We demonstrate that myeloid APCs including macrophages and myeloid dendritic cells potently induce human $IL\text{-}17^+$ T cells. Our observation may also explain why $IL\text{-}17^+$ T cells are often found in inflammatory tissues and organs. In support of this concept, we show that myeloid APCs isolated from BD patients potently stimulate $IL\text{-}17^+$ T cells. Increased circulating IFN-γ [Szegedi et al.,2003] may activate circulating APCs, allowing them to enter tissue and promote expansion of $IL\text{-}17^+$ T cells. Th1 cells can suppress Th17 cell differentiation through IFN-γ [Kolls et al., 2004; Weaver et al., 2006; Teunissen et al., 1998].

IFN-γ triggers myeloid APCs to produce IL-1 and IL-23, and in turn induce $IL\text{-}17^+$ T cells [Kryczek et al 2008]. Our data therefore demonstrate the potential mode of interaction between Th1 and $IL\text{-}17^+$ T cells in BD skin lesions: IFN-γ derived from Th1 cells promotes $IL\text{-}17^+$ T cell development through IL-1 and IL-23 in the skin lesion environment in Behcet disease. Therefore, IFN-γ may possibly play dual roles in regulating the $IL\text{-}17^+$ T cell pool: IFN-γ targets APCs to initiate and promote Th17 polarization [Teunissen et al., 1998; Kolls et al., 2004; Szabo et al., 1998] to suppress Th17 polarization.

In summary, we show that IFN-γ may promote trafficking, induction, and function of $IL\text{-}17^+$ T cells in patients with BD. This study clarify the interaction between Th1 and Th17 cells, challenges the view that Th1 cells suppress Th17 cell development, and suggests a collaborative contribution of Th1 and Th17 to autoimmune/inflammatory diseases. Ongoing research is addressing this aspect as well as attempting to define better whether $CD8^+$ $IL\text{-}17^+$ lymphocytes act as cytotoxic cells (Tc17 cells) which contribute to initiate, stabilize, or inhibit the BD process in the skin.

5. References

Acosta-Rodriguez EV., Rivino, L., Geginat, J., Jarrossay D., Gattorno, M., Lanzavecchia, A., Sallusto, F., Napolitani, G. (2007). Surface phenotype and antigenic specificity of human interleukin 17-producing T helper memory cells. *Nat Immunol,* Vol.8, pp. 639-646.

Aggarwal, S., Ghilardi, N., Xie, M. H., de Sauvage, F. J., Gurney, A. L. (2003). Interleukin-23 promotes a distinct CD4 T cell activation state characterized by the production of interleukin-17. *J. Biol. Chem.* Vol. 278, pp. 1910-1914.

Bettelli, E., Oukka, M., K. Kuchroo V. (2007) T_H-17 cells in the circle of immunity and autoimmunity. *Nat. Immunol.* Vol. 8, pp. 345-350.

Bilginer, Y., Ayaz, NA., Ozen, S. (2010). Anti-IL-1 treatment for secondary amyloidosis in an adolescent with FMF and Behçet's disease. *Clin Rheumatol.* Vol. 29 N°2, pp. 209-10.

Chi, W., Yang, P., Zhu, X., Wang, Y., Chen, L., Huang, X., Liu, X. (2010). Production of interleukin-17 in Behcet's disease is inhibited by cyclosporin A. *Mol Vis.* Vol. 16, pp. 880-6.

Clark, R. A., B. F. Chong, N. Mirchandani, K. Yamanaka, G. F. Murphy, R. K. Dowgiert, T. S. Kupper. (2006). A novel method for the isolation of skin resident T cells from normal and diseased human skin. *J. Invest. Dermatol.* Vol. 126, pp. 1059-1070.

Conrad, C., Boyman, O., Tonel, G., Tun-Kyi, A., Laggner, U., de Fougerolles, A., Kotelianski, V., Gardner, H., Nestle, F. O. (2007). α_1®$_1$ integrin is crucial for accumulation of epidermal T cells and the development of psoriasis. *Nat. Med.* Vol. 13, pp. 836-842.

Curiel, T. J., G. Coukos, L. Zou, X. Alvarez, P. Cheng, P. Mottram, M. Evdemon-Hogan, J. R. Conejo-Garcia, L. Zhang, M. Burow, (2004). Specific recruitment of regulatory T cells in ovarian carcinoma fosters immune privilege and predicts reduced survival. *Nat. Med.* Vol. 10, pp.942-949.

Curiel, T. J., Wei S, Dong H., Alvarez X., Cheng P., Mottram P., Krzysiek R., Knutson K.L., Daniel B., Zimmermann. M. C. (2003). Blockade of B7-H1 improves myeloid dendritic cell-mediated antitumor immunity. *Nat. Med.* Vol. 9, pp. 562-567.

Deknuydt, F., Bioley, G., Valmori, D., Ayyoub, M. (2009). IL-1beta and IL-2 convert human Treg into T(H)17 cells. *Clin Immunol.*Vol. 131, N°.2, pp.298-307.

Diri, E., Mat, C., Hamuryudan, V., Yurdakul, S., Hizli, N., Yazici, H. (2001). Papulopustular skin lesions are seen more frequently in patients with Behcet's syndrome who have arthritis: a controlled and masked study. *Ann Rheum Dis,* Vol. 60, pp.1074-6.

Ekinci, NS., Alpsoy, E., Karakas, AA., Yilmaz, SB., Yegin, O. (2010). IL-17A has an important role in the acute attacks of Behçet's disease. J Invest Dermatol. Vol. 130, N°. 8, pp. 2136-8.

Gudjonsson, J.E., Johnston A., Sigmundsdottir, H., Valdimarsson, H., (2004). Immunopathogenic mechanisms in psoriasis. *Clin. Exp. Immunol.* Vol. 135, pp. 1-8.

Haider, A.S., Lowes M.A., Suarez-Farinas M., Zaba L. C., Cardinale I., Khatcherian A., Novitskaya I., Wittkowski K. M., Krueger. J. G. (2008). Identification of cellular pathways of "type 1," Th17 T cells, and TNF-α and inducible nitric oxide synthase-producing dendritic cells in autoimmune inflammation through pharmacogenomic study of cyclosporine A in psoriasis. *J. Immunol.* Vol.180, pp. 1913-1920.

Hamzaoui, K., Hamzaoui, A., Guemira, F., Bessioud, M., Hamza, M., Ayed, K. (2002). Cytokine profile in Behçet's disease patients. Relationship with disease activity. *Scand J Rheumatol*, Vol. 31, pp. 205–10.

Hamzaoui, K. (2007). Paradoxical high regulatory T cell activity in Behçet's disease.*Clin Exp Rheumatol.* Vol. 25, N°. 4, (Suppl 45), pp. S107-13.

Hamzaoui, K., Houman, H., Hamzaoui, A. (2008). Serum BAFF levels and skin mRNA expression in patients with Behçet's disease. *Clin Exp Rheumatol.*Vol. 26 N°. 4 (Suppl 50), pp. S64-71.

Hamzaoui, K., Borhani Haghighi, A. (2011a). RORC and Foxp3 axis in cerebrospinal fluid of patients with Neuro-Behçet's Disease. *J Neuroimmunol.* Vol. 233, N°. 1-2, pp. 249-53.

Hamzaoui, K., Bouali, E., Ghorbel, I., Khanfir, M., Houman, H., Hamzaoui A. (2011b). Expression of Th-17 and RORγt mRNA in Behçet's Disease. *Med Sci Monit.*Vol. 17, N°. 4, PP. CR 227-34.

International Study Group for Behçet's disease: (1990). Criteria for diagnosis of Behçet's disease. *Lancet.* Vol. 335, pp. 1078-80.

Jang, WC., Nam, YH., Ahn, YC., Lee, SH., Park, SH., Choe, JY., Lee, SS., Kim, SK. (2008). Interleukin-17F gene polymorphisms in Korean patients with Behçet's disease. *Rheumatol Int.* Vol. 29, N°. 2, pp. 173-8.

Koarada S, Haruta Y, Tada Y, Ushiyama O, Morito F, Ohta A, Nagasawa K. (2004). Increased entry of $CD4^+$ T cells into the Th1 cytokine effector pathway during T-cell division following stimulation in Behcet's disease. *Rheumatology (Oxford).* 43(7): 843-51.

Kolls, J. K., A. Linden. (2004). Interleukin-17 family members and inflammation. *Immunity* 21: 467-476.

Weaver, C. T., L. E. Harrington, P. R. Mangan, M. Gavrieli, K. M. Murphy. (2006). Th17: an effector CD4 T cell lineage with regulatory T cell ties. *Immunity*, Vol. 24, pp. 677-688.

Komiyama, Y., Nakae S., Matsuki T., Nambu A., Ishigame H., Kakuta S., Sudo K., Iwakura Y. (2006). IL-17 plays an important role in the development of experimental autoimmune encephalomyelitis. *J. Immunol.* Vol. 177, pp. 566-573.

Kötter, I., Koch, S., Vonthein, R., Rückwaldt, U., Amberger, M., Günaydin, I., Zierhut, M., Stübiger, N. (2005). Cytokines, cytokine antagonists and soluble adhesion molecules in patients with ocular Behçet's disease treated with human recombinant interferon-alpha2a. Results of an open study and review of the literature. *Clin Exp Rheumatol.* Vol. 23, N°. 4 (Suppl 38), pp. S20-6.

Krause, I., Y. Molad, M. Mitrani, A. Weinberger. (2000). Pathergy reaction in Behçet's disease: lack of correlation with mucocutaneous manifestations and systemic disease expression. *Clin. Exp. Rheumatol.* Vol. 18, pp. 71-74.

Kryczek, I., Bruce, AT., Gudjonsson, JE., Johnston, A., Aphale, A., Vatan, L., Szeliga, W., Wang, Y., Liu, Y., Welling, TH., Elder, JT., Zou, W. (2008). Induction of IL-17^+ T cell trafficking and development by IFN-gamma: mechanism and pathological relevance in psoriasis. J Immunol. Vol. 181, N°.7, pp. 4733-41.

Kryczek, I., Wei, S., Gong, W., Shu, X., Szeliga, W., Vatan, L., Chen, L., Wang, G., Zou, W. (2008). Cutting edge: IFN-gamma enables APC to promote memory Th17 and abate Th1 cell development. J Immunol. Vol. 181, N°. 9, pp. 5842-6.

Kryczek, I., S. Wei, L. Zou, S. Altuwaijri, W. Szeliga, J. Kolls, A. Chang, W. Zou. (2007). Cutting edge: Th17 and regulatory T cell dynamics and the regulation by IL-2 in the tumor microenvironment. *J Immunol,* Vol. 178, pp. 6730-6733.

Kulaber, A., Tugal-Tutkun, I., Yentür, SP., Akman-Demir, G., Kaneko, F., Gül, A., Saruhan-Direskeneli, G. (2007). Pro-inflammatory cellular immune response in Behçet's disease. *Rheumatol Int,* Vol. 27, N°.12, pp. 1113-8.

Lawton G, Bhakta BB, Chamberlain A, Tenant A. (2004). The Behçet's disease activity index. *Rheumatol,* Vol. 43, pp. 73-78.

Mangan, PR., Harrington, L.E., O'Quinn, D.B., Helms, W.S.,. Bullard, D.C., Elson, C.O., Hatton, R.D., Wahl, S.M, Schoeb, T.R., Weaver, C.T. (2006). Transforming growth factor-beta induces development of the T(H)17 lineage, *Nature,* Vol. 441, pp. 231-234.

Melikoglu M, Uysal S., Krueger James G., Kaplan G, Gogus F, Yazici H, andOliver S. (2006). Characterization of the Divergent Wound-Healing Responses Occurring in the Pathergy Reaction and Normal Healthy Volunteers *J. Immunol.* 177: 6415 -21.

Keller, M., Spanou, Z., Schaerli, P., Britschgi,M., Yawalkar, N., Seitz, M., Villiger P. M., and Werner J. Pichler. (2005). T Cell-Regulated Neutrophilic Inflammation in Autoinflammatory Diseases. J Immunol, Vol. 175, pp. 7678 - 86.

Murphy, C. A., Langrish, C. L., Chen, Y., Blumenschein, W., McClanahan, T., Kastelein, R. A., Sedgwick JD., Cua, D. J. (2003). Divergent pro- and antiinflammatory roles for IL-23 and IL-12 in joint autoimmune inflammation. *J. Exp. Med.* Vol. 198, pp. 1951-1957.

Nair, R. P., Stuart, P. E., Nistor, I., R. Hiremagalore, N. V., Chia, S., Weichenthal M., Abecasis, G. R., Lim, H.W., Christophers, E., (2006). Sequence and haplotype analysis supports HLA-C as the psoriasis susceptibility 1 gene. *Am. J. Hum. Genet.* Vol. 78, pp. 827-851.

Onder, M., Gurer, MA. (2001). The multiple faces of Behçet's disease and its etiological factors. *J Eur Acad Dermatol Venereol,* Vol. 15, pp. 126–136.

Pauls, K., M. Schon, R. C. Kubitza, B. Homey, A. Wiesenborn, P. Lehmann, T. Ruzicka, C. M. Parker, M. P. Schon. Role of integrin α_E (CD103) β_7 for tissue-specific epidermal localization of $CD8^+$ T lymphocytes. *J. Invest. Dermatol.* 2001; 117: 569-575.

Saruhan-Direskeneli, G., Yentur, SP., Akman-Demir, G. Isik, N., Serdaroglu, P. (2003). Cytokines and chemokines in neuro-Behçet's disease compared to multiple sclerosis and other neurological diseases. *J Neuroimmunol;* Vol. 145,pp. 127-34.

Suzuki, N., Nara, K., Suzuki, T. (2006). Skewed Th1 responses caused by excessive expression of Txk, a member of the Tec family of tyrosine kinases in patients with Behcet's disease. *Clin Med Res.* Vol. 4. Pp.147-151.

Szabo, S.K., Hammerberg, C. Yoshida, Y., Bata-Csorgo, Z., Cooper, K. D. (1998). Identification and quantitation of interferon-γ producing T cells in psoriatic lesions: localization to both $CD4^+$ and $CD8^+$ subsets. *J. Invest. Dermatol.* Vol. 111, pp. 1072-1078.

Szegedi, A., M. Aleksza, A., Gonda, B., Irinyi, S., Sipka, J., Hunyadi, P., Antal-Szalmas. (2003). Elevated rate of Thelper1 (T_H1) lymphocytes and serum IFN-γ levels in psoriatic patients. *Immunol. Lett.* Vol. 86, pp. 277-280.

Takeuchi, M. Usui, Y., Okunuki, Y., Zhang, L., Ma, J., Yamakawa, N., Hattori, T., Kezuka, T., Sakai, J., Goto, H. (2010). Immune responses to interphotoreceptor retinoid-binding protein and S-antigen in Behcet's patients with uveitis. Invest Ophthalmol Vis Sci. Vol.51, N°. 6, pp. 3067-75.

Teunissen, M.B., Koomen, C.W., de Waal Malefyt R., Wierenga E. A., Bos J. D. (1998). Interleukin-17 and interferon-γ synergize in the enhancement of proinflammatory cytokine production by human keratinocytes. *J. Invest. Dermatol.* Vol. 111, pp. 645-649.

Odunsi Tosello, K., Souleimanian, N.E., Lele, S., P. Shrikant, Old, L.J., Valmori D., Ayyoub M. 2008. Differential expression of CCR7 defines two distinct subsets of human memory CD4(+)CD25(+) Tregs, *Clin. Immunol.* Vol. 126, pp. 291–302.

Veldhoen, M, Hocking, R.J., Atkins, C.J., Locksley, R.M., Stockinger, B. (2006). TGFbeta in the context of an inflammatory cytokine milieu supports de novo differentiation of IL-17-producing T cells, *Immunity* Vol. 24, pp. 179–189.

Weaver, C.T., Harrington, L. E., Mangan, P. R., Gavrieli, M., Murphy, K. M. Th17: an effector CD4 T cell lineage with regulatory T cell ties. *Immunity,* Vol. 24, pp. 677-688.

Wilson, N.J., Boniface, K., Chan, J.R., McKenzie, B.S., Blumenschein, W.M., Mattson, J.D., Basham, B., Smith, K., Chen, T., Morel, F. (2007). Development, cytokine profile and function of human interleukin 17-producing helper T cells. *Nat. Immunol.* Vol. 8, pp.950-957.

Yazici, H, Yurdakul, S., Fresko V. (2003) Behçet's syndrome, in: M. C Hochberg, J. A Silman, J. S Smolen, M. E Weinblatt and M. H Weisman (Eds). *Rheumatology,* pp. 1665–9. London: Mosby.

Zaba, L.C., Cardinale, I., Gilleaudeau, P., Sullivan-Whalen, M., Farinas, M. S., Fuentes-Duculan J., Novitskaya, I., Khatcherian, A., Bluth, M. J., Lowes, M. A., Krueger, J. G. (2007). Amelioration of epidermal hyperplasia by TNF inhibition is associated with reduced Th17 responses. *J. Exp. Med.* Vol.204, pp. 3183-94.

Part 4

Activate Protein C Role in Inflammatory Disease

4

Anti-Inflammatory Actions of the Anticoagulant, Activated Protein C

Christopher John Jackson and Meilang Xue
Sutton Arthritis Research Laboratories, Department of Rheumatology, Institute of Bone and Joint Research, Kolling Institute, University of Sydney at Royal North Shore Hospital, St Leonards Australia

1. Introduction

Protein C is a vitamin K–dependent zymogen, discovered in 1976 in bovine plasma (Stenflo, 1976). It is derived from the human PROC gene on chromosome 2 (2q13-q14) which contains 9 exons (Rezaie, 1993). Post-translational modifications include β-hydroxylation at Asp71, N-linked glycosylation at residues 97, 248, 313 and 329 and γ-carboxylation of 9 glutamic acid residues which forms the Gla domain at the amino terminus. Human protein C is 62kD protein and consists of 419 amino acids. The four major moieties that make up the protein C molecule are a Gla domain, two epidermal growth factor (EGF)- like regions, a small activation peptide, and an active serine protease domain (Griffin, 2005). Mature 62 000 Da human protein C is cleaved by a furin-like endoprotease that releases Lys156–Arg157 before secretion from liver cells. Protein C is activated on the endothelial surface when thrombin binds to thrombomodulin and cleaves protein C's activation peptide. This conversion to activated protein C (APC) is augmented by endothelial cell protein C receptor (EPCR) (Fukudome & Esmon, 1994). Protein C circulates in plasma at 70 nM whereas APC is present in much lower concentrations (40 pM or ~ 2.3 ng/mL) (Gruber & Griffin, 1992).
APC was first recognized as an anticoagulant. In the presence of its cofactor, protein S, APC degrades the coagulation factors Va and VIIIa and inhibits thrombin generation. The light chain provides anticoagulant activity by having highly specific protein–protein interactions with factors Va and VIIIa followed by proteolytic inactivation of factor Va by cleavage at Arg (506) and Arg (306) and of factor VIIIa by cleavage at Arg (336) and Arg (562) (Zlokovic & Griffin, 2011). In addition, APC promotes fibrinolysis by binding to plasminogen activator inhibitor which prevents inhibition of plasminogen conversion to plasmin. The significance of APC as an anticoagulant is reflected by the findings that deficiencies in protein C result in severe familial disorders of thrombosis (Baker & Bick, 1999). Replenishment of protein C/APC in patients with systemic or local hypercoagulation can reverse the abnormality.

2. Anti-inflammatory and cytoprotective functions of APC

In addition to its anticoagulant activity, APC exerts a broad range of cytoprotective and anti-inflammatory actions described below.

2.1 Inflammation

Independent of its effect on coagulation, APC has potent anti-inflammatory properties (Joyce, 2001; Mosnier & Griffin, 2003) associated with a decrease in pro-inflammatory cytokines and a reduction of leukocyte recruitment. Joyce et al (Joyce, 2001) have shown that APC directly suppresses expression of p50 and p52 nuclear factor (NF)-κB subunits in human umbilical vein endothelial cells. The NF-κB pathway is important for the expression of a wide variety of inflammatory genes including tumor necrosis factor (TNF)-α and cell adhesion molecules that are associated with diseases ranging from inflammation to cancer (Li & Verma, 2002). Direct inhibition of NF-κB is sufficient to block symptoms of many inflammatory diseases so these inhibitors have potential therapeutic value (Bell, 1915; Li & Verma, 2002; Calzado, 1914; Calzado, 2007). APC inhibits the expression and activation of NF-κB in unstimulated and stimulated monocytes (White, 2000; Xue, 2007; Yuksel, 2002), keratinocytes (Xue, 2004), endothelial cells (Franscini, 2004). APC also suppresses inflammation in vivo by inhibition of NF-κB (Cheng, 2006). In addition, APC has the ability to upregulate and activate matrix metalloproteinase (MMP)-2 (Nguyen, 2000; Xue, 2004), a MMP with anti-inflammatory properties (Itoh, 2002; McQuibban, 2002) and to suppress gelatinase B (Cheng, 2006; Xue, 2007), a MMP associated with many inflammatory conditions (Itoh, 2002; Ram, 2006). During acute inflammation, plasma APC levels are diminished (Liaw, 2004) and inflammatory cytokines such as interleukin (IL)-1β and TNF-α, as well as endotoxin, can attenuate thrombomodulin and EPCR expression which further reduces the ability of endothelial cells to generate APC. Acute inflammation is exacerbated in mice genetically predisposed to a severe protein C deficiency (Lay, 2007).

APC also regulates the immuno/inflammatory response. Monocytes treated with APC decrease the release of tissue factor (Toltl, 2008), the pro-inflammatory cytokines TNF-α (Grey, 1994), IL-1β, IL-6, and & IL-8 (Stephenson, 2006). Additionally, APC induces the release of the anti-inflammatory cytokine IL-10 from monocytes (Toltl, 2008).

APC targets CD8+ dendritic cells to reduce the mortality of endotoxemia in mice (Kerschen, 2010). Expression of EPCR in mature murine immune cells is limited to a subset of CD8+ conventional dendritic cells. Adoptive transfer of splenic CD11chiPDCA-1- dendritic cells from wild-type mice into animals with hematopoietic EPCR deficiency restored the therapeutic efficacy of APC, whereas transfer of EPCR-deficient CD11chi dendritic cells or wild-type CD11chi dendritic cells depleted of EPCR+ cells did not. These data reveal an essential role for EPCR and PAR1 on hematopoietic cells, identify EPCR-expressing dendritic immune cells as a critical target of APC therapy, and document EPCR-independent anti-inflammatory effects of APC on innate immune cells.

2.2 Cell proliferation and apoptosis

APC induces growth of cultured human umbilical vein endothelial cells (HUVEC) (Uchiba, 2004). In smooth muscle cells, APC elicits an increase in [(3)H]-thymidine incorporation (Bretschneider, 2007) and enhances proliferation and migration of human skin keratinocytes (Xue, 2005). Consistent with the stimulatory effects on cell growth, APC displays strong anti-apoptotic properties. APC decreases sepsis-induced apoptosis resulting from increased p21 and p53 proteins in mice (Sakar, 2007) and modulates Bcl-2 and Bax and inhibits caspase-3 and -8 activity which results in inhibition of apoptosis in a number of cell types (Joyce, 2001). During hypoxic stress of brain endothelial cells, APC inhibits p53, reduces pro-apoptotic Bax and maintains levels of protective Bcl-2 protein, thereby preventing the stimulation of the intrinsic apoptotic pathway (Cheng, 2003). In human skin keratinocytes, APC prevents cell apoptosis via inhibition of caspase-3 activation (Xue, 2004) and in podocytes, APC protects against glucose-induced apoptosis both in vitro and in vivo (Isermann, 2007). APC inhibits bisphosphonate-induced endothelial cell death via EPCR-induced inactivation of caspase-3 and NF-κB, and also suggests that APC has the potential to be a therapeutic drug in various vascular diseases induced by endothelial cell damage (Seol, 2011).

2.3 Barrier stabilization

Endothelial cells normally form a dynamically regulated stable barrier at the blood-tissue interface, and breakdown of this barrier is a key pathogenic factor in inflammatory disorders, such as sepsis. APC boosts the barrier via at least two different mechanisms. First, APC enhances sphingosine-1-phosphate (S-1-P) production, which signals through its G-protein coupled receptor to stabilize the cytoskeleton and reduce endothelial permeability (Feistritzer & Riewald, 2005; Finigan, 2005). Second, APC utilizes the angiopoietin (Ang)/Tie2 axis to promote endothelial barrier function (Minhas, 2010). APC significantly up-regulates gene and protein expression of Tie2 and Ang1 in a dose (0.01-10 μg/ml) and time (0.5 h - 24 h) dependent manner in HUVEC, whilst it markedly inhibits Ang2 with an IC50 of ~ 0.1 μg/ml. HUVEC permeability, measured using Evans blue dye transfer, is significantly reduced in the presence of APC and, in concordance, the tight junction associated protein, zona occludens (ZO)-1, is up regulated and localized peripherally around cells, compared to control. Smooth muscle cell migration towards APC-stimulated HUVEC is elevated compared to unstimulated cells. Blocking antibodies and small interfering (si) RNA treatment, compared to isotype or scrambled siRNA controls, show that APC requires three receptors, endothelial protein C receptor (EPCR), protease activated receptor (PAR)-1 and Tie2 to perform all these barrier stabilization functions (Minhas, 2010). We have shown that HUVEC produce protein C that acts through novel mediators to enhance their own functional integrity (Xue, 2010). When endogenous protein C or its receptor, EPCR, is suppressed by si RNA, HUVEC proliferation is decreased and apoptosis elevated. Interestingly, protein C or EPCR siRNA significantly increases HUVEC permeability, which occurs via a reduction of the Ang1/Ang2 ratio and inhibition of the peripheral localization of the tight junction protein, ZO-1. In addition, protein C or EPCR siRNA inhibits type IV collagen and MMP-2, providing the first evidence that protein C contributes to vascular basement membrane formation (Xue, 2010). Barrier stabilization is more effective when APC is derived endogenously and functions in an autocrine manner, than when the source of APC is exogenous (Feistritzer, 2006).

The barrier protective effect of APC is also relevant to epidermal keratinocytes (Xue, 2011). In response to APC, Tie2, a tyrosine kinase receptor, is rapidly activated within 30 minutes, and relocates to cell-cell contacts. APC also increases junction proteins ZO-1, claudin-1 and VE-cadherin. Inhibition of Tie2 by its peptide inhibitor or small interfering RNA abolished the barrier protective effect of APC (Xue, 2011).

3. APC cellular signalling

APC exerts its anti-inflammatory, cyto-protective and barrier stabilization effects by acting on receptors which initiates cellular signaling, as described below.

3.1 EPCR and PARs

Many of the cyto-protective actions of APC are mediated through EPCR, which itself is anti-inflammatory (Esmon, 2004). This receptor binds protein C and APC with similar affinity (Fukudome & Esmon, 1994), and protein C can be converted to APC whilst remaining bound to EPCR. EPCR is a type I transmembrane protein which shares homology with the major histocompatibility class 1/CD1 family of proteins involved in the immune response. EPCR was discovered on endothelial cells, however EPCR was subsequently found on some leukocytes (Esmon, 2004) and is strongly expressed by the basal layer of keratinocytes in skin epidermis as well as in cultured keratinocytes (Xue, 2005). Recent studies show that EPCR has important physiological functions. For example, over-expression of EPCR protects transgenic mice from endotoxin-induced injury (Li, 2005) and EPCR is essential for normal embryonic development as deletion of the EPCR gene in mice is lethal by embryonic day 10 (Gu, 2002).

Recently, EPCR has been identified as a marker of certain stem cells in mice (Balazs, 2006; Kent, 2009). EPCR is expressed at high levels within the bone marrow in hematopoietic stem cells (HSCs). Mouse bone marrow cells isolated on the basis of EPCR expression alone are highly enriched HSCs, showing levels of engraftment in vivo comparable to that of stem cells purified using the most effective conventional methods (Balazs, 2006). Moreover, they showed that hematopoietic stem cell activity is always associated with EPCR-expressing cells (Balazs, 2006). In addition, high EPCR-expressing cells are observed in basal-like tumours in breast cancer (Park, 2010).

EPCR does not mediate cell signalling, but acts as a homing receptor to allow APC to cleave PAR-1 (Riewald, 2002). The PARs are G-protein coupled receptors found on most cells. The four known PARs are activated via proteolytic cleavage by various proteases that results in an intra-molecular tethered ligand that triggers activation of a G protein and subsequent intracellular signalling (Coughlin, 2000). Thrombin activates PAR-1, PAR-3, and PAR-4, whereas other serine proteases, including APC (Riewald, 2002). but not thrombin, activate PAR-2. Subsequent functional activity of APC cleavage of PAR-2 is yet to be fully elucidated, although our experiments indicate that APC acts through PAR-2 to promote wound healing in mice (Julovi et al, personal communication) . While the majority of reports cast PAR-2 as pro-inflammatory, others show that PAR-2 agonists are beneficial in several mouse models that involve inflammation or ischemia (Milia, 2002). Among the PARs, PAR-1 is most widely expressed and has been most extensively studied. APC bound to EPCR can activate PAR-1 and promote the anti-inflammatory and anti-apoptotic actions of APC (Riewald, 2002).

Both thrombin and APC can cleave PAR-1 at identical locations. Thrombin cleavage causes platelet activation, increases vascular permeability, activates NF-κB and elevates inflammatory cytokines, all of which promote an inflammatory response. Unexpectedly, when APC cleaves PAR-1, its actions are directly opposite to that of thrombin. APC strongly inhibits vascular permeability, activation of NF-κB, endothelial adhesion molecule expression, cytokine production and monocyte migration (Riewald, 2002). Studies using endothelial cells and other cell types show that when APC activates PAR-1 in an EPCR-dependent manner, it causes alterations in gene expression profiles and exerts direct anti-apoptotic effects (Guo, 2004; Joyce, 2001). However, compared to thrombin, APC is relatively inefficient and requires ~10^4 higher concentration (Kuliopulos, 1999) to cleave PAR-1. This has raised doubts about the possibility of APC having a physiological effect by acting through PAR-1. Bae et al (Bae, 2007) have partially solved this issue by showing that APC cleaves PAR-1 on lipid rafts in endothelial cells. They subsequently identified a novel pathway whereby EPCR is associated with caveolin-1 in lipid rafts in endothelial cells (Bae, 2007). These discrete, cholesterol and sphingolipid enriched microdomains of the cell membrane provide a protective compartment for APC to act in isolation. When APC binds to EPCR in the lipid raft, caveolin-1 is replaced with PAR-1 which couples with the pertussis toxin sensitive Gi-protein to initiate a protective signalling pathway. In contrast, when thrombin cleaves PAR-1 outside the lipid raft signalling occurs via Gq and/or G12/13 which exert inflammatory effects. Interestingly, if EPCR is occupied on the lipid raft, even thrombin, can induce activation of the Gi protein and mimic the protective effects of APC (Bae, 2007).

3.2 Epidermal growth factor receptor (EGFR) and Tie2

In normal epidermis, EGFR is important for autocrine growth of this renewing tissue, suppression of terminal differentiation, promotion of cell survival, and regulation of cell migration during epidermal morphogenesis. In wounded skin, EGFR is momentarily up-

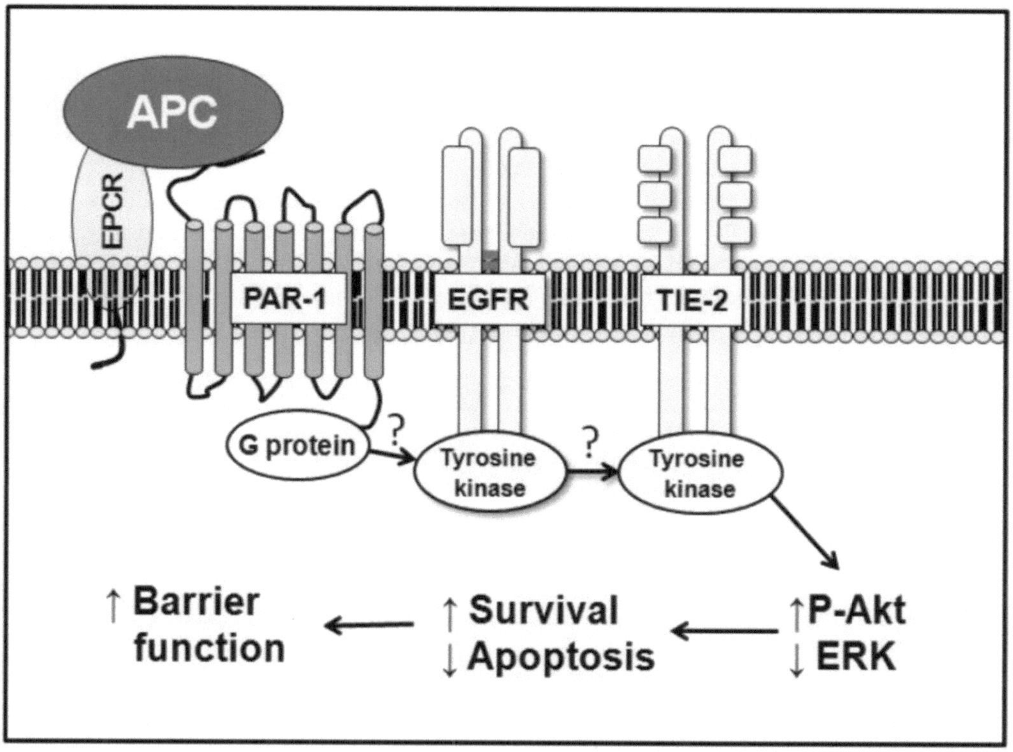

Fig. 1. Proposed signal pathway for APC's protective role on barrier function in confluent keratinocytes. APC binds to EPCR which cleaves PAR-1. G protein transactivates EGFR which may further transactivate Tie2 receptor, although the mechanism of activation is unclear. This triple receptor action results in increased ZO-1 and phosphorylation of Akt via PI3K and inhibition of ERK, leading to an increase in keratinocyte survival and barrier function. From (Xue, 2011).

regulated and is a major contributor to the proliferative and migratory aspects of wound re-epithelialization. EGFR is able to regulate cell adhesion, expression of matrix degrading proteinases, and cell migration to provide a vital contribution to the migratory and invasive potential of keratinocytes (Hudson & McCawley, 1998). APC appears to act through EGFR to regulate lymphocyte migration (Feistritzer, 2006) and wound healing (Xue, 2007). When keratinocytes are stimulated with APC, the expression and phosphorylation of EGFR is markedly increased and conversely when cells are treated with protein C siRNA, the phosphorylated form of EGFR in cell lysates is inhibited by more than 50% (Xue, 2007). Using dual immunofluorescent staining, we found that both EPCR and activated EGFR are co-localized in basal and suprabasal keratinocytes in the epidermis, which is identical to protein C localization in skin epidermis (Xue, 2007). Furthermore, APC does not activate Tie2 through its major ligand, Ang-1, in keratinocytes, but instead acts by binding to EPCR, cleaving PAR-1 and trans-activating EGFR followed by transactivation of Tie2 (Figure 1). When activation of Akt, but not ERK, is inhibited, the barrier protective effect of APC on keratinocytes is abolished. Another report has indicated that, extracellularly, APC engages EPCR, PAR-1, and EGFR in order to increase the invasiveness of MDA-MB-231 cells (Gramling, 2010).

3.3 Other receptors

EPCR-independent signaling components of the APC pathway have been identified in monocytes. Apolipoprotein E receptor 2 (ApoER2) binding of APC results in phosphorylation of Dab1 and activation of the PI3K and Akt pathway resulting in decreased tissue factor release from monocytes (Yang, 2009).

The efficacy of APC in murine endotoxemia is dependent on integrin CD11b. Genetic inactivation of CD11b, PAR1, or sphingosine kinase-1, but not EPCR, abolished the ability of APC to suppress the macrophage inflammatory response in vitro. Using a LPS-induced mouse model of lethal endotoxemia, Cao et al (Cao, 2010) showed that APC administration reduced the mortality of wild-type mice, but not CD11b-deficient mice.

Receptor	Significant Finding	Year	Reference
Tie2	APC increases angiopoietin to activate Tie2 in endothelial cells APC activates PAR-1 which transactivates Tie2 in keratinocytes	2010 2011	(Minhas, 2010) (Xue, 2011)
CD11b	APC acts through Cd11b in macrophages	2009	(Cao, 2010)
ApoER2	ApoER2 acts independent of EPCR and PAR-1 to phosphorylate Dab-1	2008	(Yang, 2009)
EGFR	APC phosphorylates EGFR in HUVEC	2005	(Montiel, 2005)
PAR-3	Prevention of neuronal cell apoptosis	2004	(Guo, 2004)
PAR-2	APC bound EPCR supports cleavage of PAR-2	2002	(Riewald, 2002)
EPCR/PAR-1	APC bound EPCR cleaves PAR-1 resulting in APCs effects	2002	(Riewald, 2002)

Table 1. Cell receptors that APC acts through to exert its anti-inflammatory and cytoprotective effects.

3.4 Intracellular signaling

The transcription factors, NF-κB and the AP-1 complex, a transcriptionally active heterodimer of Fos and Jun proteins, regulate the expression of genes involved in immune and inflammatory responses. They play a pivotal role in the regulation of inflammation (Carmi & Razin, 2007). APC prevents activation of NF-κB and AP-1 stimulated by LPS and endotoxin in human monocytes. The MAP kinase pathway is a prerequisite for growth factor stimulated mitogenesis in many cell types. Three major downstream MAP kinase cascades are mitogen- activated ERK1/2 and stress/cytokine-activated p38 and c-Jun N-terminal kinases. APC induces cell proliferation via activation of the ERK1/2 pathway in endothelial cells (Uchiba, 2004). Similarly, stimulation of smooth muscle cells with APC induces a synergistic effect on ERK-1/2 phosphorylation and DNA synthesis (Bretschneider, 2007). In human keratinocytes, blocking protein C expression or inhibiting its binding to EPCR/EGFR decreases the phosphorylation of ERK1/2 but increases p38 activation. Furthermore, inhibition of ERK completely abolishes APC's stimulatory effect on proliferation. These results indicate that keratinocyte-derived protein C promotes cell growth in an autocrine manner via EPCR, EGFR and activation of ERK1/2 (Xue, 2007). Furthermore, when activation of Akt, but not ERK, is inhibited, the barrier protective effect of APC on keratinocytes is abolished. Thus, APC activates Tie2, which selectively enhances the PI3K/Akt signalling to stimulate junctional complexes and reduce keratinocyte permeability (Xue, 2011).

4. APC in inflammatory disease

APC has therapeutic benefit in a number of other diseases, through its anticoagulant, anti-apoptotic, anti-inflammatory activities and positive effects on cell growth, migration and barrier stabilization, summarized in Figure 2. The following sections detail evidence for the potential beneficial effects of APC in a number of disorders associated with abnormal auto-immune/inflammatory responses.

4.1 Sepsis

Severe sepsis is a very serious condition characterized physiologically by an aberrant systemic inflammatory response and microvascular dysfunction. Low levels of endogenous protein C provokes endotoxic (Levi, 2003) and septic responses (Ganopolsky & Castellino, 2004). In human sepsis, there is a reduction in circulating APC which appears to be due to both decreased levels of protein C, with protein C levels strongly inversely correlating with sepsis prognosis (Fisher, Jr. & Yan, 2000) and decreased activation of protein C to APC (Liaw, 2004). Evidence from the PROWESS and ENHANCE clinical trials suggests that administration of recombinant human APC (drotrecogin alfa) reduces mortality in a subset of patients with severe sepsis (Bernard, 2004; Bernard, 2001; Marti-Carvajal, 2003). It is indicated for use in patients with sepsis involving acute organ dysfunction who have a high risk of death. Two recent case reports provide evidence that APC may also be useful to treat multi-organ failure resulting from severe malaria (Kendrick, 2006; Srinivas, 2007). However, there is evidence that APC may cause bleeding in some patients, especially children and patients who have undergone recent surgery (Marti-Carvajal, 2007). The therapeutic effect and controversies of APC in severe sepsis has been extensively reviewed (Griffin, 2002; O'Brien, 2006; Short, 2006). Commercial preparations of recombinant APC (Xigris, Ely Lilly, Indianapolis) are readily available and FDA approved.

Endogenous APC signaling is critical to protection of mice from LPS-induced septic shock (Xu, 2009). Many mechanisms have been described, but the exact manner in which APC affects sepsis patients is unclear. Therapeutic APC can regulate neutrophil migration and extravasation by direct engagement of β_1 and β_3 integrins (Elphick, 2009), suppress macrophage activation dependent on integrin CD11b/CD18 (Kerschen, 2010), control maturation and activation of $CD8^+$ DCs dependent on EPCR (Kerschen, 2010), and neutralize late-stage inflammatory mediators by degrading nuclear histones from apoptotic cells (Xu, 2009).

A recent Cochrane review suggested that APC should not be used for treating patients with severe sepsis or septic shock and that APC is associated with a higher risk of bleeding (Marti-Carvajal, 2011). Unless additional RCTs provide evidence of a treatment effect, policy-makers, clinicians and academics have been advised not promote the use of APC (Marti-Carvajal, 2011). Nonetheless, new reports continue to show that patients with septic shock who were treated with APC had a reduced in-hospital mortality compared with those not treated with APC (Sadaka, 2011).

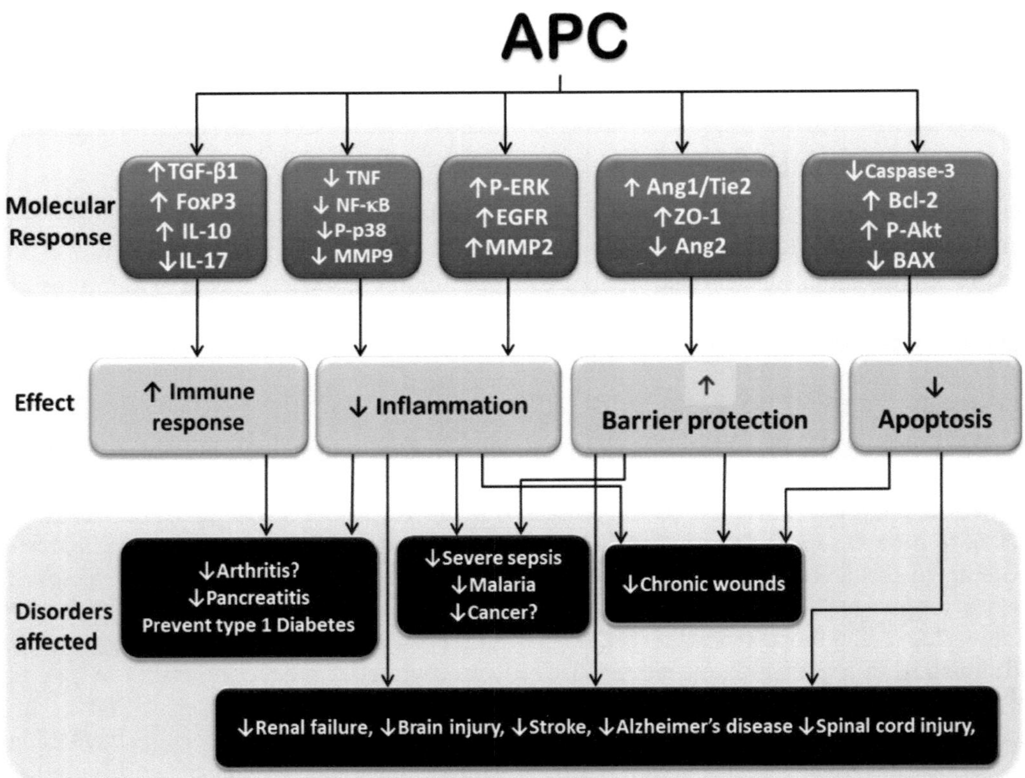

Fig. 2. The diverse biological effects of APC. APC exerts numerous molecular effects which lead to cellular responses which cause protective effects in a number of diseases. Ang= angiopoietin; EGFR= epidermal growth factor receptor; IL=interleukin; MMP=matrix metalloproteinase; TGF=transforming growth factor; TNF=tumour necrosis factor-α; ZO=zona occludens; Bcl=B-cell lymphoma; BAX=Bcl-2–associated X protein.

4.2 Spinal cord injury (SCI)

SCI can be induced by a physical insult resulting in an inflammatory response that leads to tissue destruction and life-long disabilities. Therapeutic intervention in SCI is largely being directed at reducing or alleviating inflammation (Okajima, 2004). In rat models, the inflammatory response occurs due to infiltration by neutrophils and release of TNF-α (Taoka, 2000). Taoka et al (Taoka, 1997) demonstrated that a P-selectin mediated interaction between activated neutrophils and endothelial cells may be a critical step in endothelial cell damage leading to spinal cord injury in rats. These authors (Taoka, 1998) originally showed that rats subjected to compression-trauma induced SCI and treated with APC have a marked reduction in motor disturbances (Taoka, 1998), however, 12 years later this paper was retracted by the authors (2011). APC significantly reduces motor disturbances and micro-infarctions of the spinal cord in rats subjected to ischemia/reperfusion-induced SCI (Hirose, 2000). The increased tissue levels of TNF-α and neutrophils in the injured part of the spinal cord were significantly reduced in animals that received APC.

APC has direct neuroprotective effects, independent of its anticoagulant activity (Zlokovic, 2005). In a rabbit model of ischemic spinal cord injury, APC eases the functional deficits and increases the number of motor neurons (Yamauchi, 2006). Interestingly, APC induces insulin-like growth factor (IGF)-1, IGF-1 receptor and the downstream p-Akt which might partially explain the neuroprotective effects of APC after transient spinal cord ischemia in rabbit.

4.3 Brain injury and stroke

Elevated plasma protein C levels are linked to a lower incidence of ischemic stroke in humans (Folsom, 1999) and conversely, lower circulating APC levels are found in patients with post-infection ischemic stroke compared to the control subjects (Macko, 1996). These data imply that the protein C pathway may protect against stroke. In a murine model of focal cerebral ischemia, APC significantly improved cerebral blood flow in the ischemic hemisphere and markedly reduced the volume of brain injury caused by middle cerebral vein occlusion. These effects were dependent on EPCR and PAR-1 and seemingly independent of APC's anticoagulant effects (Fernandez, 2003; Guo, 2004; Shibata, 2001).

APC directly prevents apoptosis in hypoxic human brain endothelium through inhibition of p53, normalization of the pro-apoptotic Bax/Bcl-2 ratio, and reduction of caspase-3 signalling (Guo, 2004). APC's cytoprotection of endothelial cells in vitro requires EPCR and PAR-1(Guo, 2004; Mosnier & Griffin, 2003). APC can also directly protect perturbed neurons from cell injury and apoptosis. In vitro, APC reduces apoptosis in mouse cortical neurons treated with N-methyl-D-aspartate (NMDA) and staurosporine (Guo, 2004). Interestingly, PAR-1 and PAR-3 are required for this effect. Intra-cerebral APC infusion dose-dependently reduces NMDA excitotoxic injury in mice (Guo, 2004). Overall, APC maintains the patency of ischemic vasculature by inhibiting hypoxia-induced endothelial cell apoptosis and also directly protects the integrity and functionality of the neuronal network.

Periventricular leukomalacia is the dominant form of brain injury in premature infants, characterized by white matter injury. The underlying pathogenic mechanisms include hypoperfusion, procoagulant activity, apoptotic cell death, microglial activation and inflammation associated with maternal and/or fetal infection (Genc, 2006). They hypothesized that APC, which modulates many of these processes, is a promising therapeutic agent for periventricular leukomalacia.

4.4 Alzheimer's disease

Alzheimer's disease is characterized by elevated levels of amyloid β peptide (Aβ) in the brain that are associated with neuronal and vascular toxicity and is the major cause of dementia with advancing age. Inflammation, Aβ deposition in the brain parenchyma and vessels, blood-brain barrier dysfunction, oxidative stress, formation of advanced end glycation products and endothelial and neural cell death have all been implicated in the pathogenesis of Alzheimer's disease (Zlokovic, 2005). It has been proposed that APC could be useful in treating Alzheimer's disease, since it has anti-inflammatory, anti-oxidant, profibrinolytic, neurovascular protectant and pro-angiogenic properties (Genc, 2007). Furthermore, APC exerts anti-inflammatory and anti-apoptotic activities directly on endothelial and neural cells (Griffin, 2006). APC protects against neurovascular injury in experimental stroke models, protects endothelial barrier integrity and decreases fibrin deposition (Griffin, 2006). Similar to its anti-inflammatory effect on other cells, APC may inhibit the activation status of the microglia that plays a key role in neuroinflammation.

4.5 Acute kidney injury

In a rat model of endotoxemia, rat APC significantly improved peritubular capillary flow and reduced leukocyte adhesion and rolling, 3 hours after treatment with LPS (Gupta, 2007). After 24 hr, APC treatment significantly improved renal blood flow. In addition, APC modulated the renin-angiotensin system by reducing mRNA expression levels of angiotensin converting enzyme-1, angiotensinogen in the kidney (Gupta, 2007). Thus, APC can suppress LPS-induced acute renal failure by modulating factors involved in vascular inflammation.

Ischemia/reperfusion-induced renal injury is an important pathologic mechanism leading to acute renal failure (Thadhani, 1996). In a rat model, intravenous administration of APC markedly reduces ischemia/reperfusion -induced renal dysfunction and tubular necrosis, whereas heparin or inactive APC has no effect (Mizutani, 2000). Furthermore, APC significantly inhibited the ischemia/reperfusion -induced decrease in renal tissue blood flow, the increase in the vascular permeability, and renal levels of TNF-α, IL-8, and myeloperoxidase. Leukocytopenia produced effects similar to those of APC. These findings strongly suggested that APC has a protective effect against ischemia/reperfusion-induced renal injury by inhibiting activation of leukocytes rather than inhibiting coagulation (Okajima, 2004). Recently, Isemann et al (Isermann, 2007) have shown that APC protects against diabetic nephropathy by inhibiting endothelial and podocyte apoptosis. In a rat model of sepsis by cecal ligation and puncture (CLP), treatment with APC significantly inhibited sepsis-induced elevations in creatinine, LDH levels, and improved renal architecture. Furthermore, sepsis-induced inhibition of interferon (INF)-γ and increase in IL-1β and IL-10 were attenuated by APC treatment. The authors suggested that APC confers a survival advantage by reducing systemic inflammation and, in doing so, preserves organ function (Keller, 2011).

4.6 Lung disorders

In a mouse model of acute lung injury, APC inhalation attenuates LPS-induced amplification of neutrophils and macrophages in bronchoalveolar lavage fluid as well as VCAM-1 protein levels in lung tissue (Kotanidou, 2006). In a murine model of asthma, inhalation of APC significantly inhibits the expression of T helper 2 (Th2) cytokines, IgE, eosinophilic inflammation, and hyper-responsiveness in bronchiolar lavage fluid (Yuda, 2004). Electromobility shift assays show that translation of signal transducer and activator of transcription 6 (STAT6) and NF-κB to the nucleus is reduced in lung samples from mice treated with inhaled APC. Although APC is thought to have a short half-life of ~ 20 mins, it can be detected in mice bronchoalveolar lavage fluid 24 h after inhalation. Thus, APC inhalation might offer a long-acting alternative route of administration to the lungs to attenuate pulmonary inflammation in acute lung injury.

It is unclear whether APC has any beneficial effect in humans with inflammatory lung diseases. Nick et al (Nick, 2004) performed a double-blinded, placebo-controlled study of APC in a human model of endotoxin-induced pulmonary inflammation and showed that APC significantly reduced leukocyte accumulation to the airspaces, independent of pulmonary cytokine or chemokine release. Bronchoalveolar lavage fluid neutrophils of patients receiving APC demonstrated decreased chemotaxis ex vivo but no change in cytokine release, cell survival, or apoptosis. The major components of the protein C pathway, including thrombomodulin, protein C and EPCR are all expressed by human airway epithelial cells (Hataji, 2002). Activation of protein C is reduced in sputum of patients with bronchial asthma compared to control subjects, which may contribute to exacerbation of the inflammatory response in the airway of asthmatic patients (Hataji, 2002). However, Schouten et al (Schouten, 2011) showed that endogenous protein C has strong effects on the host response to lethal influenza A infection, on the one hand inhibiting pulmonary coagulopathy and inflammation, but on the other hand facilitating neutrophil influx and protein leak and accelerating mortality.

4.7 Acute pancreatitis

Acute pancreatitis is a local inflammatory process that leads to a systemic inflammatory response and multiple organ failure (Kirschenbaum & Astiz, 2005). Disseminated intravascular coagulation and thromboembolism are related to overall morbidity of this disease which provides a setting in which APC could play a therapeutic role. Ottesen et al (Ottesen, 1999) found a decrease in levels of protein C in animals with acute pancreatitis. In a rodent model of pancreatitis (Alsfasser, 2006), treatment with APC reduces inflammation in the pancreas and lungs and significantly improves survival compared to controls (86% vs 38%; P=.05). This animal model exhibits severe consumptive coagulopathy, however APC's anti-coagulation properties did not worsen this condition. In another study, when APC was given 6 hours after the induction of pancreatitis, it significantly reduced acinar necrosis, tissue edema, fat necrosis, IL-6 and TNF-α and inflammatory infiltration compared to controls. Inhibition of expression of pancreatic p38 MAPK and JNK and upregulation of ERK1/2 expression by APC treatment protects against pancreatic injury, thus ameliorating severity of the disease (Chen, 2007).

4.8 Type 1 Diabetes (T1D)

T1D is a chronic progressive autoimmune disease that affects genetically prone individuals. The physiological destruction of β-cells is a crucial event for disease onset (Mathis, 2001). Inflammation and auto-immunity play an important role in the destruction of pancreatic islet β-cells in T1D, with apoptosis being the dominant form of β-cell death in both animal models of diabetes and humans. Replacement of the β-cells by transplantation of islet cells is a radical therapy for human T1D. A major problem with this therapy is the large loss of viability of islet cells during the procedure. APC's strong anti-inflammatory and anti-apoptotic properties appear to be beneficial in preventing destruction of islet cells. Exogenous administration of APC significantly reduces loss of functional islet mass after intraportal transplantation in diabetic mice (Contreras, 2004). Animals given APC exhibit better glucose control, higher glucose disposal rates and higher arginine-stimulated acute insulin release (Contreras, 2004). These effects are associated with a reduction in plasma proinsulin, intrahepatic fibrin deposition, and islet apoptosis early after the transplant. APC treatment is also associated with a significant reduction of proinflammatory cytokine release and prevents endothelial cell activation and dysfunction. This study suggests that APC therapy will improve the take-rate of the transplanted islet cells and thus decrease the number of the cells required for human pancreatic islet transplantation (Contreras, 2004).

Interestingly, plasma levels of protein C/APC are reduced in humans with T1D (Gruden, 1997; Vukovich & Schernthaner, 1986). In addition, soluble EPCR, which binds to APC and inhibits its activity, is increased in T1D (Wu, 2000). These data together indicate that circulating APC activity is markedly reduced in T1D. Whether replenishment of APC levels will benefit patients with T1D is yet to be resolved. However, APC exhibits great potential in preventing glucose-induced apoptosis in endothelial cells and podocytes (Isermann, 2007).

4.9 Rheumatoid Arthritis (RA)

RA is a chronic autoimmune disease characterized by persistent inflammation of multiple synovial joints which results in progressive tissue destruction of bone and cartilage. Protein C/APC is present in RA synovial tissues and co-localizes with MMP-2 in endothelial and synovial lining cells (Buisson-Legendre, 2004). EPCR is also strongly expressed by synovial tissue in patients with RA and co-localizes with CD68 positive staining cells, indicating that these cells are largely macrophage/monocytes (Xue, 2007). Inhibiting the activation of monocytes/macrophages reduces the severity of arthritis in patients with RA and in animal models of RA (Bondeson, 1999; Kwasny-Krochin, 2002). APC inhibits activation of normal monocytes by preventing their migration and production of proinflammatory cytokines/chemokines, such as TNF-α and macrophage migration inhibitory factor levels (Schmidt-Supprian, 2000). When monocytes from RA patients are pre-treated with APC, their migration towards monocyte chemoattractant protein-1 (MCP-1) is inhibited in a dose-dependent manner (Xue, 2007). Pre-incubation of these cells with RCR252, an antibody which blocks APC binding to EPCR, abolishes this inhibitory effect of APC, indicating that APC acts through EPCR to inhibit the chemotactic response of RA monocytes. MMP-9 regulation may be at least one downstream effector of APC's inhibition of monocyte migration. When added to purified monocytes from RA patients, APC dose-dependently inhibits the production of MMP-9 (Xue, 2007). MMP-9 not only allows cell migration but also exerts direct pro-inflammatory effects, such as activation of cytokines which would enhance the beneficial effect of APC in RA.

NF-κB is activated in synovium from RA patients (Marok, 1996) and in cultured RA synovial fibroblasts (Fujisawa, 1996). Inhibition of NF-κB activity strongly reduces the severity of disease in animal models of arthritis by inhibiting leukocyte infiltration (Blackwell, 2004). High levels of NF-κB activity are present in RA monocytes under basal conditions. APC (20 μg/ml) dramatically inhibits the active form of NF-κB in both control and LPS stimulated monocytes from RA patients. Downstream of NF-κB is one of the most potent inflammatory cytokines in RA, TNF-α (Xue, 2007). Specific inhibition of TNF-α using biological agents such as the monoclonal antibody, Adalimumab (marketed as Humira), is proving very successful in treating moderate to severe RA in adults who have had a poor response to other anti-rheumatic drugs. Monocytes/macrophages are the primary source of TNF-α which, after release, promotes the proinflammatory activity of these and other surrounding cells. APC significantly decreases TNF-α both in control and LPS-stimulated RA monocytes (Xue, 2007). Thus, APC may mimic the action of the "biological" agents, through inhibition of TNF-α. However, by acting on multiple targets, APC may be more effective.

4.10 Cancer

APC can activate signaling molecules to promote MDA-MB-231 breast cancer cell and endothelial cell motility (Gramling, 2010). However, accumulating evidence suggests that the APC pathway limits cancer progression. Acquired protein C deficiency is observed in cancer patients, especially in patients using certain types of chemotherapy (Feffer, 1989; Mewhort-Buist, 2008; Rogers, 1988; Woodley-Cook, 2006). The loss of expression of thrombomodulin (or increase in its soluble form), a receptor required to convert protein C to APC, on cancer cells correlates with advanced stage and poor prognosis (Hanly, 2006; Hanly & Winter, 2007; Lindahl, 1993). Low levels of thrombomodulin also increase the invasive ability of cancer cells in vitro (Matsushita, 1998) and is significantly correlated with a high relapse rate in breast cancer (Kim, 1997). It is likely that low thrombomodulin levels induce metastasis due to reduced endogenous APC levels, although several alternative mechanisms have also been proposed (Hanly & Winter, 2007). Additionally, EPCR, the specific receptor for APC is detected in several cell lines derived from various types of cancer (Van Sluis, 2010). For example, EPCR is expressed on human breast cancer cells, with an extremely high frequency (Tsuneyoshi, 2001). EPCR on the vascular wall inhibits cancer cell adhesion and transmigration (Bezuhly, 2009; Lindahl, 1993). Finally, significant resistance to APC was found in women with a lymph-node-positive breast carcinoma (Bezuhly, 2009; Lindahl, 1993; Nijziel, 2003). In a mouse model, endogenous APC has been found to limit cancer cell extravasation via sphingosine-1-phosphate receptor-1 and VE-cadherin-dependent vascular barrier enhancement. Van Sluis et al (Van Sluis, 2011) showed that in the absence of endogenous APC, fibrinogen depletion does not prevent cancer cell dissemination and secondary tumor formation in immune-competent mice. Overall, they show that endogenous APC is essential for immune-mediated cancer cell elimination (Van Sluis, 2011). The exact mechanisms on how about prevents cancer are not clear. However, recently, a number of studies have shown that activation of PAR1 are involved in limiting of tumour cell migration and invasion/metastasis in vitro and in vivo (Kamath, 2001; Nierodzik, 1998; Villares, 2011) and intact barrier function can effectively prevent tumour cell migration and metastasis. APC can enhance both endothelial and epithelial barrier functions via activation of PAR1 which may partly explain the underlying mechanisms(Minhas, 2010; Xue, 2011).

4.11 Skin injuries

Chronic wounds are a common health problem. There are many different factors which lead to a chronic wound, including advancing age, persistent inflammatory stimuli, tissue hypoxia, diabetes mellitus, immunodeficiency, a smoking history or the use of certain medications, but they can affect patients at any race or economic background. The common types of chronic wounds include: peripheral ulcers, which are the most frequent cause of lower limb amputation in patients with type I and type II diabetes (Levin, 1993); decubitus ulcers, a result of prolonged, unrelieved pressure over a bony prominence and venous stasis ulcers, where venous congestion of the lower extremities results in local hypoxia (Trent, 2005). With the current diabetes epidemic and increasing aging population, chronic wounds are a serious concern to the health system. They require dedicated care including regular dressings, frequent clinic appointments and when complications arise, hospital admission potentially requiring surgery or even amputation. The "state-of-the-art" treatments for chronic wounds are expensive and have limited success. Cutaneous wound repair can be divided into a series of overlapping phases including formation of fibrin clot, inflammatory response, granulation tissue formation, which includes re-epithelialization and angiogenesis, and matrix remodeling. Re-epithelialization is an important component of wound repair as it serves to restore the barrier function of skin. Newly formed blood vessels provide nutrition and oxygen to the growing tissue and allow leukocytes to enter the site of injury. A chronic wound or ulcer occurs when the co-coordinated cellular and biochemical response to injury are disrupted.

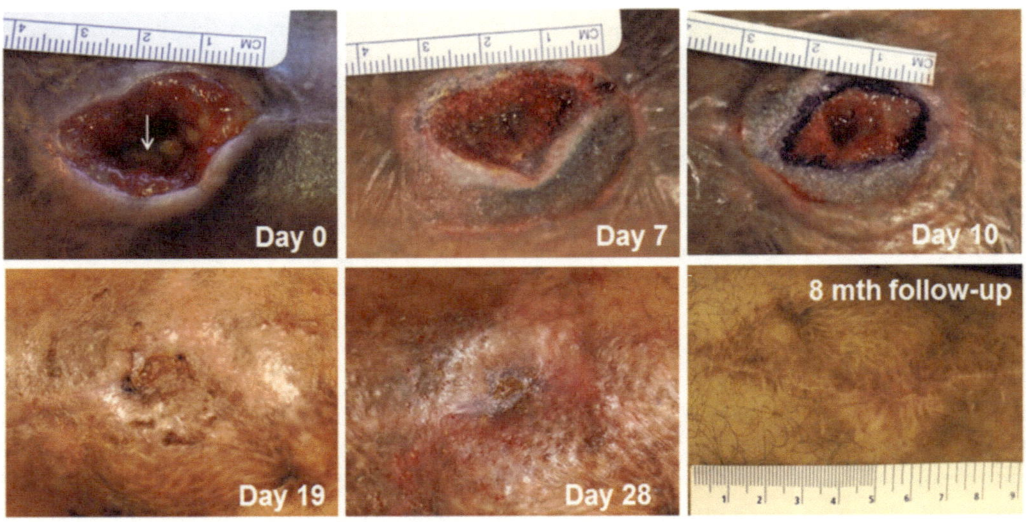

Fig. 3. APC treatment used in conjunction with topical negative pressure (TNP) to treat a recalcitrant orthopaedic wound present for 2 years. APC and TNP were applied on day 0 and twice a week until day 19. Day 0 shows exposed bone (arrow) and day 7 shows healthy granulation tissue covering bone. Wound is fully healed by day 28 and remained healed at 8 months follow-up. Taken from Wijewardana et al, Int J Lower Extrem Wounds in press, 2011.

The role of inflammation in wound healing is under debate. Many researchers believe that the inflammatory phase is vital for wound healing to proceed, however, there is evidence to suggest otherwise. Whereas normal adult healing results in a fibrous scar, early fetal wounds which have very little, if any, inflammatory response, exhibit scarless healing with complete restoration of the normal skin architecture. Scar formation exacerbates when inflammation is provoked in fetal wounds, suggesting that the absence of inflammation contributes to the rapid and flawless repair of these wounds (Szpaderska & DiPietro, 2005). Compared to dermal wounds, oral wounds have substantially lower levels of macrophage, neutrophil, and T-cell infiltration and heal rapidly with minimal inflammation and often with minimal scar formation (Szpaderska, 2003). Redd et al (Redd, 2004) studied wound healing in the PU.1 null mouse, which is genetically incapable of raising an inflammatory response because several haematopoietic lineages, including macrophages and neutrophils, are absent or severely delayed in their differentiation. Wounds in these animals rapidly repair with increased vascularity at the wound site and faster reepithelialisation of the wound surface, as well as being scarless (Redd, 2004). They hypothesised that the lower the level of some growth factors in adult wounds the closer it would mimic scar-free healing in the embryo. This is relevant to many chronic wounds which are often associated with excess inflammation and become locked in this inflammatory phase. Thus, APC's anti-inflammatory effects may actually benefit, rather than hinder, the healing of chronic wounds.

Keratinocytes and endothelial cells are two major cell types in skin and play critical roles in the healing of skin injury. Keratinocytes of the epidermis provide the major cellular component of the outermost barrier to the environment. When the skin is broken, a critical response is triggered to restore its protective function. Within 24 hours of wounding, keratinocytes from the wound margins begin to migrate and invade the wound bed, where they proliferate to form the new epithelium. We have shown that protein C is produced by skin keratinocytes, especially those in the basal layer (Xue, 2007). This endogenous protein C is activated on the cell surface, with the resulting APC stimulating a wound healing phenotype in keratinocytes (Xue, 2005; Xue, 2007). Furthermore, the autocrine actions of APC are necessary for normal keratinocyte growth and function (Xue, 2007). APC stimulates proliferation, MMP-2 activity, migration and prevents apoptosis in skin keratinocytes, all vital processes of re-epithelialization (Xue, 2005; Xue, 2004). Endothelial migration and proliferation are vital to generate new blood vessels for wound healing. APC stimulates endothelial cell proliferation and induces tube-like structure formation in vitro (Uchiba, 2004) and cell migration (Brueckmann, 2003). In the chick chorioallantoic membrane (CAM) assay, APC stimulates angiogenesis and re-epithelialization. In vivo, APC induces corneal angiogenesis in a mouse model (Uchiba, 2004). APC also stimulates the proliferation of smooth muscle cells (Bretschneider, 2007), which would contribute to the formation of mature blood vessels. In a full-thickness rat skin-healing model, a single topical application of APC enhances wound healing compared to saline control at least partly via stimulating angiogenesis and re-epithelialisation (Jackson, 2005).

Recent evidence suggests that APC will be effective in humans with chronic wounds. An open label pilot study was conducted on 4 patients whose wounds were not improving, despite standard wound treatment for 4 months or greater (Whitmont, 2008). APC was applied topically to wounds once weekly for 4 weeks. All 4 patients showed rapid positive response to treatment which was maintained during a 4 month follow-up period. Overall, there was more than 80% reduction in wound size. The treatment was well tolerated with no significant side effects or complications experienced. In another recent study, APC treatment was used in conjunction with topical negative pressure (TNP), to treat recalcitrant long-standing orthopaedic wounds (Wijewardana et al, Combination of activated protein C and topical negative pressure vacuum therapy rapidly regenerates granulation tissue over exposed bone to heal recalcitrant orthopaedic wounds, in press, 2011, Int J Lower Extrem Wounds). One example is a 47 year old male with no significant co-morbidities who had tibial and fibula fractures following an assault and being hit in the leg by a baseball bat, 2 years prior to presentation. The fractures required open reduction and fixation with plates and screws. Two months post-operatively he developed an infection and breakdown of the wound. He was started on antibiotic treatment and had wash out of the wound and scraping of the bone which showed osteomyelitis. Antibiotic treatment was continued but failed to control the infection so all metal-ware was removed and the wound was debrided. There was malunion of the bone and after 3 months the plates and screws were replaced and the wound was covered with a fasciocutaneous flap. After one month, he again developed infection and breakdown of the flap. For the following year he had continued treatment with antibiotics, conventional and TNP dressings, however the wound remained non-healing. He was then treated with APC plus topical negative pressure and after 7 days a layer of healthy granulation tissue covered the bone and almost filled the entire wound space (Figure 3). By day 10 re-epithelialization had occurred on top of the dermis around the perimeter of the wound and by day 19 the wound had completely healed. Follow up at 8 month showed the wound had continued to remain intact

By dampening inflammation and accelerating angiogenesis and re-epithellialisation, APC is also likely to minimize scar formation, which holds great potential for burn victims and those susceptible to keloid scarring. Patients with burn injuries and inhalation trauma have a significant increase in thrombin generation in the airways compared with control patients, as reflected by increased lavage fluid levels of thrombin-antithrombin complexes and fibrin degradation products, and decreased lavage fluid levels of APC and antithrombin (Hofstra, 2011).

5. Engineered protein C/APC

The stereospecific interactions of APC with factors Va and VIIIa involve both the APC enzymatic active-site region and residues that are not part of the immediate APC active site. These residues are termed 'exosites' on the APC active enzyme surface and can be mutated to diminish the anticoagulant activity of APC without altering the cell-signaling activity of the molecule (Bae, 2007; Gale, 2002; Kerschen, 2007; Mosnier, 2004). Replacement of a cluster of five positively charged residues by alanine residues (ie. 5A-APC) on the top surface of the APC heavy-chain protease domain restructures this crucial positively charged exosite, causing >98% loss of the anticoagulant activity of human APC while leaving intact APC cell-signaling activities on different cell types within the neurovascular unit (Mosnier, 2007; Mosnier, 2009). Replacement of three of these five residues (i.e. lysine residues 191–193) by three alanine residues produces the 3K3A-APC variant (Deane, 2009; Guo, 2009; Wang, 2009) which has a similar effect to the 5A-APC variant, causing loss of >92% of APC anticoagulant activity. These engineered variants provide APC for therapeutic purposes in which the risk of serious bleeding caused by the anticoagulant activity of APC is diminished while the cytoprotective effects of APC are preserved. In preclinical animal models of ALS (Zhong, 2009), stroke (Guo, 2009; Wang, 2009), brain injury (Walker, 2010) and sepsis {Kerschen, 2007 KERSCHEN2007 /id} and cytoprotective function (Ni, 2011) these APC variants show beneficial effects that were equivalent to, or sometimes greater than, the wild-type recombinant APC. Bir et al (Bir, 2011) demonstrated that 5A-APC could attenuate lung damage caused by P. aeruginosa in critically ill patients. In addition, 5A-APC inhibits the inflammatory response of conventional dendritic cells independent of EPCR and suppresses IFN-gamma production by natural killer-like dendritic cells (Kerschen, 2010). Recently, an APC variant (APC-L38D/N329Q) was generated with minimal anticoagulant activity, but 5-fold enhanced endothelial barrier protective function and 30-fold improved anti-apoptotic function when compared with wild type APC (Ni, 2011).

An APC variant with minimal cell-signaling activity but with substantially increased anticoagulant activity, E149A-APC, has been useful for proof of concept studies and for antithrombotic indications (Mosnier, 2009). E149A-APC has superior antithrombotic activity in a mouse model of arterial thrombosis compared to wt-APC, but has no benefit in an endotoxemia sepsis model where wild type (wt)-APC or the 5A-APC variant reduced mortality {Kerschen, 2007 KERSCHEN2007 /id} (Mosnier, 2009).

6. Conclusion

APC, an anticoagulant with anti-inflammatory, anti-apoptotic, proliferative and barrier stabilization properties, has not only emerged as a therapeutic agent for use in selected patients with severe sepsis, but also appears to have considerable benefit in chronic wounds and a number of other autoimmune/inflammatory diseases. The in vitro, preclinical and limited clinical data for these diseases indicate that APC holds a remarkable promise. Further insights into the mechanisms of action of APC will be required for the translation of preclinical study results to the bedside.

More than three decades since the discovery of APC, we are only beginning to learn of its biological diversity. The clinical evidence for APC as a treatment for severe sepsis is perplexing (Marti-Carvajal, 2007; Marti-Carvajal, 2011). Strong evidence indicates that APC will benefit other disorders involving various organ injuries including kidney injury, spinal cord injury, respiratory function and stroke. Blinded and controlled clinical trials will elucidate its clinical protective effects in these disorders. With the recent discovery that the largest organ of the body, the skin, positively responds to APC, it is likely that APC will accelerate healing of skin injuries and disorders.

7. References

Retraction for yuji taoka et Al., (2011). "activated protein C reduces the severity of compression-induced spinal cord injury in rats by inhibiting activation of leukocytes". *J.Neurosci.* Vol.31, No.23, pp. 8697

Alsfasser, G., Warshaw, A.L., Thayer, S.P., Antoniu, B., Laposata, M., Lewandrowski, K.B., & Fernandez-del, C.C. (2006). Decreased inflammation and improved survival with recombinant human activated protein C treatment in experimental acute pancreatitis. *Arch.Surg.* Vol.141, No.7, pp. 670-676

Bae, J.S., Yang, L., Manithody, C., & Rezaie, A.R. (2007). Engineering a disulfide bond to stabilize the calcium binding loop of activated protein C eliminates its anticoagulant but not protective signaling properties. *J.Biol.Chem.* Vol.282, No.35, pp.25493-25500

Bae, J.S., Yang, L., Manithody, C., & Rezaie, A.R. (2007). The ligand occupancy of endothelial protein C receptor switches the protease-activated receptor 1-dependent signaling specificity of thrombin from a permeability-enhancing to a barrier-protective response in endothelial cells. *Blood.* Vol.110, No.12, pp. 3909-3916

Bae, J.S., Yang, L., & Rezaie, A.R. (2007). Receptors of the protein C activation and activated protein C signaling pathways are colocalized in lipid rafts of endothelial cells. *Proc.Natl.Acad.Sci.U.S.A.* Vol.104, No.8, pp. 2867-2872

Baker, W.F. & Bick, R.L. (1999). Treatment of hereditary and acquired thrombophilic disorders. *Semin.Thromb.Hemostasis.* Vol.25, No.4, pp. 387-405

Balazs, A.B., Fabian, A.J., Esmon, C.T., & Mulligan, R.C. (2006). Endothelial protein C receptor (CD201) explicitly identifies hematopoietic stem cells in murine bone marrow. *Blood.* Vol.107, No.6, pp. 2317-2321

Bernard, G.R., Margolis, B.D., Shanies, H.M., Ely, E.W., Wheeler, A.P., Levy, H., Wong, K., & Wright, T.J. (2004). Extended Evaluation of Recombinant Human Activated Protein C United States Trial (ENHANCE US): A Single-Arm, Phase 3B, Multicenter Study of Drotrecogin Alfa (Activated) in Severe Sepsis. *Chest.* Vol.125, No.6, pp. 2206-2216

Bernard, G.R., Vincent, J.L., Laterre, P.F., LaRosa, S.P., Dhainaut, J.F., Lopez-Rodriguez, A., Steingrub, J.S., Garber, G.E., Helterbrand, J.D., Ely, E.W., & Fisher, C.J. (2001). Efficacy and Safety of Recombinant Human Activated Protein C for Severe Sepsis. *New Engl. J Med.* Vol.344, No.10, pp. 699-709

Bezuhly, M., Cullen, R., Esmon, C.T., Morris, S.F., West, K.A., Johnston, B., & Liwski, R.S. (2009). Role of activated protein C and its receptor in inhibition of tumor metastasis. *Blood.* Vol.113, No.14, pp. 3371-3374

Bir, N., Lafargue, M., Howard, M., Goolaerts, A., Roux, J., Carles, M., Cohen, M.J., Iles, K.E., Fernandez, J.A., Griffin, J.H., & Pittet, J.F. (2011). Cytoprotective-selective Activated Protein C Attenuates P. aeruginosa-induced Lung Injury in Mice. *Am.J.Respir.Cell Mol.Biol.* Epub ahead of print

Blackwell, N.M., Sembi, P., Newson, J.S., Lawrence, T., Gilroy, D.W., & Kabouridis, P.S. (2004). Reduced infiltration and increased apoptosis of leukocytes at sites of inflammation by systemic administration of a membrane-permeable IkappaBalpha repressor. *Arthritis Rheum.* Vol.50, No.8, pp. 2675-2684

Bondeson, J., Browne, K.A., Brennan, F.M., Foxwell, B.M.J., & Feldmann, M. (1999). Selective Regulation of Cytokine Induction by Adenoviral Gene Transfer of I{kappa}B{alpha} into Human Macrophages: Lipopolysaccharide-Induced, But Not Zymosan-Induced, Proinflammatory Cytokines Are Inhibited, But IL-10 Is Nuclear Factor-{kappa}B Independent. *J. Immunol.* Vol.162, No.5, pp. 2939-2945

Bretschneider, E., Uzonyi, B., Weber, A.A., Fischer, J.W., Pape, R., Lotzer, K., & Schror, K. (2007). Human vascular smooth muscle cells express functionally active endothelial cell protein C receptor. *Circ.Res.* Vol.100, No.2, pp. 255-262

Brueckmann, M., Marx, A., Martin, W.H., Liebe, V., Lang, S., Kaden, J.J., Zieger, W., Borggrefe, M., Huhle, G., & Konstantin, H.K. (2003). Stabilization of monocyte chemoattractant protein-1-mRNA by activated protein C. *Thromb.Haemost.* Vol.89, No.1, pp. 149-160

Buisson-Legendre, N., Smith, S., March, L., & Jackson, C. (2004). Elevation of activated protein C in synovial joints in rheumatoid arthritis and its correlation with matrix metalloproteinase 2. *Arthritis Rheum.* Vol.50, No.7, pp. 2151-2156

Calzado, M.A., Bacher, S., & Schmitz, M.L. (2007). NF-kappaB inhibitors for the treatment of inflammatory diseases and cancer. *Curr.Med.Chem.* Vol.14, No.3, pp.367-376

Calzado, M.A., Bacher, S., & Schmitz, M.L. (2007). NF-kappaB inhibitors for the treatment of inflammatory diseases and cancer. *Curr.Med.Chem.* Vol.14, No.3, pp. 367-376

Cao, C., Gao, Y., Li, Y., Antalis, T.M., Castellino, F.J., & Zhang, L. (2010). The efficacy of activated protein C in murine endotoxemia is dependent on integrin CD11b. *J. Clin Invest.* Vol.120, No.6, pp. 1971-1980

Carmi, I. & Razin, E. (2007). The role played by key transcription factors in activated mast cells. *Immunol.Rev.* Vol.217:280-91., No.280-291

Chen, P., Zhang, Y., Qiao, M., & Yuan, Y. (2007). Activated protein C, an anticoagulant polypeptide, ameliorates severe acute pancreatitis via regulation of mitogen-activated protein kinases. *J.Gastroenterol.* Vol.42, No.11, pp. 887-896

Cheng, T., Liu, D., Griffin, J.H., Fernandez, J.A., Castellino, F., Rosen, E.D., Fukudome, K., & Zlokovic, B.V. (2003). Activated protein C blocks p53-mediated apoptosis in ischemic human brain endothelium and is neuroprotective. *Nat.Med.* Vol.9, No.3, pp. 338-342

Cheng, T., Petraglia, A.L., Li, Z., Thiyagarajan, M., Zhong, Z., Wu, Z., Liu, D., Maggirwar, S.B., Deane, R., Fernandez, J.A., LaRue, B., Griffin, J.H., Chopp, M., & Zlokovic, B.V. (2006). Activated protein C inhibits tissue plasminogen activator-induced brain hemorrhage. *Nat. Med.* Vol.12, No.11, pp. 1278-1285

Contreras, J.L., Eckstein, C., Smyth, C.A., Bilbao, G., Vilatoba, M., Ringland, S.E., Young, C., Thompson, J.A., Fernandez, J.A., Griffin, J.H., & Eckhoff, D.E. (2004). Activated protein C preserves functional islet mass after intraportal transplantation: a novel link between endothelial cell activation, thrombosis, inflammation, and islet cell death. *Diabetes.* Vol.53, No.11, pp. 2804-2814

Coughlin, S.R. (2000). Thrombin signalling and protease-activated receptors [In Process Citation]. *Nature.* Vol.407, No.6801, pp. 258-264

Deane, R., LaRue, B., Sagare, A.P., Castellino, F.J., Zhong, Z., & Zlokovic, B.V. (2009). Endothelial protein C receptor-assisted transport of activated protein C across the mouse blood-brain barrier. *J.Cereb.Blood Flow Metab.* Vol.29, No.1, pp. 25-33

Elphick, G.F., Sarangi, P.P., Hyun, Y.M., Hollenbaugh, J.A., Ayala, A., Biffl, W.L., Chung, H.L., Rezaie, A.R., McGrath, J.L., Topham, D.J., Reichner, J.S., & Kim, M. (2009). Recombinant human activated protein C inhibits integrin-mediated neutrophil migration. *Blood.* Vol.113, No.17, pp. 4078-4085

Esmon, C.T. (2004). Crosstalk between inflammation and thrombosis. *Maturitas.* Vol.47, No.4, pp. 305-314

Esmon, C.T. (2004). Structure and functions of the endothelial cell protein C receptor. *Crit Care Med.* Vol.32, No.5 Suppl, pp. S298-S301

Feffer, S.E., Carmosino, L.S., & Fox, R.L. (989). Acquired protein C deficiency in patients with breast cancer receiving cyclophosphamide, methotrexate, and 5-fluorouracil. *Cancer.* Vol.63, No.7, pp. 1303-1307

Feistritzer, C., Mosheimer, B.A., Sturn, D.H., Riewald, M., Patsch, J.R., & Wiedermann, C.J. (2006). Endothelial protein C receptor-dependent inhibition of migration of human lymphocytes by protein C involves epidermal growth factor receptor. *J.Immunol.* Vol.176, No.2, pp. 1019-1025

Feistritzer, C. & Riewald, M. (2005). Endothelial barrier protection by activated protein C through PAR1-dependent sphingosine 1-phosphate receptor-1 crossactivation. *Blood.* Vol.105, No.8, pp. 3178-3184

Feistritzer, C., Schuepbach, R.A., Mosnier, L.O., Bush, L.A., Di, C.E., Griffin, J.H., & Riewald, M. (2006). Protective signaling by activated protein C is mechanistically linked to protein C activation on endothelial cells. *J. Biol. Chem.* Vol.281, No.29, pp. 20077-20084

Fernandez, J.A., Xu, X., Liu, D., Zlokovic, B.V., & Griffin, J.H. (2003). Recombinant murine-activated protein C is neuroprotective in a murine ischemic stroke model. *Blood Cells Mol.Dis.* Vol.30, No.3, pp. 271-276

Finigan, J.H., Dudek, S.M., Singleton, P.A., Chiang, E.T., Jacobson, J.R., Camp, S.M., Ye, S.Q., & Garcia, J.G. (2005). Activated protein C mediates novel lung endothelial barrier enhancement: Role of sphingosine 1-phosphate receptor transactivation. *J.Biol.Chem.* Vol.280, No.17, pp.17286-17293

Fisher, C.J., Jr. & Yan, S.B. (2000). Protein C levels as a prognostic indicator of outcome in sepsis and related diseases. *Crit Care Med.* Vol.28, No.9 Suppl, pp. S49-S56

Folsom, A.R., Rosamond, W.D., Shahar, E., Cooper, L.S., Aleksic, N., Nieto, F.J., Rasmussen, M.L., & Wu, K.K. (1999). Prospective study of markers of hemostatic function with risk of ischemic stroke. The Atherosclerosis Risk in Communities (ARIC) Study Investigators. *Circulation.* Vol.100, No.7, pp. 736-742

Franscini, N., Bachli, E.B., Blau, N., Leikauf, M.S., Schaffner, A., & Schoedon, G. (2004). Gene expression profiling of inflamed human endothelial cells and influence of activated protein C. *Circulation.* Vol.110, No.18, pp. 2903-2909

Fujisawa, K., Aono, H., Hasunuma, T., Yamamoto, K., Mita, S., & Nishioka, K. (1996). Activation of transcription factor NF-kappa B in human synovial cells in response to tumor necrosis factor alpha. *Arthritis Rheum.* Vol.39, No.2, pp. 197-203

Fukudome, K. & Esmon, C.T. (1994). Identification, cloning, and regulation of a novel endothelial cell protein c activated protein c receptor. *J. Biol. Chem.* Vol.269, No.42, pp. 26486-26491

Gale, A.J., Tsavaler, A., & Griffin, J.H. (2002). Molecular characterization of an extended binding site for coagulation factor Va in the positive exosite of activated protein C. *J. Biol. Chem.* Vol.277, No.32, pp. 28836-28840

Ganopolsky, J.G. & Castellino, F.J. (2004). A Protein C Deficiency Exacerbates Inflammatory and Hypotensive Responses in Mice During Polymicrobial Sepsis in a Cecal Ligation and Puncture Model. *Am. J. Pathol.* Vol.165, No.4, pp. 1433-1446

Genc, K. (2007). The rationale for activated protein C treatment in perinatal white matter injury. *Med.Hypotheses.* Vol.68, No.6, pp. 1418-1419

Genc, K. (2007). Activated protein C: therapeutic implications for Alzheimer's disease. *Med Hypotheses.* Vol.69, No.3, pp. 701-702

Gramling, M.W., Beaulieu, L.M., & Church, F.C. (2010). Activated protein C enhances cell motility of endothelial cells and MDA-MB-231 breast cancer cells by intracellular signal transduction. *Exp.Cell Res.* Vol.316, No.3, pp. 314-328

Grey, S.T., Tsuchida, A., Hau, H., Orthner, C.L., Salem, H.H., & Hancock, W.W. (1994). Selective inhibitory effects of the anticoagulant activated protein C on the responses of human mononuclear phagocytes to LPS, IFN-gamma, or phorbol ester. *J. Immunol.* Vol.153, No.8, pp. 3664-3672

Griffin, J.H., Fernandez, J.A., Gale, A.J., & Mosnier, L.O. (2005). Activated protein C. *J.Thromb.Haemost.2007.Vol.5,No.suppl 1, pp.*73-80.

Griffin, J.H., Fernandez, J.A., Mosnier, L.O., Liu, D., Cheng, T., Guo, H., & Zlokovic, B.V. (2006). The promise of protein C. *Blood Cells Mol.Dis.* Vol.36, No.2, pp. 211-216

Griffin, J.H., Zlokovic, B., & Fernandez, J.A. (2002). Activated protein C: potential therapy for severe sepsis, thrombosis, and stroke. *Semin.Hematol.* Vol.39, No.3, pp. 197-205

Gruber, A. & Griffin, J.H. (1992). Direct detection of activated protein C in blood from human subjects. *Blood.* Vol.79, No.9, pp. 2340-2348

Gruden, G., Olivetti, C., Cavallo-Perin, P., Bazzan, M., Stella, S., Tamponi, G., & Pagano, G. (1997). Activated protein C resistance in type I diabetes. *Diabetes Care.* Vol.20, No.3, pp. 424-425

Gu, J.M., Crawley, J.T.B., Ferrell, G., Zhang, F., Li, W., Esmon, N.L., & Esmon, C.T. (2002). Disruption of the Endothelial Cell Protein C Receptor Gene in Mice Causes Placental Thrombosis and Early Embryonic Lethality. *J. Biol. Chem.* Vol.277, No.45, pp. 43335-43343

Guo, H., Gu, F., Li, W., Zhang, B., Niu, R., Fu, L., Zhang, N., & Ma, Y. (2009). Reduction of protein kinase C zeta inhibits migration and invasion of human glioblastoma cells. *J.Neurochem.* Vol.109, No.1, pp. 203-213

Guo, H., Liu, D., Gelbard, H., Cheng, T., Insalaco, R., Fernandez, J.A., Griffin, J.H., & Zlokovic, B.V. (2004). Activated protein C prevents neuronal apoptosis via protease activated receptors 1 and 3. *Neuron.* Vol.41, No.4, pp. 563-572

Guo, H., Singh, I., Wang, Y., Deane, R., Barrett, T., Fernandez, J.A., Chow, N., Griffin, J.H., & Zlokovic, B.V. (2009). Neuroprotective activities of activated protein C mutant with reduced anticoagulant activity. *Eur J Neurosci.* Vol.29, No.6, pp. 1119-1130

Guo, H., Liu, D., Gelbard, H., Cheng, T., Insalaco, R., Fernandez, J.A., Griffin, J.H., & Zlokovic, B.V. (2004). Activated Protein C Prevents Neuronal Apoptosis via Protease Activated Receptors 1 and 3. *Neuron.* Vol.41, No.4, pp. 563-572

Gupta, A., Rhodes, G.J., Berg, D.T., Gerlitz, B., Molitoris, B.A., & Grinnell, B.W. (2007). Activated protein C ameliorates LPS-induced acute kidney injury and downregulates renal INOS and angiotensin 2. Am.J.Physiol. Renal Physiol. Vol.293, No.1, pp. F245-F254

Hanly, A.M., Redmond, M., Winter, D.C., Brophy, S., Deasy, J.M., Bouchier-Hayes, D.J., & Kay, E.W. (2006). Thrombomodulin expression in colorectal carcinoma is protective and correlates with survival. *Br J Cancer.* Vol.94, No.9, pp. 1320-1325

Hanly, A.M. & Winter, D.C. (2007). The role of thrombomodulin in malignancy. *Semin Thromb Hemost.* Vol.33, No.7, pp. 673-679

Hataji, O., Taguchi, O., Gabazza, E.C., Yuda, H., Fujimoto, H., Suzuki, K., & Adachi, Y. (2002). Activation of protein C pathway in the airways. *Lung.* Vol.180, No.1, pp. 47-59

Hirose, K., Okajima, K., Taoka, Y., Uchiba, M., Tagami, H., Nakano, K., Utoh, J., Okabe, H., & Kitamura, N. (2000). Activated protein C reduces the ischemia/reperfusion-induced spinal cord injury in rats by inhibiting neutrophil activation. *Ann Surg.* Vol.232, No.2, pp. 272-280

Hofstra, J.J., Vlaar, A.P., Knape, P., Mackie, D.P., Determann, R.M., Choi, G., van Der, P.T., Levi, M., & Schultz, M.J. (2011). Pulmonary Activation of Coagulation and Inhibition of Fibrinolysis After Burn Injuries and Inhalation Trauma. *J Trauma.* Epub ahead of print

Hudson, L.G. & McCawley, L.J. (1998). Contributions of the epidermal growth factor receptor to keratinocyte motility. *Microsc.Res.Tech.* Vol.43, No.5, pp. 444-455

Isermann, B., Vinnikov, I.A., Madhusudhan, T., Herzog, S., Kashif, M., Blautzik, J., Corat, M.A.F., Zeier, M., Blessing, E., Oh, J., Gerlitz, B., Berg, D.T., Grinnell, B.W.,

Chavakis, T., Esmon, C.T., Weiler, H., Bierhaus, A., & Nawroth, P.P. (2007). Activated protein C protects against diabetic nephropathy by inhibiting endothelial and podocyte apoptosis. *Nat Med.* Vol.13, No.11, pp. 1349-1358

Itoh, T., Matsuda, H., Tanioka, M., Kuwabara, K., Itohara, S., & Suzuki, R. (2002). The role of matrix metalloproteinase-2 and matrix metalloproteinase-9 in antibody-induced arthritis. *J.Immunol.* Vol.169, No.5, pp. 2643-2647

Jackson, C.J., Xue, M., Thompson, P., Davey, R.A., Whitmont, K., Smith, S., Buisson-Legendre, N., Sztynda, T., Furphy, L.J., Cooper, A., Sambrook, P., & March, L. (2005). Activated protein C prevents inflammation yet stimulates angiogenesis to promote cutaneous wound healing. *Wound.Repair Regen.* Vol.13, No.3, pp. 284-294

Joyce, D.E., Gelbert, L., Ciaccia, A., DeHoff, B., & Grinnell, B.W. (2001). Gene expression profile of antithrombotic protein c defines new mechanisms modulating inflammation and apoptosis. *J.Biol.Chem.* Vol.276, No.14, pp. 11199-11203

Kamath, L., Meydani, A., Foss, F., & Kuliopulos, A. (2001). Signaling from protease-activated receptor-1 inhibits migration and invasion of breast cancer cells. *Cancer Res.* Vol.61, No.15, pp. 5933-5940

Keller, S.A., Moore, C.C., Evans, S.L., McKillop, I.H., & Huynh, T. (2011). Activated protein C alters inflammation and protects renal function in sepsis. *J Surg.Res.* Vol.168, No.1, pp. e103-e109

Kendrick, B.J., Gray, A.G., Pickworth, A., & Watters, M.P. (2006). Drotrecogin alfa (activated) in severe falciparum malaria. *Anaesthesia.* Vol.61, No.9, pp. 899-902

Kent, D.G., Copley, M.R., Benz, C., Wohrer, S., Dykstra, B.J., Ma, E., Cheyne, J., Zhao, Y., Bowie, M.B., Zhao, Y., Gasparetto, M., Delaney, A., Smith, C., Marra, M., & Eaves, C.J. (2009). Prospective isolation and molecular characterization of hematopoietic stem cells with durable self-renewal potential. *Blood.* Vol.113, No.25, pp. 6342-6350

Kerschen, E., Hernandez, I., Zogg, M., Jia, S., Hessner, M.J., Fernandez, J.A., Griffin, J.H., Huettner, C.S., Castellino, F.J., & Weiler, H. (2010). Activated protein C targets CD8+ dendritic cells to reduce the mortality of endotoxemia in mice. *J Clin Invest.* Vol.120, No.9, pp. 3167-3178

Kerschen, E.J., Fernandez, J.A., Cooley, B.C., Yang, X.V., Sood, R., Mosnier, L.O., Castellino, F.J., Mackman, N., Griffin, J.H., & Weiler, H. (2007). Endotoxemia and sepsis mortality reduction by non-anticoagulant activated protein C. *J Exp Med.* Vol.204, No.10, pp. 2439-2448

Kim, S.J., Shiba, E., Ishii, H., Inoue, T., Taguchi, T., Tanji, Y., Kimoto, Y., Izukura, M., & Takai, S. (1997). Thrombomodulin is a new biological and prognostic marker for breast cancer: an immunohistochemical study. *Anticancer Res.* Vol.17, No.3C, pp. 2319-2323

Kirschenbaum, L. & Astiz, M. (2005). Acute pancreatitis: a possible role for activated protein C? *Crit Care.* Vol.9, No.3, pp. 243-244

Kotanidou, A., Loutrari, H., Papadomichelakis, E., Glynos, C., Magkou, C., Armaganidis, A., Papapetropoulos, A., Roussos, C., & Orfanos, S.E. (2006). Inhaled activated protein C attenuates lung injury induced by aerosolized endotoxin in mice. *Vascul.Pharmacol.* Vol.45, No.2, pp. 134-140

Kuliopulos, A., Covic, L., Seeley, S.K., Sheridan, P.J., Helin, J., & Costello, C.E. (1999). Plasmin desensitization of the PAR1 thrombin receptor: kinetics, sites of truncation, and implications for thrombolytic therapy. *Biochemistry.* Vol.38, No.14, pp. 4572-4585

Kwasny-Krochin, B., Bobek, M., Kontny, E., Gluszko, P., Biedron, R., Chain, B.M., Maslinski, W., & Marcinkiewicz, J. (2002). Effect of taurine chloramine, the product of activated neutrophils, on the development of collagen-induced arthritis in DBA 1/J mice. *Amino.Acids.* Vol.23, No.4, pp. 419-426

Lay, A.J., Donahue, D., Tsai, M.J., & Castellino, F.J. (2007). Acute inflammation is exacerbated in mice genetically predisposed to a severe protein C deficiency. *Blood.* Vol.109, No.5, pp. 1984-1991

Levi, M., Dorffler-Melly, J., Reitsma, P., Buller, H., Florquin, S., van der Poll, T., & Carmeliet, P. (2003). Aggravation of endotoxin-induced disseminated intravascular coagulation and cytokine activation in heterozygous protein-C-deficient mice. *Blood.* Vol.101, No.12, pp. 4823-4827

Levin, M.E. (1993). Diabetic foot ulcers: pathogenesis and management. *J.ET Nurs.* Vol.20, No.5, pp. 191-198

Li, Q. & Verma, I.M. (2002). NF-kappaB regulation in the immune system. *Nat.Rev.Immunol.* Vol.2, No.10, pp. 725-734

Li, W., Zheng, X., Gu, J., Hunter, J., Ferrell, G.L., Lupu, F., Esmon, N.L., & Esmon, C.T. (2005). Overexpressing endothelial cell protein C receptor alters the hemostatic balance and protects mice from endotoxin. *J Thromb.Haemost.* Vol.3, No.7, pp. 1351-1359

Liaw, P.C., Esmon, C.T., Kahnamoui, K., Schmidt, S., Kahnamoui, S., Ferrell, G., Beaudin, S., Julian, J.A., Weitz, J.I., Crowther, M., Loeb, M., & Cook, D.J. (2004). Patients with severe sepsis vary markedly in their ability to generate activate protein C. *Blood.* Vol.104, No,13, pp 3958-3964

Lindahl, A.K., Boffa, M.C., & Abildgaard, U. (1993). Increased plasma thrombomodulin in cancer patients. *Thromb Haemost.* Vol.69, No.2, pp. 112-114

Macko, R.F., Ameriso, S.F., Gruber, A., Griffin, J.H., Fernandez, J.A., Barndt, R., Quismorio, F.P., Jr., Weiner, J.M., & Fisher, M. (1996). Impairments of the protein C system and fibrinolysis in infection-associated stroke. *Stroke.* Vol.27, No.11, pp. 2005-2011

Marok, R., Winyard, P.G., Coumbe, A., Kus, M.L., Gaffney, K., Blades, S., Mapp, P.I., Morris, C.J., Blake, D.R., Kaltschmidt, C., & Baeuerle, P.A. (1996). Activation of the transcription factor nuclear factor-kappa-b in human inflamed synovial tissue. *Arthritis Rheum.* Vol.39, No.4, pp. 583-591

Marti-Carvajal, A., Salanti, G., & Cardona, A.F. (2003). Human recombinant activated protein C for severe sepsis. *Cochrane.Database.Syst.Rev.* Vol.5,CD004388

Marti-Carvajal, A., Salanti, G., & Cardona, A.F. (2007). Human recombinant activated protein C for severe sepsis. *Cochrane.Database.Syst.Rev.* Vol.3, CD004388

Marti-Carvajal, A.J., Sola, I., Lathyris, D., & Cardona, A.F. (2011). Human recombinant activated protein C for severe sepsis. *Cochrane.Database.Syst.Rev.* Vol.4,.CD004388

Mathis, D., Vence, L., & Benoist, C. (2001). [beta]-Cell death during progression to diabetes. *Nature.* Vol.414, No.6865, pp. 792-798

Matsushita, Y., Yoshiie, K., Imamura, Y., Ogawa, H., Imamura, H., Takao, S., Yonezawa, S., Aikou, T., Maruyama, I., & Sato, E. (1998). A subcloned human esophageal squamous cell carcinoma cell line with low thrombomodulin expression showed increased invasiveness compared with a high thrombomodulin-expressing clone--thrombomodulin as a possible candidate for an adhesion molecule of squamous cell carcinoma. *Cancer Lett.* Vol.127, No.1-2, pp. 195-201

McQuibban, G.A., Gong, J.H., Wong, J.P., Wallace, J.L., Clark-Lewis, I., & Overall, C.M. (2002). Matrix metalloproteinase processing of monocyte chemoattractant proteins generates CC chemokine receptor antagonists with anti-inflammatory properties in vivo. *Blood.* Vol.100, No.4, pp. 1160-1167

Mewhort-Buist, T.A., Liaw, P.C., Patel, S., Atkinson, H.M., Berry, L.R., & Chan, A.K. (2008). Treatment of endothelium with the chemotherapy agent vincristine affects activated protein C generation to a greater degree in newborn plasma than in adult plasma. *Thromb Res.* Vol.122, No.3, pp. 418-426

Milia, A.F., Salis, M.B., Stacca, T., Pinna, A., Madeddu, P., Trevisani, M., Geppetti, P., & Emanueli, C. (2002). Protease-activated receptor-2 stimulates angiogenesis and accelerates hemodynamic recovery in a mouse model of hindlimb ischemia. *Circ.Res.* Vol.91, No.4, pp. 346-352

Minhas, N., Xue, M., Fukudome, K., & Jackson, C.J. (2010). Activated protein C utilizes the angiopoietin/Tie2 axis to promote endothelial barrier function. *FASEB J.* Vol.24, No.3, pp. 873-881

Mizutani, A., Okajima, K., Uchiba, M., & Noguchi, T. (2000). Activated protein C reduces ischemia/reperfusion-induced renal injury in rats by inhibiting leukocyte activation. *Blood.* Vol.95, No.12, pp. 3781-3787

Montiel, M., de la Blanca, E.P., & Jimenez, E. (2005). Angiotensin II induces focal adhesion kinase/paxillin phosphorylation and cell migration in human umbilical vein endothelial cells. *Biochem.Biophys.Res.Commun.* Vol.327, No.4, pp. 971-978

Mosnier, L.O., Gale, A.J., Yegneswaran, S., & Griffin, J.H. (2004). Activated protein C variants with normal cytoprotective but reduced anticoagulant activity. *Blood.* Vol.104, No.6, pp 1740-1744

Mosnier, L.O. & Griffin, J.H. (2003). Inhibition of staurosporine-induced apoptosis of endothelial cells by activated protein C requires protease-activated receptor-1 and endothelial cell protein C receptor. *Biochem.J.* Vol.373, No.Pt 1, pp. 65-70

Mosnier, L.O., Yang, X.V., & Griffin, J.H. (2007). Activated protein C mutant with minimal anticoagulant activity, normal cytoprotective activity, and preservation of thrombin activable fibrinolysis inhibitor-dependent cytoprotective functions. *J.Biol.Chem.* Vol.282, No.45, pp. 33022-33033

Mosnier, L.O., Zampolli, A., Kerschen, E.J., Schuepbach, R.A., Banerjee, Y., Fernandez, J.A., Yang, X.V., Riewald, M., Weiler, H., Ruggeri, Z.M., & Griffin, J.H. (2009). Hyperantithrombotic, noncytoprotective Glu149Ala-activated protein C mutant. *Blood.* Vol.113, No.23, pp. 5970-5978

Nguyen, M., Arkell, J., & Jackson, C.J. (3000). Activated protein C directly activates human endothelial gelatinase A. *J. Biol. Chem.*Vol.275, No.13, pp. 9095-9098

Ni, A.F., O'Donnell, J.S., Johnson, J.A., Brown, L., Gleeson, E.M., Smith, O.P., & Preston, R.J. (2011). Activated protein C N-linked glycans modulate cytoprotective signaling function on endothelial cells. *J. Biol. Chem.* Vol.286, No.2, pp. 1323-1330

Nick, J.A., Coldren, C.D., Geraci, M.W., Poch, K.R., Fouty, B.W., O'Brien, J., Gruber, M., Zarini, S., Murphy, R.C., Kuhn, K., Richter, D., Kast, K.R., & Abraham, E. (2004). Recombinant human activated protein C reduces human endotoxin-induced pulmonary inflammation via inhibition of neutrophil chemotaxis. *Blood.* Vol.104, No.13, pp 3878-3885

Nierodzik, M.L., Chen, K., Takeshita, K., Li, J.J., Huang, Y.Q., Feng, X.S., D'Andrea, M.R., ndrade-Gordon, P., & Karpatkin, S. (1998). Protease-activated receptor 1 (PAR-1) is required and rate-limiting for thrombin-enhanced experimental pulmonary metastasis. *Blood.* Vol.92, No.10, pp. 3694-3700

Nijziel, M.R., van, O.R., Christella, M., Thomassen, L.G., van Pampus, E.C., Hamulyak, K., Tans, G., & Rosing, J. (2003). Acquired resistance to activated protein C in breast cancer patients. *Br.J Haematol.* Vol.120, No.1, pp. 117-122

O'Brien, L.A., Gupta, A., & Grinnell, B.W. (2006). Activated protein C and sepsis. *Front Biosci.* Vol.11, No.1, pp. 676-698

Okajima, K. (2004). Regulation of inflammatory responses by activated protein C: the molecular mechanism(s) and therapeutic implications. *Clin.Chem.Lab Med.* Vol.42, No.2, pp. 132-141

Ottesen, L.H., Bladbjerg, E.M., Osman, M., Lausten, S.B., Jacobsen, N.O., Gram, J., & Jensen, S.L. (1999). Protein C activation during the initial phase of experimental acute pancreatitis in the rabbit. *Dig.Surg.* Vol.16, No.6, pp. 486-495

Park, S.Y., Lee, H.E., Li, H., Shipitsin, M., Gelman, R., & Polyak, K. (2010). Heterogeneity for Stem CellGÇôRelated Markers According to Tumor Subtype and Histologic Stage in Breast Cancer. *Clin. Cancer Res.* Vol.16, No.3, pp. 876-887

Ram, M., Sherer, Y., & Shoenfeld, Y. (2006). Matrix metalloproteinase-9 and autoimmune diseases. *J Clin Immunol.* Vol.26, No.4, pp. 299-307

Redd, M.J., Cooper, L., Wood, W., Stramer, B., & Martin, P. (2004). Wound healing and inflammation: embryos reveal the way to perfect repair. *Philos.Trans.R.Soc.Lond B Biol.Sci.* Vol.359, No.1445, pp. 777-784

Rezaie, A.R., Neuenschwander, P.F., Morrissey, J.H., & Esmon, C.T. (1993). Analysis of the functions of the first epidermal growth factor-like domain of factor X. *J.Biol.Chem.* Vol.268, No.11, pp. 8176-8180

Riewald, M., Petrovan, R.J., Donner, A., Mueller, B.M., & Ruf, W. (2002). Activation of endothelial cell protease activated receptor 1 by the protein C pathway. *Science.* Vol.296, No.5574, pp. 1880-1882

Rogers, J.S., Murgo, A.J., Fontana, J.A., & Raich, P.C. (1988). Chemotherapy for breast cancer decreases plasma protein C and protein S. *J Clin Oncol.* Vol.6, No.2, pp. 276-281

Sadaka, F., O'Brien, J., Migneron, M., Stortz, J., Vanston, A., & Taylor, R.W. (2011). Activated protein C in septic shock: a propensity-matched analysis. *Crit Care.* Vol.15, No.2, pp. R89-

Sakar, A., Vatansever, S., Sepit, L., Ozbilgin, K., & Yorgancioglu, A. (2007). Effect of recombinant human activated protein C on apoptosis-related proteins. *Eur.J Histochem.* Vol.51, No.2, pp. 103-109

Schmidt-Supprian, M., Murphy, C., While, B., Lawler, M., Kapurniotu, A., Voelter, W., Smith, O., & Bernhagen, J. (2000). Activated protein C inhibits tumor necrosis factor and macrophage migration inhibitory factor production in monocytes. *Eur Cytokine Netw.* Vol.11, No.3, pp. 407-413

Schouten, M., de Boer, J.D., van der Sluijs, K.F., Roelofs, J.J., van, '., V, Levi, M., Esmon, C.T., & van Der, P.T. (2011). Impact of Endogenous Protein C on Pulmonary Coagulation and Injury During Lethal H1N1 Influenza in Mice. *Am J Respir.Cell Mol Biol.* Vol.44, No.3, pp. 377-383

Seol, J.W., Lee, Y.J., Jackson, C.J., Sambrook, P.N., & Park, S.Y. (2011). Activated protein C inhibits bisphosphonate-induced endothelial cell death via the endothelial protein C receptor and nuclear factor-kappaB pathways. *Int J Mol Med.* Vol.27, No.6, pp. 835-840

Shibata, M., Kumar, S.R., Amar, A., Fernandez, J.A., Hofman, F., Griffin, J.H., & Zlokovic, B.V. (2001). Anti-inflammatory, antithrombotic, and neuroprotective effects of activated protein C in a murine model of focal ischemic stroke. *Circulation.* Vol.103, No.13, pp. 1799-1805

Short, M.A., Schlichting, D., & Qualy, R.L. (2006). From bench to bedside: a review of the clinical trial development plan of drotrecogin alfa (activated). *Curr.Med.Res.Opin.* Vol.22, No.12, pp. 2525-2540

Srinivas, R., Agarwal, R., & Gupta, D. (2007). Severe sepsis due to severe falciparum malaria and leptospirosis co-infection treated with activated protein C. *Malar.J.* Vol.6, No.6, pp.42

Stenflo, J. (1976). A new vitamin K-dependent protein. Purification from bovine plasma and preliminary characterization. *J.Biol.Chem.* Vol.251, No.2, pp. 355-363

Stephenson, D.A., Toltl, L.J., Beaudin, S., & Liaw, P.C. (2006). Modulation of monocyte function by activated protein C, a natural anticoagulant. *J.Immunol.* Vol.177, No.4, pp. 2115-2122

Szpaderska, A.M. & DiPietro, L.A. (2005). Inflammation in surgical wound healing: friend or foe? *Surgery.* Vol.137, No.5, pp. 571-573

Szpaderska, A.M., Zuckerman, J.D., & DiPietro, L.A. (2003). Differential injury responses in oral mucosal and cutaneous wounds. *J.Dent.Res.* Vol.82, No.8, pp. 621-626

Taoka, Y., Okajima, K., Uchiba, M., & Johno, M. (2000). Neuroprotection by recombinant thrombomodulin. *Thromb Haemost.* Vol.83, No.3, pp. 462-468

Taoka, Y., Okajima, K., Uchiba, M., Murakami, K., Harada, N., Johno, M., & Naruo, M. (1998). Activated protein C reduces the severity of compression-induced spinal cord injury in rats by inhibiting activation of leukocytes. *J Neurosci.* Vol.18, No.4, pp. 1393-1398

Taoka, Y., Okajima, K., Uchiba, M., Murakami, K., Kushimoto, S., Johno, M., Naruo, M., Okabe, H., & Takatsuki, K. (1997). Role of neutrophils in spinal cord injury in the rat. *Neuroscience.* Vol.79, No.4, pp. 1177-1182

Thadhani, R., Pascual, M., & Bonventre, J.V. (1996). Acute renal failure. *N.Engl.J.Med.* Vol.334, No.22, pp. 1448-1460

Toltl, L.J., Beaudin, S., & Liaw, P.C. (2008). Activated protein C up-regulates IL-10 and inhibits tissue factor in blood monocytes. *J.Immunol.* Vol.181, No.3, pp. 2165-2173

Trent, J.T., Falabella, A., Eaglstein, W.H., & Kirsner, R.S. (2005). Venous ulcers: pathophysiology and treatment options. *Ostomy.Wound Manage.* Vol.51, No.5, pp. 38-54

Tsuneyoshi, N., Fukudome, K., Horiguchi, S., Ye, X., Matsuzaki, M., Toi, M., Suzuki, K., & Kimoto, M. (2001). Expression and anticoagulant function of the endothelial cell protein C receptor (EPCR) in cancer cell lines. *Thromb Haemost.* Vol.85, No.2, pp. 356-361

Uchiba, M., Okajima, K., Oike, Y., Ito, Y., Fukudome, K., Isobe, H., & Suda, T. (2004). Activated protein C induces endothelial cell proliferation by mitogen-activated protein kinase activation in vitro and angiogenesis in vivo. *Circ Res.* Vol.95, No.1, pp. 34-41

Van Sluis, G.L., Bruggemann, L.W., Esmon, C.T., Kamphuisen, P.W., Richel, D.J., Buller, H.R., Van Noorden, C.J., & Spek, C.A. (2011). Endogenous activated protein C is essential for immune-mediated cancer cell elimination from the circulation. *Cancer Lett.* Vol.306, No.1, pp. 106-110

Van Sluis, G.L., Buller, H.R., & Spek, C.A. (2010). The role of activated protein C in cancer progression. *Thromb Res.* Vol.125 Suppl 2, No.S138-S142

Villares, G.J., Zigler, M., Dobroff, A.S., Wang, H., Song, R., Melnikova, V.O., Huang, L., Braeuer, R.R., & Bar-Eli, M. (2011). Protease activated receptor-1 inhibits the Maspin tumor-suppressor gene to determine the melanoma metastatic phenotype. *Proc Natl Acad Sci U.S.A.* Vol.108, No.2, pp. 626-631

Vukovich, T.C. & Schernthaner, G. (1986). Decreased protein C levels in patients with insulin-dependent type I diabetes mellitus. *Diabetes.* Vol.35, No.5, pp. 617-619

Walker, C.T., Marky, A.H., Petraglia, A.L., Ali, T., Chow, N., & Zlokovic, B.V. (2010). Activated protein C analog with reduced anticoagulant activity improves functional recovery and reduces bleeding risk following controlled cortical impact. *Brain Res.* Vol.1347, No.125-131

Wang, Y., Thiyagarajan, M., Chow, N., Singh, I., Guo, H., Davis, T.P., & Zlokovic, B.V. (2009). Differential neuroprotection and risk for bleeding from activated protein C with varying degrees of anticoagulant activity. *Stroke.* Vol.40, No.5, pp. 1864-1869

White, B., Schmidt, M., Murphy, C., Livingstone, W., O'Toole, D., Lawler, M., O'Neill, L., Kelleher, D., Schwarz, H.P., & Smith, O.P. (2000). Activated protein C inhibits lipopolysaccharide-induced nuclear translocation of nuclear factor kappaB (NF-kappaB) and tumour necrosis factor alpha (TNF-alpha) production in the THP-1 monocytic cell line. *Br.J.Haematol.* Vol.110, No.1, pp. 130-134

Whitmont, K., Reid, I., Tritton, S., March, L., Xue, M., Lee, M., Fulcher, G., Sambrook, P., Slobedman, E., Cooper, A., & Jackson, C. (2008). Treatment of chronic leg ulcers with topical activated protein C. *Arch.Dermatol.* Vol.144, No.11, pp. 1479-1483

Woodley-Cook, J., Shin, L.Y., Swystun, L., Caruso, S., Beaudin, S., & Liaw, P.C. (2006). Effects of the chemotherapeutic agent doxorubicin on the protein C anticoagulant pathway. *Mol Cancer Ther.* Vol.5, No.12, pp. 3303-3311

Wu, J., Zhou, Z., Ye, S., Dai, H., Ma, L., Xu, X., & Li, X. (2000). [Detection of soluble endothelial protein C receptor (sEPCR) in patients with CHD, DM and SLE]. *Zhonghua Xue.Ye.Xue.Za Zhi.* Vol.21, No.9, pp. 472-474

Xu, J., Ji, Y., Zhang, X., Drake, M., & Esmon, C.T. (2009). Endogenous activated protein C signaling is critical to protection of mice from lipopolysaccaride-induced septic shock. *J Thromb Haemost.* Vol.7, No.5, pp. 851-856

Xu, J., Zhang, X., Pelayo, R., Monestier, M., Ammollo, C.T., Semeraro, F., Taylor, F.B., Esmon, N.L., Lupu, F., & Esmon, C.T. (2009). Extracellular histones are major mediators of death in sepsis. *Nat Med.* Vol.15, No.11, pp. 1318-1321

Xue, M., Campbell, D., Sambrook, P.N., Fukudome, K., & Jackson, C.J. (2005). Endothelial protein C receptor and protease-activated receptor-1 mediate induction of a wound-healing phenotype in human keratinocytes by activated protein C. *J. Invest. Dermatol.* Vol.125, No.6, pp. 1279-1285

Xue, M., Chow, S.O., Dervish, S., Chan, Y.K., Julovi, S.M., & Jackson, C.J. (2011). Activated protein C enhances human keratinocyte barrier integrity via sequential activation of epidermal growth factor receptor and Tie2. *J. Biol. Chem.* Vol.286, No.8, pp. 6742-6750

Xue, M., March, L., Sambrook, P.N., Fukudome, F., & Jackson, C.J. (2007). Endothelial protein C receptor is over-expressed in rheumatoid arthritic (RA) synovium and mediates the anti-inflammatory effects of activated protein C in RA monocytes. *Ann.Rheum.Dis.* Vol.66, No.12, pp.1574-1580

Xue, M., March, L., Sambrook, P.N., & Jackson, C.J. (2007). Differential regulation of matrix metalloproteinase 2 and matrix metalloproteinase 9 by activated protein C: relevance to inflammation in rheumatoid arthritis. *Arthritis Rheum.* Vol.56, No.9, pp. 2864-2874

Xue, M., Minhas, N., Chow, S.O., Dervish, S., Sambrook, P.N., March, L., & Jackson, C.J. (2010). Endogenous protein C is essential for the functional integrity of human endothelial cells. *Cell Mol Life Sci.* Vol.67, No.9, pp.1537-1546

Xue, M., Thompson, P., Kelso, I., & Jackson, C. (2004). Activated protein C stimulates proliferation, migration and wound closure, inhibits apoptosis and upregulates MMP-2 activity in cultured human keratinocytes. *Exp Cell Res.* Vol.299, No.1, pp. 119-127

Xue, M., Campbell, D., & Jackson, C.J. (2007). Protein C is an autocrine growth factor for human skin keratinocytes. *J. Biol. Chem.* Vol.282, No.18, pp. 13610-13616

Yamauchi, T., Sakurai, M., Abe, K., Takano, H., & Sawa, Y. (2006). Neuroprotective effects of activated protein C through induction of insulin-like growth factor-1 (IGF-1), IGF-1 receptor, and its downstream signal phosphorylated serine-threonine kinase after spinal cord ischemia in rabbits. *Stroke.* Vol.37, No.4, pp. 1081-1086

Yang, X.V., Banerjee, Y., Fernandez, J.A., Deguchi, H., Xu, X., Mosnier, L.O., Urbanus, R.T., de Groot, P.G., White-Adams, T.C., McCarty, O.J., & Griffin, J.H. (2009). Activated protein C ligation of ApoER2 (LRP8) causes Dab1-dependent signaling in U937 cells. *Proc. Nat. Acad. Sci. U.S.A.* Vol.106, No.1, pp. 274-279

Yuda, H., Adachi, Y., Taguchi, O., Gabazza, E.C., Hataji, O., Fujimoto, H., Tamaki, S., Nishikubo, K., Fukudome, K., D'Alessandro-Gabazza, C.N., Maruyama, J., Izumizaki, M., Iwase, M., Homma, I., Inoue, R., Kamada, H., Hayashi, T., Kasper, M., Lambrecht, B.N., Barnes, P.J., & Suzuki, K. (2004). Activated protein C inhibits bronchial hyperresponsiveness and Th2 cytokine expression in mice. *Blood.* Vol.103, No.6, pp. 2196-2204

Yuksel, M., Okajima, K., Uchiba, M., Horiuchi, S., & Okabe, H. (2002). Activated protein C inhibits lipopolysaccharide-induced tumor necrosis factor-alpha production by inhibiting activation of both nuclear factor-kappa B and activator protein-1 in human monocytes. *Thromb.Haemost.* Vol.88, No.2, pp. 267-273

Zhong, Z., Ilieva, H., Hallagan, L., Bell, R., Singh, I., Paquette, N., Thiyagarajan, M., Deane, R., Fernandez, J.A., Lane, S., Zlokovic, A.B., Liu, T., Griffin, J.H., Chow, N., Castellino, F.J., Stojanovic, K., Cleveland, D.W., & Zlokovic, B.V. (2009). Activated protein C therapy slows ALS-like disease in mice by transcriptionally inhibiting SOD1 in motor neurons and microglia cells. *J. Clin. Invest.* Vol.119, No.11, pp. 3437-3449

Zlokovic, B.V. (2005). Neurovascular mechanisms of Alzheimer's neurodegeneration. *Trends Neurosci.* Vol.28, No.4, pp. 202-208

Zlokovic, B.V. & Griffin, J.H. (2011). Cytoprotective protein C pathways and implications for stroke and neurological disorders. *Trends Neurosci.* Vol.34, No.4, pp. 198-209

Part 5

Role of TrkA Receptor in Inflammation

5

Expression and Role of the TrkA Receptor in Pulmonary Inflammatory Diseases

Véronique Freund-Michel[1,2], Bernard Muller[1,2] and Nelly Frossard[3,4]

[1]*INSERM U1045 "Centre de Recherche Cardio-thoracique de Bordeaux", Bordeaux*

[2]*University Bordeaux Segalen, Bordeaux*

[3]*UMR 7200 CNRS "Laboratoire d'Innovation Thérapeutique", Strasbourg*

[4]*University of Strasbourg, Strasbourg*

France

1. Introduction

The nerve growth factor NGF belongs to the neurotrophin family and was described for the first time more than fifty years ago by Rita Levi-Montalcini and collaborators (Levi-Montalcini et al., 1995; Levi-Montalcini & Hamburger, 1951), who showed its major role in neuronal growth and survival. NGF effects are mediated by activation of two receptor types: the low-affinity p75 receptor for neurotrophins ($p75^{NTR}$) and the high-affinity tropomyosin-related kinase A (TrkA) receptor (Freund-Michel & Frossard, 2008a). The $p75^{NTR}$ receptor belongs to the death receptor family and its activation by NGF at nanomolar concentrations leads either to pro- or anti-apoptotic signalling pathways. The $p75^{NTR}$ receptor is not selective for NGF as it can also bind pro-neurotrophins and the other neurotrophins at the same nanomolar concentrations (Chao, 2003). Inversely, the TrkA receptor is selective for NGF and belongs to the tyrosine-kinase receptor family. Its activation by NGF at picomolar concentrations activates signalling pathways inducing cell proliferation, differentiation and survival in particular through activation of phosphatidylinositol-3 kinase (PI3K), small protein G Ras, phospholipase Cβ (PLCβ) and mitogen-activated protein kinases (MAPK) (Freund-Michel & Frossard, 2008a).

The role of NGF in neuronal growth and survival has been widely studied and led to consider NGF as a promising therapeutic target in several pathologies of the nervous system, in particular neurodegenerative diseases (Prakash et al., 2010). In addition, many studies have suggested that NGF also plays the role of an inflammatory mediator, in particular in the lung (Freund-Michel & Frossard, 2008a). Indeed, numerous sources of NGF have been described in the lung, including infiltrated inflammatory cells, sensory nerves, and many lung structural cells such as fibroblasts, epithelial, endothelial, and airway or pulmonary vascular smooth muscle cells (Ricci et al., 2004b). These cells have been shown to release more NGF in inflammatory conditions, and may thus participate in increased NGF levels observed in pulmonary inflammatory diseases. In parallel, many studies have shown an active role of NGF in pulmonary inflammation, airway sensory nerve plasticity, airway and vascular hyperreactivity and remodelling (Freund-Michel & Frossard, 2008a). Most of these NGF effects occur through activation of the TrkA receptor, thus highlighting the pivotal role played by this receptor in pulmonary inflammatory diseases.

The aim of the present chapter is to describe the role of the TrkA receptor activated by NGF in pulmonary inflammatory diseases. We will first present the TrkA receptor by describing its discovery, its structure and activity as well as its major signalling pathways. We will then focus on the TrkA receptor in the lung, by describing its pulmonary expression and review its involvement in NGF-mediated effects in the lung. We will describe in particular how the TrkA receptor participates to NGF-induced inflammation, airway and vascular hyperreactivity and remodelling in the lung, focusing on two major pulmonary diseases: asthma and pulmonary hypertension.

2. Presentation of the TrkA receptor

The TrkA receptor belongs to the Trk receptor family, together with TrkB and TrkC receptors. Each Trk receptor binds with a picomolar affinity to a preferred ligand: NGF for TrkA, BDNF (brain-derived neurotrophic factor) and NT-4/5 (neurotrophin-4/5) for TrkB, and NT-3 (neurotrophin-3) for TrkC (Chao, 2003). However, some crosstalks have been described, in particular for NT-3 being able to bind TrkA and TrkB receptors but at higher concentrations (Ryden & Ibanez, 1996).

2.1 Discovery of the TrkA receptor

A proto-oncogene was identified in 1986 by Martin-Zanca and co-workers in human colon carcinomas (Martin-Zanca et al., 1986). This proto-oncogene, resulting from fusion between genes encoding for a tyrosine-kinase domain and a non muscular tropomyosin, was named NTRK or trk for « tropomyosin-related kinase ». Three isoforms were identified and named NTRK1 (or TRKA), NTRK2 (or TRKB) and NTRK3 (or TRKC), with proteins encoded by these genes named Trk (TrkA, TrkB and TrkC) (Martin-Zanca et al., 1986). Expression of Trk proteins was later also detected in thyroid carcinomas and other cancers such as melanomas or breast cancers, as well as in non cancer tissues, in particular in the nervous system (Greco et al., 1997). In 1991, the TrkA protein was identified as the high affinity receptor for NGF (Kaplan et al., 1991a; Klein et al., 1991).

2.2 Structure of the TrkA receptor

The human TrkA receptor is encoded by a gene of 23kb located on chromosome 1q21-q22 (Weier et al., 1995). This gene contains 16 introns of 70bp to 3.3kb and 17 exons of 18 to 394bp (Indo et al., 1997), with the 9 first exons encoding for the extracellular part of the receptor (Metsis, 2001). The TrkA protein contains 790 amino acids with a molecular weight of 140 kDa (Meakin & Shooter, 1992), and is composed of an intracellular domain containing a tyrosine-kinase intrinsic activity, a unique transmembrane helix, and an extracellular domain dedicated to NGF binding (Wiesmann & de Vos, 2001). This extracellular domain is highly glycosylated, which is essential for activation of TrkA signalling pathways (Friedman & Greene, 1999).

Alternative splicing leads to several isoforms of the TrkA receptor. TrkA I and TrkA II splice variants differ only in the presence or absence of a 6 amino acid sequence. However, even if TrkA II expression is restricted to the nervous system, whereas TrkA I is more ubiquitously expressed (Clary & Reichardt, 1994), no differences in NGF binding or in TrkA function have been identified between these two isoforms (Barker et al., 1993). More recently, a novel hypoxia-regulated TrkA III splice variant has also been described: this isoform is expressed on internal membranes (Tacconelli et al., 2005) and exhibits oncogenic activity (Farina et al., 2009). Finally, a metalloproteinase-dependent cleavage of TrkA extracellular domain has been described, with release of a soluble fragment whose function remains unknown (Cabrera et al., 1996). In parallel, this cleavage induces activation of TrkA intracellular kinase domain, thus providing a TrkA NGF-independent activation, which may contribute to TrkA-dependent effects *in vivo* (Diaz-Rodriguez et al., 1999).

2.3 Activation and signalling pathways of the TrkA receptor

As classically described for other tyrosine-kinase receptors, NGF binds to the extracellular domain of the TrkA receptor and induces its dimerization thereby activating its intracellular tyrosine kinase domain (Kaplan et al., 1991b). Each kinase domain induces phosphorylation of three tyrosine residues (Y670, Y674 and Y675) on the contralateral kinase domain (Mitra, 1991), thus leading to enhancement of kinase activity and further phosphorylation of three other tyrosine residues outside the kinase domain (Y490, Y751 and Y785) (Stephens et al., 1994). These newly phosphorylated tyrosine residues are then recognized by proteins through their SH2 (Src homology domain 2) domains. The adapter protein Shc (Src homology 2-containing protein) interacts with the phosphorylated Y490 residue, phosphatidyl-inositol 3-kinase (PI3K) interacts with the phosphorylated Y751 residue, and phospholipase Cγ (PLCγ) interacts with the phosphorylated Y785 residue, thereby initiating three main signalling pathways that have been widely studied in particular in neuronal cells (Skaper, 2008). However, some recent studies also show activation of these TrkA signalling pathways in non neuronal cells, and in particular in the airways (for reviews: Freund-Michel & Frossard, 2008a; Prakash et al., 2010).

2.3.1 Ras/Raf pathway

Shc intracellular binding to the TrkA receptor leads to phosphorylation of its tyrosine residues and further recognition by the adapter protein Grb-2 (growth factor receptor bound protein-2) through SH3 (Src homology domain 3) domains. Grb-2 then binds to the factor sos (factor son of sevenless) to induce recruitment of the small G protein Ras to the cell membrane and its activation (Segal & Greenberg, 1996). This translocation to the cell membrane enables Ras-induced activation of the Raf kinase and therefore phosphorylation of Raf and activation of the MAPK (mitogen-activated protein kinase) ERK1/2 (extracellular-regulated protein kinase 1/2), leading to activation of survival mechanisms and proliferation (Freund-Michel et al., 2006). Concomitant activation of Rap1, another small

G protein, can potentiate Ras activation and enhance activation of the ERK1/2 pathway (York et al., 2000).

2.3.2 PI3K pathway

PI3K intracellular binding to the TrkA receptor leads to its phosphorylation and activation. PI3K then induces synthesis of phosphatidyl-inositol 3,4-bisphosphate that recruits PDK-1 (phosphoinositide-dependent kinase-1) to the cell membrane and induces activation of PKB (protein-kinase B, also called Akt) (Ashcroft et al., 1999). PKB then leads to activation of gene transcription, either through activation of the small G protein Rac and the MAPK pathway (Kita et al., 1998; Yamaguchi et al., 2001), or through activation of the atypical PKC zeta in a MAPK-independent manner (Wooten et al., 1994). In addition, PKB can lead to activation of proteins belonging to the IAP (inhibitors of apoptosis) family that are involved in cell survival (Wiese et al., 1999). Finally, a Ras-dependent activation of PI3K has also been described, through direct interaction between Ras and PI3K in a complex also containing the adapter protein Gab-1 (Grb2-associated binder-1) after activation of Shc and Grb-2 (Holgado-Madruga et al., 1997; Korhonen et al., 1999).

2.3.3 PLC/PKC pathway

PLCγ is activated by its interaction with the TrkA receptor and its phosphorylation by TrkA intrinsic kinase domains. PLCγ then induces cleavage of phosphatidyl inositol 4,5-bisphosphate into inositol trisphosphate (IP_3) and diacylglycerol (DAG). DAG activates protein-kinase C (PKC) to activate the MAPK pathway, with in particular activation of JNK (c-jun N-terminal kinase) and p38 (Patapoutian & Reichardt, 2001). IP_3 binds to its receptor localized on the endoplasmic reticulum and induces calcium release into the cell cytoplasm, thus contributing to PKC activation (Obermeier et al., 1993).

2.4 Transactivation of the TrkA receptor by G protein-coupled receptors

Neurotrophin-independent activation of Trk receptors, and in particular of the TrkA receptor, has been evidenced in rat neuronal cells after adenosine treatment (Lee & Chao, 2001). Activation of the adenosine A_{2A} receptor, a G protein-coupled receptor (GPCR), induces activation of a kinase belonging to the Src family that is then able to phosphorylate the TrkA receptor and activate the PI3K/PKB pathway (Lee & Chao, 2001; Lee et al., 2002a). This effect has also been evidenced with another GPCR agonist, the pituitary adenylate cyclase-activating peptide (PACAP), being able to induce TrkA transactivation and specific activation of the PI3K/PKB pathway in absence of NGF (Lee et al., 2002b). Since neuroprotective effects of adenosine and PACAP had been previously demonstrated, it has been suggested that this TrkA transactivation mechanism may contribute to these neuroprotective effects through activation of PI3K/PKB (Lee et al., 2002b). However more recent studies suggested that this TrkA transactivation mechanism occurred on newly synthesized TrkA receptors that were not already expressed at the cell membrane (Rajagopal et al., 2004).

2.5 Trafficking of the TrkA receptor

NGF activation of the TrkA receptor expressed on neurons can activate signalling pathways close to the nucleus through a specific mechanism called retrograde transport (Heerssen &

Segal, 2002). Once activated by NGF, the TrkA receptor is internalized, mainly through activation of three mechanisms: clathrine-dependent internalization, caveolae-dependent internalization, or macroendocytosis (Philippidou et al., 2011; Zweifel et al., 2005). All these mechanisms are involved in TrkA internalization and depend i) on the cell type studied, ii) on the concentration of NGF, and iii) on the amplitude of the signal generated by TrkA activation (Zweifel et al., 2005). Once internalized, only a few number of TrkA receptors are transported close to the nucleus, using early endosomes characterized by expression of the small G protein Rab5 and its effector EEA1 (Early endosome antigen 1) (Delcroix et al., 2003). TrkA retrograde transport is dependent upon activation of the PI3K-PKB pathway (Delcroix et al., 2003; Kuruvilla et al., 2000; York et al., 2000). Most of internalized TrkA receptors are either degraded through targeting to lysosomes (Jullien et al., 2002; Saxena et al., 2005) or to the proteasome after ubuquitination (Georgieva et al., 2011; Takahashi et al., 2011), or recycled at the cell membrane (Chen et al., 2005).

3. TrkA expression in the lung

Neurotrophin expression was first described in the central and peripheral nervous systems, participating to nerve growth and survival through activation of Trk and $p75^{NTR}$ receptors. However, neurotrophins and their receptors were later also described in a variety of non-neuronal tissues, and in particular in the lung (Lomen-Hoerth & Shooter, 1995).

3.1 *In vitro* studies

3.1.1 Inflammatory cells

NGF expression, which was first reported in T lymphocytes (Ehrhard et al., 1993a), was later also described in a variety of inflammatory cells including B lymphocytes (Torcia et al., 1996), mast cells (Leon et al., 1994), eosinophils (Solomon et al., 1998) and macrophages (Ricci et al., 2000b). Expression of the TrkA receptor was shown on mast cells (Tam et al., 1997), Th2 lymphocytes (Ehrhard et al., 1993a; Lambiase et al., 1997), B lymphocytes (Torcia et al., 1996), eosinophils (Hahn et al., 2006; Nassenstein et al., 2003; Noga et al., 2002), monocytes and macrophages (Ehrhard et al., 1993b; Otten et al., 1994), and basophils (Burgi et al., 1996).

3.1.2 Airway structural cells

Many airway structural cells such as fibroblasts (Antonelli et al., 2005; Olgart & Frossard, 2001), epithelial cells (Fox et al., 2001; Pons et al., 2001), airway smooth muscle cells (Freund et al., 2002), pulmonary endothelial and vascular smooth muscle cells (Freund-Michel et al., 2009) are sources of NGF (**Fig. 1**). Investigation of TrkA expression on these cells showed TrkA expression in particular on pulmonary fibroblasts (Micera et al., 2001), airway smooth muscle cells (Dagnell et al., 2007; Freund-Michel et al., 2006; Freund-Michel & Frossard, 2008b), airway epithelial cells (Othumpangat et al., 2009), and pulmonary endothelial and vascular smooth muscle cells (Freund-Michel et al., 2010) (**Fig. 1**).

3.2 *In vivo* studies

Expression of TrkA mRNA was initially evidenced in rat and human lung homogenates (Barbacid et al., 1991; Lomen-Hoerth & Shooter, 1995). Expression of TrkA protein was then shown by immunohistochemistry in isolated human alveolar macrophages (Ricci et al., 2000b), in isolated extrapulmonary arteries (Ricci et al., 2000a), and was later also evidenced on human airway and vascular smooth muscles, on alveolar cells, on airway sensory nerves, as well as on infiltrated inflammatory cells, in particular macrophages, mast cells and lymphocytes (Kassel et al., 2001; Olgart Hoglund et al., 2002; Ricci et al., 2004b). Similar TrkA expression was shown in the mouse lung (Hikawa et al., 2002; Nassenstein et al., 2006).

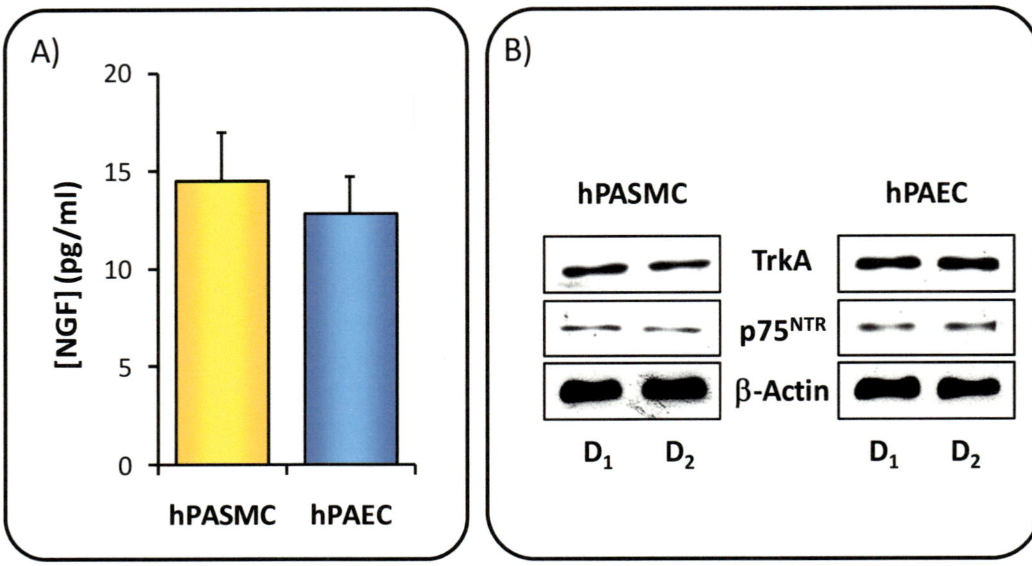

Fig. 1. Expression of NGF and its receptors in human pulmonary vascular cells

A) NGF protein levels (pg/ml) secreted after 24h by human pulmonary arterial smooth muscle cells (hPASMC) or human pulmonary arterial endothelial cells (hPAEC) in primary culture were assessed by ELISA in the culture cell supernatant. Data are means ± S.E.M. of n=3 experiments performed in triplicates with cells from two different donors. B) TrkA and $p75^{NTR}$ proteins were detected by Western blotting in cultured hPASMC or hPAEC from two different donors (D1 and D2), with rabbit polyclonal anti-human TrkA or $p75^{NTR}$ antibodies as specific protein bands of 140 and 75 kDa respectively. β-Actin probed in the same blots was used to control for protein loading.

4. NGF effects in the lung mediated by activation of the TrkA receptor

NGF is able to stimulate inflammatory cells infiltrated in the bronchial mucosa, promoting in particular their activation and survival in the airways (Freund-Michel & Frossard, 2008a). NGF also displays its role of growth factor on airway nerves, in particular on sensory airway nerves (Hoyle et al., 1998), and is able to stimulate other airway structural cells such as pulmonary fibroblasts or airway smooth muscle cells (Freund-Michel & Frossard, 2008a). Some of these effects involve activation of the TrkA receptor expressed on these cells **(Fig. 2)**.

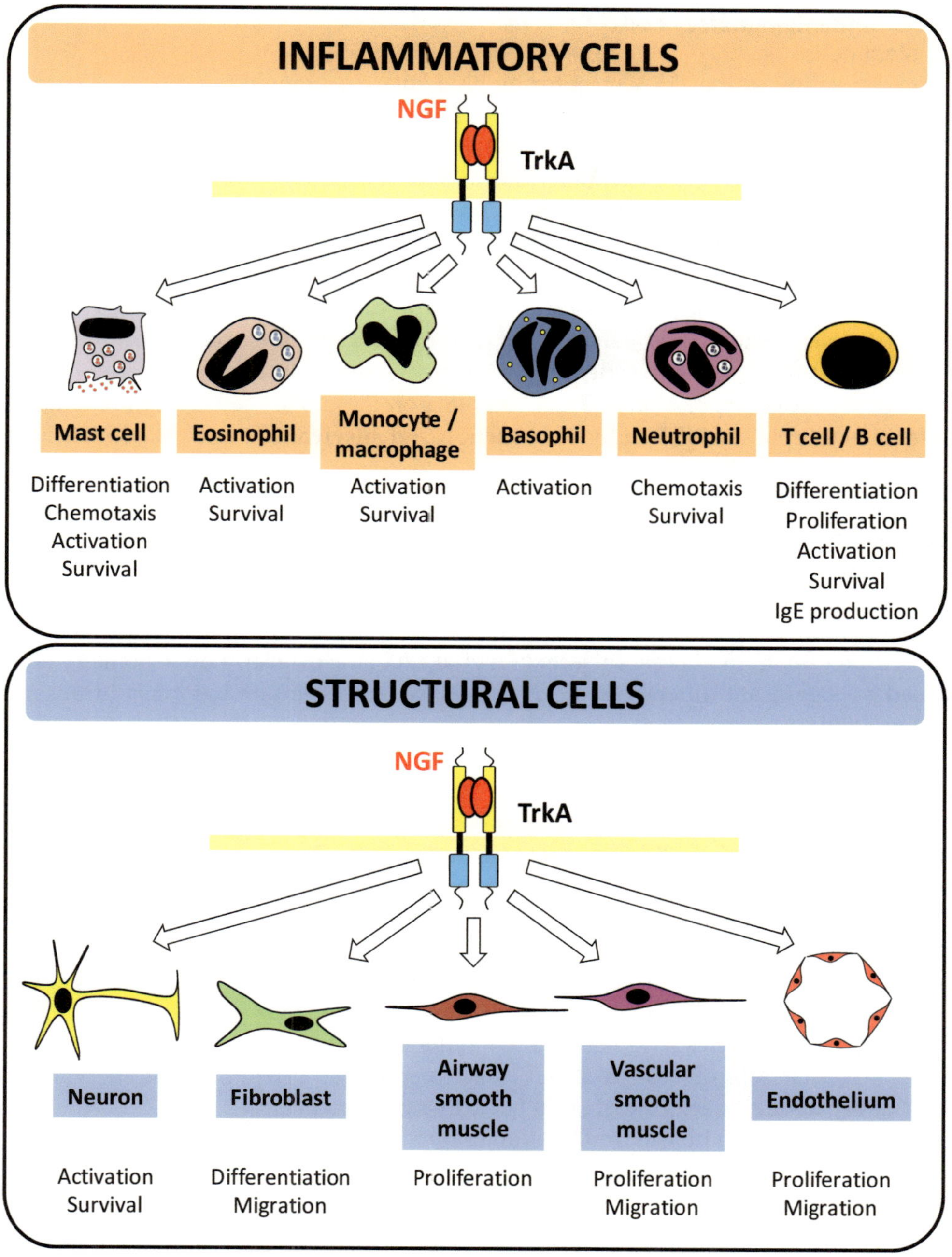

Fig. 2. NGF effects in the lung mediated via activation of the TrkA receptor

NGF-induced activation of the TrkA receptor participates to attraction and activation of inflammatory cells in the lung and may therefore contribute to lung inflammation. The TrkA receptor is also expressed on lung structural cells and participates to NGF-induced effects that may contribute to altered reactivity and remodelling processes existing in pulmonary inflammatory diseases.

4.1 TrkA and inflammatory cells

4.1.1 Mast cells

In vitro, activation of the TrkA receptor by NGF induces granule formation in immature mast cells and therefore contributes to their differentiation (Kim et al., 2008). In addition, NGF is a chemotactic factor for mast cells through both MAPK and PI3K signalling pathways following TrkA activation (Sawada et al., 2000). TrkA activation is also involved in NGF-induced degranulation of mast cells and mediators release such as for example chemokines (Ahamed et al., 2004), or serotonin (Kawamoto et al., 2002). Finally, NGF acts as a key factor to promote mast cell survival through TrkA-induced suppression of apoptosis (Kawamoto et al., 1995). *In vivo,* a correlation between NGF levels in bronchoalveolar lavage (BAL) fluids and the number of mast cells infiltrated in the bronchial mucosa has been evidenced in asthmatic patients after allergenic challenge (Kassel et al., 2001). Expression of TrkA receptors on these mast cells therefore suggests a role for this receptor in NGF-induced attraction and survival of these cells in the lung *in vivo* (Kassel et al., 2001).

4.1.2 Basophils

In vitro, NGF potentiates mediator release from human basophils as well as primes the cells to produce leukotriene C4, and these effects are TrkA-dependent (Burgi et al., 1996). NGF can also modulate IgE-mediated responses in human basophils, and these effects are enhanced on cells from allergic subjects (Sin et al., 2001). However, flow cytometry studies revealed no significant differences in TrkA receptor expression on basophils in this study (Sin et al., 2001).

4.1.3 T and B cells

Although various effects of NGF have been described on T lymphocytes, few studies have investigated the role of the TrkA receptor in these effects. Only one study by Ehrhard and co-workers clearly demonstrates involvement of the TrkA receptor in NGF-induced activation of T lymphocytes *in vitro* (Ehrhard et al., 1994). *In vivo,* NGF effects on T lymphocytes remain controversial, since two studies conducted in a mouse model of asthma failed to show NGF-related effects on T cells (Braun et al., 1998; Path et al., 2002). However, in a transgenic mouse tissue-specifically overexpressing NGF in the lung, increased numbers of T lymphocytes have been shown in the lung after allergenic challenge (Quarcoo et al., 2004). The role of NGF and its TrkA receptor on T lymphocytes in pulmonary inflammatory diseases needs therefore to be further clarified *in vivo.*

NGF has been shown to induce proliferation of B lymphocytes *in vitro,* and this effect occurs through activation of the TrkA receptor and its signalling pathways involving PLCγ, PI3K and MAPK (Melamed et al., 1996). NGF-induced activation of the TrkA receptor also participates to B cell survival through PI3K-dependent activation of PKC zeta (Kronfeld et al., 2002). *In vivo,* in mice lacking TrkA in non-neuronal tissues, all major immune system cell populations were present in normal numbers and distributions, excepted for B lymphocytes, demonstrating that endogenous NGF modulates B cell development through activation of the TrkA receptor (Coppola et al., 2004). Moreover, during allergic airway inflammation in the mouse *in vivo,* NGF contributes to B cell differentiation into plasma cells and activates the TrkA receptor to enhance plasma cell survival and production of immunoglobulins E (Abram et al., 2009).

4.1.4 Eosinophils

In vitro, eosinophil degranulation is promoted by NGF-induced activation of the TrkA receptor, inducing release of inflammatory mediators such as interleukin-4 (Noga et al., 2002). *In vitro* NGF treatment of eosinophils from patients with allergic bronchial asthma increases viability of these cells, and this effect is correlated to increased expression of the TrkA receptor on eosinophils (Nassenstein et al., 2003). In addition, coculture of lung eosinophils with airway epithelial cells resulted in enhanced epithelial neurotrophin production, as well as in prolonged survival of eosinophils (Hahn et al., 2006). Complete inhibition of eosinophil survival in the presence of the TrkA kinase inhibitor K252a confirmed the important role of the TrkA receptor in eosinophil survival (Hahn et al., 2006).

4.1.5 Monocytes / macrophages

NGF induces TrkA activation in monocytes *in vitro* to trigger a respiratory burst, the major component of monocyte cytotoxic activity (Ehrhard et al., 1993b). Activation of the TrkA receptor by NGF also promotes monocytes survival (la Sala et al., 2000). TrkA transactivation mechanisms with GPCR ligands, recently evidenced in monocytes, contribute to pro-inflammatory activities such as for example synthesis of reactive oxygen species (El Zein et al., 2007, 2010). Expression of the TrkA receptor was shown to decrease during *in vitro* differentiation of monocytes to macrophages, suggesting a maturation-dependent regulation of TrkA expression in these cells (Ehrhard et al., 1993b).
NGF was reported to activate macrophages *in vitro* in the process of inflammatory and immune actions, inducing phagocytosis, parasite killing, and production of inflammatory cytokines in a TrkA dependent-manner (Barouch et al., 2001; Susaki et al., 1996). *In vivo*, TrkA expression was reported on human alveolar macrophages (Ricci et al., 2004b; Ricci et al., 2000b), and the TrkA receptor and its binding protein SH2-Bβ participate to activation of alveolar macrophages *in vivo* in a guinea pig model of asthma (Li et al., 2009).

4.1.6 Neutrophils

In a murine model of rhinitis induced by toluene diisocyanate exposure, a massive increased number of neutrophils in the nasal mucosa correlates to increased levels of NGF (Wilfong & Dey, 2004 & 2005). Neutrophil infiltration was inhibited after *in vivo* pre-treatment with the TrkA kinase inhibitor K252a, thus showing the important role of the TrkA receptor on neutrophil attraction in the nasal mucosa (Wilfong & Dey, 2004).

4.2 TrkA and airway structural cells

A role for the TrkA receptor has been evidenced in NGF-induced effects on airway sensory nerves. In particular, NGF induces release of neuropeptides such as substance P by airway neurons, and this effect is TrkA-dependent (de Vries et al., 2006; Dinh et al., 2004). A similar effect has been reported in nasal sensory neurons (Wilfong & Dey, 2004). NGF induces proliferation of airway smooth muscle cells through activation of the TrkA receptor (Freund-Michel et al., 2006). We also showed that NGF multiple stimulation of these cells induce internalization and degradation of the TrkA receptor followed by upregulated re-synthesis of functional TrkA receptors and increased proliferative effect (Freund-Michel & Frossard, 2008b). In ongoing studies, we have recently found that NGF induces proliferation and migration of human pulmonary endothelial and vascular smooth muscle cells *in vitro*, and that these effects are inhibited by pre-treatment with the TrkA kinase inhibitor K252a, thus suggesting a role for the TrkA receptor in these NGF-mediated effects (Freund-Michel et al., 2009) (**Fig. 3**).

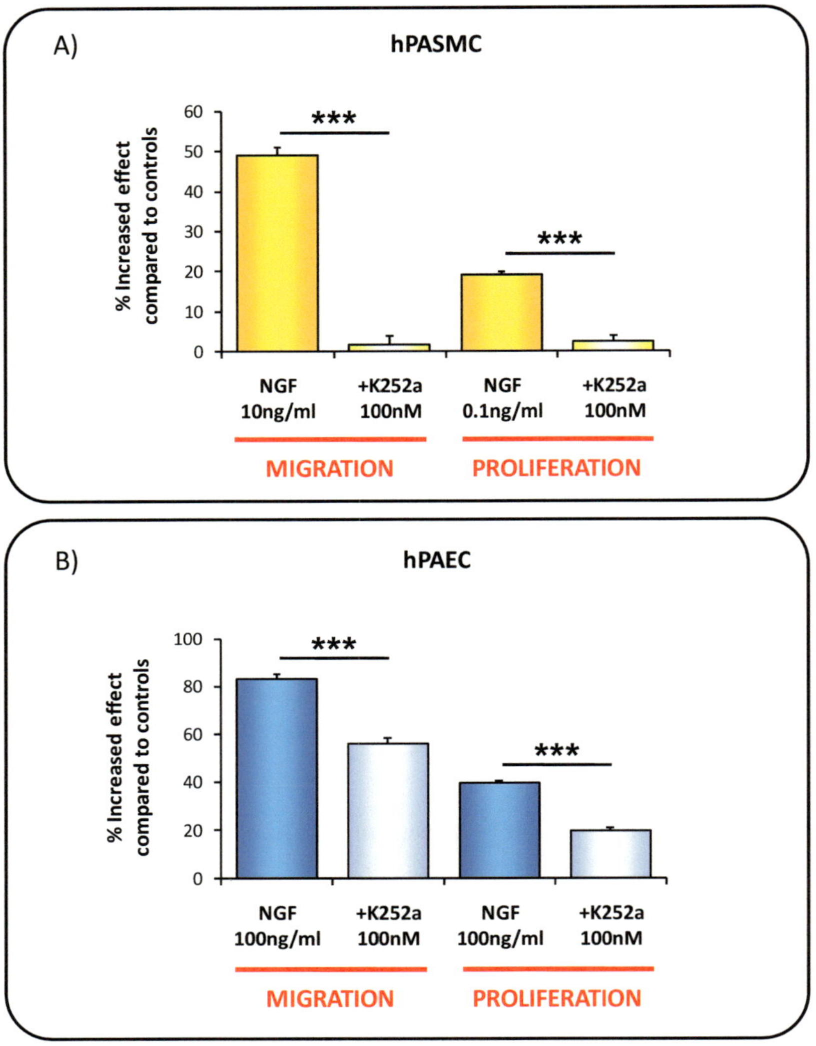

Fig. 3. Involvement of the TrkA receptor in NGF-induced effects on human pulmonary vascular cells.

Effect of NGF (0.1, 10 or 100 ng/ml) after 24h on A) human pulmonary arterial smooth muscle cells (hPASMC) or B) human pulmonary arterial endothelial cells (hPAEC) in primary culture. Cell proliferation was assessed by the BrdU technique and cell migration was evaluated by the Transwell assay. Data are presented as the maximal percentage of increased proliferation or migration compared to untreated control cells. NGF effect was evaluated in the presence or absence of the TrkA kinase inhibitor K252a (100nM, 30min pre-treatment followed by 24h concomitant treatment with NGF). ***: $P<0.001$ versus NGF alone with n=5 independent experiments performed in triplicates with cells from two different donors.

5. Role of the TrkA receptor in pulmonary inflammatory diseases

Circulating NGF levels are increased in human allergic and inflammatory diseases (Bonini et al., 1996). A local increase in NGF secretion has also been evidenced in BAL fluid from asthmatic patients (Kassel et al., 2001; Olgart Hoglund et al., 2002). In addition, our ongoing studies show that pulmonary arteries from patients suffering from pulmonary hypertension secondary to chronic obstructive pulmonary diseases (COPD) secrete more NGF than pulmonary arteries from control donors (Freund-Michel et al., 2010). Asthma and pulmonary hypertension share in common three major features occurring either in airways or in pulmonary arteries: inflammation, tissue hyperreactivity and remodelling (Barnes, 2010; Broide et al., 2011; Hassoun et al., 2009; Humbert, 2010). Several *in vitro* and *in vivo* studies suggest that NGF may play a role in these three physiopathological mechanisms, in particular through activation of the TrkA receptor (**Fig. 4**).

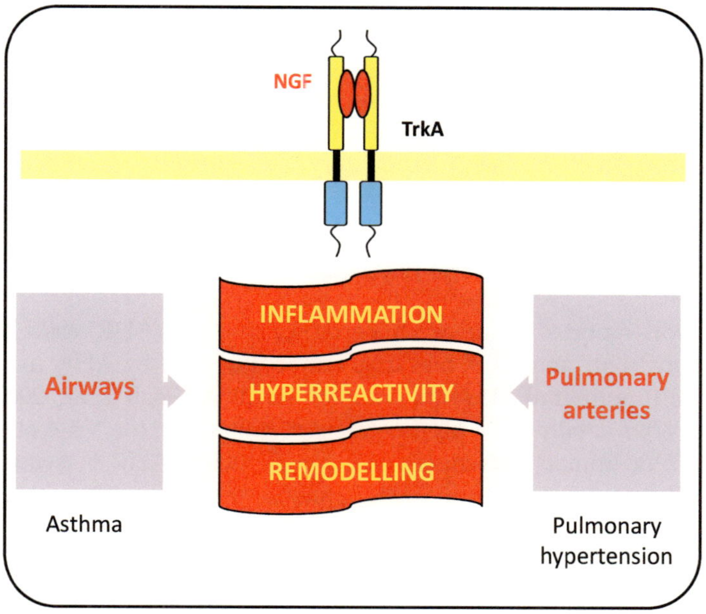

Fig. 4. Potential role of the TrkA receptor in asthma and pulmonary hypertension

In vitro and *in vivo* studies suggest that activation of the TrkA receptor by NGF contributes to inflammation as well as tissue remodelling and altered reactivity, three features occurring in particular in airways and in pulmonary arteries and playing a major role in the physiopathology of asthma and pulmonary hypertension.

5.1 NGF, TrkA and inflammation

5.1.1 Asthma

In a mouse model of asthma, NGF inhibition induced by blocking antibodies administered *in vivo* decreases airway inflammation (Braun et al., 1998; Path et al., 2002). On the contrary, allergen sensitization and challenge in a transgenic mouse tissue specifically overexpressing NGF in the lung displays greater airway inflammation (Path et al., 2002; Quarcoo et al., 2004). *In vivo* administration of a pan-Trk receptor decoy in a mouse model of asthma reduces interleukin-(IL-)4 and IL-5 cytokine levels (Nassenstein et al., 2006). Substance P is one of the neuropeptides released by airway sensory nerves that participates to neurogenic inflammation in asthma (Quarcoo et al., 2004). *In vivo* treatment with the TrkA kinase inhibitor K252a prevents the increase in substance P observed in a guinea pig model of asthma (de Vries et al., 2006). *In vivo* pre-treatment with TrkA blocking antibodies decreases IL-1β and IL-4 levels in the BAL fluid after allergen sensitization and challenge in the guinea pig (Li et al., 2009). Similar results are observed with TrkA blocking antibodies in a mouse model of asthma (Ni et al., 2010). Altogether, these results show a major role of NGF in airway inflammation through activation of its TrkA receptor.

5.1.2 Pulmonary hypertension

We recently showed that NGF stimulates secretion of inflammatory cytokines such as IL-1β and tumor necrosis factor-α from rat and human pulmonary arteries (Freund-Michel et al., 2010). Moreover, *in vivo* treatment with anti-NGF blocking antibodies in animal models of pulmonary hypertension prevents the increased secretion of these inflammatory cytokines from diseased pulmonary arteries (Freund-Michel et al., unpublished data). Contribution of the TrkA receptor in these mechanisms remains to be determined, but our preliminary data support a role for NGF in the inflammatory mechanisms associated to pulmonary hypertension.

5.2 NGF, TrkA and tissue hyperresponsiveness

5.2.1 Asthma

A role for NGF was reported in airway hyperresponsiveness (AHR) associated to asthma, since pre-treatment with anti-NGF blocking antibodies reduces AHR in various animal models of asthma (Braun et al., 1998; de Vries et al., 2006; Glaab et al., 2003). In addition, AHR is observed after *in vitro* NGF pre-treatment of guinea pig (de Vries et al., 2001), ferret (Wu & Dey, 2006) or human bronchi (Frossard et al., 2005). AHR is reduced *in vivo* after administration of a pan-Trk receptor decoy in a mouse model of asthma (Nassenstein et al., 2006), or of the TrkA kinase inhibitor K252a in a guinea pig model of asthma (de Vries et al., 2006), thus showing involvement of the TrkA receptor in NGF-induced AHR.

5.2.2 Pulmonary hypertension

In the systemic circulation, neurotrophins play a role in the control of vascular tone (Caporali & Emanueli, 2009), and a role for NGF has been suggested in systemic arterial hypertension (Sherer et al., 1998). Neurotrophins and their receptors are expressed on pulmonary arteries (Ricci et al., 2000a), and their expression is increased in the lung of spontaneously hypertensive rats (Ricci et al., 2004a). A role for neurotrophins in the control of the pulmonary arterial tone was recently proposed, through activation of the $p75^{NTR}$ receptor (Xu et al., 2008). BDNF and NT-3 induce relaxation of porcine pulmonary arterial rings, through activation of the endothelial nitric oxide synthase (Meuchel et al., 2011). Suppression of TrkB or TrkC expression via siRNA as well as functional blockade of $p75^{NTR}$ suggest a role of both Trk and $p75^{NTR}$ receptors in these effects (Meuchel et al., 2011). In our ongoing studies in rat or human pulmonary arteries, we show that NGF does not induce rat or human pulmonary arterial contraction or relaxation by itself. However, NGF pre-treatment induces pulmonary arterial hyperresponsiveness to contractile agents such as phenylephrine or prostaglandin F2α (Freund-Michel et al., 2010). Our preliminary data suggest that this effect may be due in part to activation of the TrkA receptors and increased intracellular calcium concentrations. These mechanisms are in accordance with the preliminary data recently described for BDNF and NT-3 by Prakash and co-workers (Prakash et al., 2010). Altogether, these results therefore suggest that neurotrophins, through activation of both Trk and $p75^{NTR}$ receptors, participate in both endothelial dysfunction and smooth muscle hyperreactivity observed in pulmonary hypertension.

5.3 NGF, TrkA and tissue remodelling

5.3.1 Asthma

Airway remodelling in asthma is characterized by a sub-epithelial fibrosis with an increased proliferation of fibroblasts and a thickening of the basement membrane, hypervascularisation, sensory hyperinnervation, oedema, and hypertrophy and hyperplasia of the smooth muscle layer (Bara et al., 2010). *In vitro*, NGF activates the TrkA receptor to induce migration of pulmonary fibroblasts (Kohyama et al., 2002) and regulation of extracellular matrix synthesis (Khan et al., 2002; Takahashi et al., 2000). These results therefore suggest a role for the TrkA receptor in NGF-induced airway sub-epithelial fibrosis *in vivo* (Hoyle et al., 1998). We also reported that NGF induces proliferation of the airway smooth muscle through activation of the TrkA receptor and may therefore participate to hyperplasia of the smooth muscle layer *in vivo* (Freund-Michel et al., 2006). Activation of the TrkA receptor by NGF also stimulates vascular cells from other origins than the lung to induce migration and proliferation of endothelial cells (Cantarella et al., 2002; Dolle et al., 2005; Lecht et al.,2010 ; Rahbek et al., 2005) as well as migration of vascular smooth muscle cells (Donovan et al., 1995; Kraemer et al., 1999). In addition, NGF stimulates angiogenesis *in vivo* through activation of the TrkA receptor (Cantarella et al., 2002; Caporali & Emanueli, 2009). NGF is also able to stimulate synthesis of angiogenic factors such as vascular endothelial growth factor (VEGF) from various cells through activation of its TrkA receptor (Nakamura et al., 2011). Altogether, these results suggest that activation of the TrkA receptor participates to NGF-mediated hypervascularisation in the lung (Hoyle et al., 1998).

5.3.2 Pulmonary hypertension

Vascular remodelling in pulmonary hypertension is characterized by increased proliferation, decreased apoptosis and increased migration of pulmonary vascular cells (Humbert et al., 2004). NGF-induced activation of the TrkA receptor contributes to migration and proliferation of vascular cells from other origins than the lung and stimulates angiogenesis (see paragraph above). Our recent results show that NGF induces proliferation and migration of pulmonary vascular cells through activation of the TrkA receptor (see paragraph 4.2 and Fig. 3) (Freund-Michel et al., 2010). Therefore, our findings support a role for NGF and its TrkA receptor in pulmonary vascular remodelling in this disease.

6. Therapeutic perspectives and conclusion

In regard of the different results presented in this review, NGF seems to play a major role in altered inflammatory, remodelling and reactivity processes occurring in pulmonary inflammatory diseases such as asthma or pulmonary hypertension. The TrkA receptor is involved in many NGF effects in the lung and targeting NGF or its TrkA receptor may be a new therapeutic perspective in these diseases.

Outside the lung, blockade of NGF is of therapeutic interest in other areas, in particular in pain therapy (Hefti et al., 2006). Humanized monoclonal antibodies against NGF or against TrkA, as well as small molecules acting as TrkA antagonists or as TrkA kinase inhibitors have been developed and are currently under investigation (Ma et al., 2010; Martin et al., 2011; McNamee et al., 2010; Ueda et al., 2010; Watson et al., 2008) **(Fig. 5)**. In particular, tanezumab, a recombinant humanized monoclonal antibody against NGF, has been recently tested in clinical trials in osteoarthritic pain and chronic lower back pain and demonstrated good efficacy (Cattaneo, 2010; Lane et al., 2010). Such strategies may be applied in the near future to target NGF or its receptors in pulmonary inflammatory diseases such as asthma or pulmonary hypertension in which NGF and its TrkA receptor play an important role.

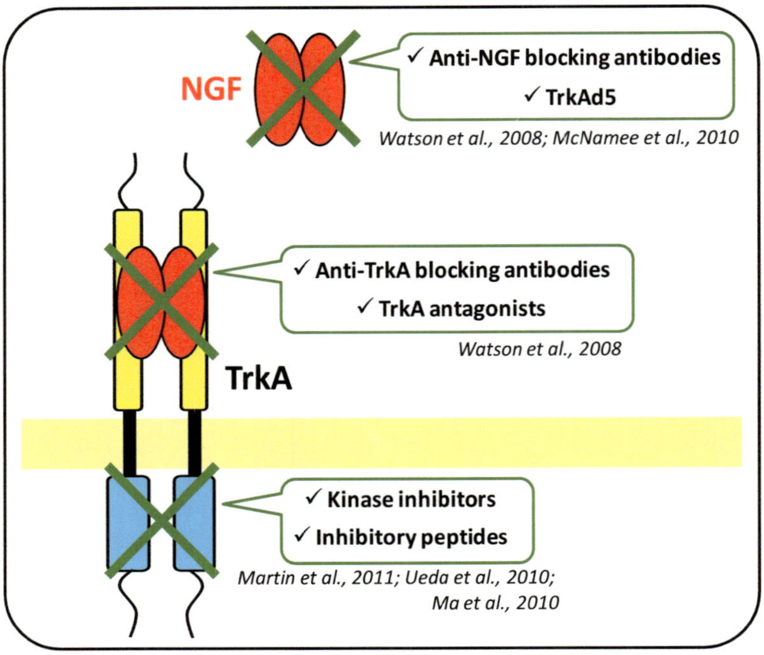

Fig. 5. Potential therapeutic strategies to target the TrkA receptor in pulmonary inflammatory diseases.
To trap circulating NGF and prevent its binding to the TrkA receptor, tools such as anti-NGF blocking antibodies or soluble chimeric TrkA receptors have been developed. Other tools have been developed to target the TrkA receptor itself, either by blocking NGF binding to its extracellular part with antagonists or anti-TrkA antibodies, or by blocking TrkA kinase activity with kinase inhibitors.

7. References

Abram, M., Wegmann, M., Fokuhl, V., Sonar, S., Luger, E.O., Kerzel, S., Radbruch, A., Renz, H. & Zemlin, M. (2009). Nerve growth factor and neurotrophin-3 mediate survival of pulmonary plasma cells during the allergic airway inflammation. *Journal of Immunology*, Vol.182, No.8, pp. 4705-4712, ISSN 0022-1767.

Ahamed, J., Venkatesha, R.T., Thangam, E.B. & Ali, H. (2004). C3a enhances nerve growth factor-induced NFAT activation and chemokine production in a human mast cell line, HMC-1. *Journal of Immunology*, Vol.172, No.11, pp. 6961-6968, ISSN 0022-1767.

Antonelli, A., Lapucci, G., Vigneti, E., Bonini, S. & Aloe, L. (2005). Human lung fibroblast response to NGF, IL-1beta, and dexamethsone. *Lung*, Vol.183, No.5, pp. 337-351, ISSN 0341-2040.

Ashcroft, M., Stephens, R.M., Hallberg, B., Downward, J. & Kaplan, D.R. (1999). The selective and inducible activation of endogenous PI 3-kinase in PC12 cells results in efficient NGF-mediated survival but defective neurite outgrowth. *Oncogene*, Vol.18, No.32, pp. 4586-4597, ISSN 0950-9232.

Bara, I., Ozier, A., Tunon de Lara, J.M., Marthan, R. & Berger, P. (2010). Pathophysiology of bronchial smooth muscle remodelling in asthma. *European Respiratory Journal*, Vol.36, No.5, pp. 1174-1184, ISSN 0903-1936.

Barbacid, M., Lamballe, F., Pulido, D. & Klein, R. (1991). The trk family of tyrosine protein kinase receptors. *Biochimica et Biophysica Acta-Cancer Reviews*, Vol.1072, No.2-3, pp. 115-127, ISSN 1879-2561.

Barker, P.A., Lomen-Hoerth, C., Gensch, E.M., Meakin, S.O., Glass, D.J. & Shooter, E.M. (1993). Tissue-specific alternative splicing generates two isoforms of the trkA receptor. *Journal of Biological Chemistry*, Vol.268, No.20, pp. 15150-15157, ISSN 0021-9258.

Barnes, P.J. (2010). New therapies for asthma: is there any progress? *Trends in Pharmacological Sciences*, Vol.31, No.7, pp. 335-343, ISSN 0165-6147.

Barouch, R., Kazimirsky, G., Appel, E. & Brodie, C. (2001). Nerve growth factor regulates TNF-alpha production in mouse macrophages via MAP kinase activation. *Journal of Leukocyte Biology*, Vol.69, No.6, pp. 1019-1026, ISSN 0741-5400.

Bonini, S., Lambiase, A., Bonini, S., Angelucci, F., Magrini, L., Manni, L. & Aloe, L. (1996). Circulating nerve growth factor levels are increased in humans with allergic diseases and asthma. *Proceedings of the National Academy of Sciences of the United States of America*, Vol.93, No.20, pp. 10955-10960, ISSN 0027-8424.

Braun, A., Appel, E., Baruch, R., Herz, U., Botchkarev, V., Paus, R., Brodie, C. & Renz, H. (1998). Role of nerve growth factor in a mouse model of allergic airway inflammation and asthma. *European Journal of Immunology*, Vol.28, No.10, pp. 3240-3251, ISSN 1521-4141.

Broide, D.H., Finkelman, F., Bochner, B.S. & Rothenberg, M.E. (2011). Advances in mechanisms of asthma, allergy, and immunology in 2010. *Journal of Allergy and Clinical Immunology*, Vol.127, No.3, pp. 689-695, ISSN 0105-4538.

Burgi, B., Otten, U.H., Ochensberger, B., Rihs, S., Heese, K., Ehrhard, P.B., Ibanez, C.F. & Dahinden, C.A. (1996). Basophil priming by neurotrophic factors. Activation through the trk receptor. *Journal of Immunology*, Vol.157, No.12, pp. 5582-5588, ISSN 0022-1767.

Cabrera, N., Diaz-Rodriguez, E., Becker, E., Martin-Zanca, D. & Pandiella, A. (1996). TrkA receptor ectodomain cleavage generates a tyrosine-phosphorylated cell-associated fragment. *Journal of Cell Biology*, Vol.132, No.3, pp. 427-436, ISSN 0021-9525.

Cantarella, G., Lempereur, L., Presta, M., Ribatti, D., Lombardo, G., Lazarovici, P., Zappala, G., Pafumi, C. & Bernardini, R. (2002). Nerve growth factor-endothelial cell interaction leads to angiogenesis in vitro and in vivo. *FASEB Journal*, Vol.16, No.10, pp. 1307-1309, ISSN 0892-6638.

Caporali, A. & Emanueli, C. (2009). Cardiovascular actions of neurotrophins. *Physiological Reviews*, Vol.89, No.1, pp. 279-308, ISSN 0031-9333.

Cattaneo, A. (2010). Tanezumab, a recombinant humanized mAb against nerve growth factor for the treatment of acute and chronic pain. *Current Opinion in Molecular Therapeutics*, Vol.12, No.1, pp. 94-106, ISSN 1464-8431.

Chao, M.V. (2003). Neurotrophins and their receptors: a convergence point for many signalling pathways. *Nature Reviews. Neuroscience*, Vol.4, No.4, pp. 299-309, ISSN 1471-0048.

Chen, Z.Y., Ieraci, A., Tanowitz, M. & Lee, F.S. (2005). A novel endocytic recycling signal distinguishes biological responses of Trk neurotrophin receptors. *Molecular Biology of the Cell*, Vol.16, No.12, pp. 5761-5772, ISSN 1059-1524.

Clary, D.O. & Reichardt, L.F. (1994). An alternatively spliced form of the nerve growth factor receptor TrkA confers an enhanced response to neurotrophin 3. *Proceedings of the National Academy of Sciences of the United States of America*, Vol.91, No.23, pp. 11133-11137, ISSN 0027-8424.

Coppola, V., Barrick, C.A., Southon, E.A., Celeste, A., Wang, K., Chen, B., Haddad el, B., Yin, J., Nussenzweig, A., Subramaniam, A. & Tessarollo, L. (2004). Ablation of TrkA function in the immune system causes B cell abnormalities. *Development*, Vol.131, No.20, pp. 5185-5195, ISSN 1011-6370.

Dagnell, C., Kemi, C., Klominek, J., Eriksson, P., Skold, C.M., Eklund, A., Grunewald, J. & Olgart Hoglund, C. (2007). Effects of neurotrophins on human bronchial smooth muscle cell migration and matrix metalloproteinase-9 secretion. *Translational Research*, Vol.150, No.5, pp. 303-310, ISSN 1931-5244.

de Vries, A., Engels, F., Henricks, P.A., Leusink-Muis, T., McGregor, G.P., Braun, A., Groneberg, D.A., Dessing, M.C., Nijkamp, F.P. & Fischer, A. (2006). Airway hyper-responsiveness in allergic asthma in guinea-pigs is mediated by nerve growth factor via the induction of substance P: a potential role for trkA. *Clinical and Experimental Allergy*, Vol.36, No.9, pp. 1192-1200, ISSN 0954-7894.

de Vries, A., van Rijnsoever, C., Engels, F., Henricks, P.A. & Nijkamp, F.P. (2001). The role of sensory nerve endings in nerve growth factor-induced airway hyperresponsiveness to histamine in guinea-pigs. *British Journal of Pharmacology*, Vol.134, No.4, pp. 771-776, ISSN 0007-1188.

Delcroix, J.D., Valletta, J.S., Wu, C., Hunt, S.J., Kowal, A.S. & Mobley, W.C. (2003). NGF signaling in sensory neurons: evidence that early endosomes carry NGF retrograde signals. *Neuron*, Vol.39, No.1, pp. 69-84, ISSN 0896-6273.

Diaz-Rodriguez, E., Cabrera, N., Esparis-Ogando, A., Montero, J.C. & Pandiella, A. (1999). Cleavage of the TrkA neurotrophin receptor by multiple metalloproteases generates signalling-competent truncated forms. *European Journal of Neuroscience*, Vol.11, No.4, pp. 1421-1430, ISSN 1460-9568.

Dinh, Q.T., Groneberg, D.A., Peiser, C., Springer, J., Joachim, R.A., Arck, P.C., Klapp, B.F. & Fischer, A. (2004). Nerve growth factor-induced substance P in capsaicin-insensitive vagal neurons innervating the lower mouse airway. *Clinical and Experimental Allergy*, Vol.34, No.9, pp. 1474-1479, ISSN 0954-7894.

Dolle, J.P., Rezvan, A., Allen, F.D., Lazarovici, P. & Lelkes, P.I. (2005). Nerve growth factor-induced migration of endothelial cells. *Journal of Pharmacology and Experimental Therapeutics*, Vol.315, No.3, pp. 1220-1227, ISSN 0022-3565.

Donovan, M.J., Miranda, R.C., Kraemer, R., McCaffrey, T.A., Tessarollo, L., Mahadeo, D., Sharif, S., Kaplan, D.R., Tsoulfas, P., Parada, L. & et al. (1995). Neurotrophin and neurotrophin receptors in vascular smooth muscle cells. Regulation of expression in response to injury. *American Journal of Pathology*, Vol.147, No.2, pp. 309-324, ISSN 0002-9440.

Ehrhard, P.B., Erb, P., Graumann, U. & Otten, U. (1993a). Expression of nerve growth factor and nerve growth factor receptor tyrosine kinase Trk in activated CD4-positive T-cell clones. *Proceedings of the National Academy of Sciences of the United States of America*, Vol.90, No.23, pp. 10984-10988, ISSN 0027-8424.

Ehrhard, P.B., Erb, P., Graumann, U., Schmutz, B. & Otten, U. (1994). Expression of functional trk tyrosine kinase receptors after T cell activation. *Journal of Immunology*, Vol.152, No.6, pp. 2705-2709, ISSN 0022-1767.

Ehrhard, P.B., Ganter, U., Stalder, A., Bauer, J. & Otten, U. (1993b). Expression of functional trk protooncogene in human monocytes. *Proceedings of the National Academy of Sciences of the United States of America*, Vol.90, No.12, pp. 5423-5427, ISSN 0027-8424.

El Zein, N., Badran, B.M. & Sariban, E. (2007). The neuropeptide pituitary adenylate cyclase activating protein stimulates human monocytes by transactivation of the Trk/NGF pathway. *Cellular Signalling*, Vol.19, No.1, pp. 152-162, ISSN 0898-6568.

El Zein, N., D'Hondt, S. & Sariban, E. (2010). Crosstalks between the receptors tyrosine kinase EGFR and TrkA and the GPCR, FPR, in human monocytes are essential for receptors-mediated cell activation. *Cellular Signalling*, Vol.22, No.10, pp. 1437-1447, ISSN 0898-6568.

Farina, A.R., Tacconelli, A., Cappabianca, L., Cea, G., Panella, S., Chioda, A., Romanelli, A., Pedone, C., Gulino, A. & Mackay, A.R. (2009). The alternative TrkAIII splice variant targets the centrosome and promotes genetic instability. *Molecular and Cellular Biology*, Vol.29, No.17, pp. 4812-4830, ISSN 0270-7306.

Fox, A.J., Patel, H.J., Barnes, P.J. & Belvisi, M.G. (2001). Release of nerve growth factor by human pulmonary epithelial cells: role in airway inflammatory diseases. *European Journal of Pharmacology*, Vol.424, No.2, pp. 159-162, ISSN 0014-2999.

Freund-Michel, V., Bertrand, C. & Frossard, N. (2006). TrkA signalling pathways in human airway smooth muscle cell proliferation. *Cellular Signalling*, Vol.18, No.5, pp. 621-627, ISSN 0898-6568.

Freund-Michel, V. & Frossard, N. (2008a). The nerve growth factor and its receptors in airway inflammatory diseases. *Pharmacology and Therapeutics*, Vol.117, No.1, pp. 52-76, ISSN 0163-7258.

Freund-Michel, V. & Frossard, N. (2008b). Overexpression of functional TrkA receptors after internalization in human airway smooth muscle cells. *Biochimica et Biophysica Acta, Molecular and Cellular Research*, Vol.1783, No.10, pp. 1964-1971, ISSN 0167-4889.

Freund-Michel, V., Salagierska, M., Dubois, M., Guibert, C., Courtois, A., Marthan, R. & Muller, B. (2009). Potential role of the nerve growth factor NGF in pulmonary hypertension. European Respiratory Society annual congress, *European Respiratory Journal*, Vol.34, Suppl.53, A4330, ISSN 0903-1936, Vienna, Austria, September 2009.

Freund-Michel, V., Laroumanie, F., Salagierska, M., Dubois, M., Courtois, A., Autissier, M., Guibert, C., Savineau, J.P., Marthan, R. & Muller B. (2010). Nerve growth factor expression and function in pulmonary arterial hypertension. European Respiratory Society annual congress, *European Respiratory Journal*, Vol.36, Suppl.54, P1080, ISSN 0903-1936, Barcelona, Spain, September 2010.

Freund, V., Pons, F., Joly, V., Mathieu, E., Martinet, N. & Frossard, N. (2002). Upregulation of nerve growth factor expression by human airway smooth muscle cells in inflammatory conditions. *European Respiratory Journal*, Vol.20, No.2, pp. 458-463, ISSN 0903-1936.

Friedman, W.J. & Greene, L.A. (1999). Neurotrophin signaling via Trks and p75. *Experimental Cell Research*, Vol.253, No.1, pp. 131-142, ISSN 0014-4827.

Frossard, N., Naline, E., Olgart Hoglund, C., Georges, O. & Advenier, C. (2005). Nerve growth factor is released by IL-1beta and induces hyperresponsiveness of the human isolated bronchus. *European Respiratory Journal*, Vol.26, No.1, pp. 15-20, ISSN 0903-1936.

Georgieva, M.V., de Pablo, Y., Sanchis, D., Comella, J.X. & Llovera, M. (2011). Ubiquitination of TrkA by Nedd4-2 regulates receptor lysosomal targeting and mediates receptor signaling. *Journal of Neurochemistry*, Vol.117, No.3, pp. 479-493, ISSN 0022-3042.

Glaab, T., Hoymann, H.G., Hecht, M., Korolewitz, R., Tschernig, T., Hohlfeld, J.M., Krug, N. & Braun, A. (2003). Effect of anti-nerve growth factor on early and late airway responses in allergic rats. *Allergy*, Vol.58, No.9, pp. 900-904, ISSN 0105-4538.

Greco, A., Miranda, C., Pagliardini, S., Fusetti, L., Bongarzone, I. & Pierotti, M.A. (1997). Chromosome 1 rearrangements involving the genes TPR and NTRK1 produce structurally different thyroid-specific TRK oncogenes. *Genes, Chromosomes and Cancer*, Vol.19, No.2, pp. 112-123, ISSN 1098-2264.

Hahn, C., Islamian, A.P., Renz, H. & Nockher, W.A. (2006). Airway epithelial cells produce neurotrophins and promote the survival of eosinophils during allergic airway inflammation. *Journal of Allergy and Clinical Immunology*, Vol.117, No.4, pp. 787-794, ISSN 0105-4538.

Hassoun, P.M., Mouthon, L., Barbera, J.A., Eddahibi, S., Flores, S.C., Grimminger, F., Jones, P.L., Maitland, M.L., Michelakis, E.D., Morrell, N.W., Newman, J.H., Rabinovitch, M., Schermuly, R., Stenmark, K.R., Voelkel, N.F., Yuan, J.X. & Humbert, M. (2009). Inflammation, growth factors, and pulmonary vascular remodeling. *Journal of the American College of Cardiology*, Vol.54, No.1 Suppl, pp. S10-19, ISSN 0735-1097.

Heerssen, H.M. & Segal, R.A. (2002). Location, location, location: a spatial view of neurotrophin signal transduction. *Trends in Neurosciences*, Vol.25, No.3, pp. 160-165, ISSN 0166-2236.

Hefti, F.F., Rosenthal, A., Walicke, P.A., Wyatt, S., Vergara, G., Shelton, D.L. & Davies, A.M. (2006). Novel class of pain drugs based on antagonism of NGF. *Trends in Pharmacological Sciences*, Vol.27, No.2, pp. 85-91, ISSN 0165-6147.

Hikawa, S., Kobayashi, H., Hikawa, N., Kusakabe, T., Hiruma, H., Takenaka, T., Tomita, T. & Kawakami, T. (2002). Expression of neurotrophins and their receptors in peripheral lung cells of mice. *Histochemistry and Cell Biology*, Vol.118, No.1, pp. 51-58, ISSN 0948-6143.

Holgado-Madruga, M., Moscatello, D.K., Emlet, D.R., Dieterich, R. & Wong, A.J. (1997). Grb2-associated binder-1 mediates phosphatidylinositol 3-kinase activation and the promotion of cell survival by nerve growth factor. *Proceedings of the National Academy of Sciences of the United States of America*, Vol.94, No.23, pp. 12419-12424, ISSN 0027-8424.

Hoyle, G.W., Graham, R.M., Finkelstein, J.B., Nguyen, K.P., Gozal, D. & Friedman, M. (1998). Hyperinnervation of the airways in transgenic mice overexpressing nerve growth factor. *American Journal of Respiratory Cell and Molecular Biology*, Vol.18, No.2, pp. 149-157, ISSN 1044-1549.

Humbert, M. (2010). Pulmonary arterial hypertension and chronic thromboembolic pulmonary hypertension: pathophysiology. *European Respiratory Review*, Vol.19, No.115, pp. 59-63, ISSN 0905-9180.

Humbert, M., Morrell, N.W., Archer, S.L., Stenmark, K.R., MacLean, M.R., Lang, I.M., Christman, B.W., Weir, E.K., Eickelberg, O., Voelkel, N.F. & Rabinovitch, M. (2004). Cellular and molecular pathobiology of pulmonary arterial hypertension. *Journal of the American College of Cardiology*, Vol.43, No.12 Suppl S, pp. 13S-24S, ISSN 0735-1097.

Indo, Y., Mardy, S., Tsuruta, M., Karim, M.A. & Matsuda, I. (1997). Structure and organization of the human TRKA gene encoding a high affinity receptor for nerve growth factor. *Japanese Journal of Human Genetics*, Vol.42, No.2, pp. 343-351, ISSN 0916-8478.

Jullien, J., Guili, V., Reichardt, L.F. & Rudkin, B.B. (2002). Molecular kinetics of nerve growth factor receptor trafficking and activation. *Journal of Biological Chemistry*, Vol.277, No.41, pp. 38700-38708, ISSN 0021-9258.

Kaplan, D.R., Hempstead, B.L., Martin-Zanca, D., Chao, M.V. & Parada, L.F. (1991a). The trk proto-oncogene product: a signal transducing receptor for nerve growth factor. *Science*, Vol.252, No.5005, pp. 554-558, ISSN 0036-8075.

Kaplan, D.R., Martin-Zanca, D. & Parada, L.F. (1991b). Tyrosine phosphorylation and tyrosine kinase activity of the trk proto-oncogene product induced by NGF. *Nature*, Vol.350, No.6314, pp. 158-160, ISSN 0028-0836.

Kassel, O., de Blay, F., Duvernelle, C., Olgart, C., Israel-Biet, D., Krieger, P., Moreau, L., Muller, C., Pauli, G. & Frossard, N. (2001). Local increase in the number of mast cells and expression of nerve growth factor in the bronchus of asthmatic patients after repeated inhalation of allergen at low-dose. *Clinical and Experimental Allergy*, Vol.31, No.9, pp. 1432-1440, ISSN 0954-7894.

Kawamoto, K., Aoki, J., Tanaka, A., Itakura, A., Hosono, H., Arai, H., Kiso, Y. & Matsuda, H. (2002). Nerve growth factor activates mast cells through the collaborative interaction with lysophosphatidylserine expressed on the membrane surface of activated platelets. *Journal of Immunology*, Vol.168, No.12, pp. 6412-6419, ISSN 0022-1767.

Kawamoto, K., Okada, T., Kannan, Y., Ushio, H., Matsumoto, M. & Matsuda, H. (1995). Nerve growth factor prevents apoptosis of rat peritoneal mast cells through the trk proto-oncogene receptor. *Blood*, Vol.86, No.12, pp. 4638-4644, ISSN 0006-4971.

Khan, K.M., Falcone, D.J. & Kraemer, R. (2002). Nerve growth factor activation of Erk-1 and Erk-2 induces matrix metalloproteinase-9 expression in vascular smooth muscle cells. *Journal of Biological Chemistry*, Vol.277, No.3, pp. 2353-2359, ISSN 0021-9258.

Kim, J.Y., Kim, D.Y. & Ro, J.Y. (2008). Granule formation in NGF-cultured mast cells is associated with expressions of pyruvate kinase type M2 and annexin I proteins. *International Archives of Allergy and Immunology*, Vol.146, No.4, pp. 287-297, ISSN 1018-2438.

Kita, Y., Kimura, K.D., Kobayashi, M., Ihara, S., Kaibuchi, K., Kuroda, S., Ui, M., Iba, H., Konishi, H., Kikkawa, U., Nagata, S. & Fukui, Y. (1998). Microinjection of activated phosphatidylinositol-3 kinase induces process outgrowth in rat PC12 cells through the Rac-JNK signal transduction pathway. *Journal of Cell Science*, Vol.111 (Pt 7), pp. 907-915, ISSN 0021-9533.

Klein, R., Jing, S.Q., Nanduri, V., O'Rourke, E. & Barbacid, M. (1991). The trk proto-oncogene encodes a receptor for nerve growth factor. *Cell*, Vol.65, No.1, pp. 189-197, ISSN 0092-8674.

Kohyama, T., Liu, X., Wen, F.Q., Kobayashi, T., Abe, S., Ertl, R. & Rennard, S.I. (2002). Nerve growth factor stimulates fibronectin-induced fibroblast migration. *Journal of Laboratory and Clinical Medicine*, Vol.140, No.5, pp. 329-335, ISSN 0022-2143.

Korhonen, J.M., Said, F.A., Wong, A.J. & Kaplan, D.R. (1999). Gab1 mediates neurite outgrowth, DNA synthesis, and survival in PC12 cells. *Journal of Biological Chemistry*, Vol.274, No.52, pp. 37307-37314, ISSN 0021-9258.

Kraemer, R., Nguyen, H., March, K.L. & Hempstead, B. (1999). NGF activates similar intracellular signaling pathways in vascular smooth muscle cells as PDGF-BB but elicits different biological responses. *Arteriosclerosis, Thrombosis, and Vascular Biology*, Vol.19, No.4, pp. 1041-1050, ISSN 1079-5642.

Kronfeld, I., Kazimirsky, G., Gelfand, E.W. & Brodie, C. (2002). NGF rescues human B lymphocytes from anti-IgM induced apoptosis by activation of PKCzeta. *European Journal of Immunology*, Vol.32, No.1, pp. 136-143, ISSN 1521-4141.

Kuruvilla, R., Ye, H. & Ginty, D.D. (2000). Spatially and functionally distinct roles of the PI3-K effector pathway during NGF signaling in sympathetic neurons. *Neuron*, Vol.27, No.3, pp. 499-512, ISSN 0896-6273.

la Sala, A., Corinti, S., Federici, M., Saragovi, H.U. & Girolomoni, G. (2000). Ligand activation of nerve growth factor receptor TrkA protects monocytes from apoptosis. *Journal of Leukocyte Biology*, Vol.68, No.1, pp. 104-110, ISSN 0741-5400.

Lambiase, A., Bracci-Laudiero, L., Bonini, S., Bonini, S., Starace, G., D'Elios, M.M., De Carli, M. & Aloe, L. (1997). Human CD4+ T cell clones produce and release nerve growth factor and express high-affinity nerve growth factor receptors. *Journal of Allergy and Clinical Immunology*, Vol.100, No.3, pp. 408-414, ISSN 0105-4538.

Lane, N.E., Schnitzer, T.J., Birbara, C.A., Mokhtarani, M., Shelton, D.L., Smith, M.D. & Brown, M.T. (2010). Tanezumab for the treatment of pain from osteoarthritis of the knee. *New England Journal of Medicine*, Vol.363, No.16, pp. 1521-1531, ISSN 0028-4793.

Lecht, S., Arien-Zakay, H., Wagenstein, Y., Inoue, S., Marcinkiewicz, C., Lelkes, P.I. & Lazarovici, P. (2010) Transient signaling of Erk1/2, Akt and PLCgamma induced by nerve growth factor in brain capillary endothelial cells. *Vascular Pharmacology*, Vol.53, No.3-4, pp. 107-114, ISSN 1537-1891.

Lee, F.S. & Chao, M.V. (2001). Activation of Trk neurotrophin receptors in the absence of neurotrophins. *Proceedings of the National Academy of Sciences of the United States of America*, Vol.98, No.6, pp. 3555-3560, ISSN 0027-8424.

Lee, F.S., Rajagopal, R. & Chao, M.V. (2002a). Distinctive features of Trk neurotrophin receptor transactivation by G protein-coupled receptors. *Cytokine and Growth Factor Reviews*, Vol.13, No.1, pp. 11-17, ISSN 1359-6101.

Lee, F.S., Rajagopal, R., Kim, A.H., Chang, P.C. & Chao, M.V. (2002b). Activation of Trk neurotrophin receptor signaling by pituitary adenylate cyclase-activating polypeptides. *Journal of Biological Chemistry*, Vol.277, No.11, pp. 9096-9102, ISSN 0021-9258.

Leon, A., Buriani, A., Dal Toso, R., Fabris, M., Romanello, S., Aloe, L. & Levi-Montalcini, R. (1994). Mast cells synthesize, store, and release nerve growth factor. *Proceedings of the National Academy of Sciences of the United States of America*, Vol.91, No.9, pp. 3739-3743, ISSN 0027-8424.

Levi-Montalcini, R., Dal Toso, R., della Valle, F., Skaper, S.D. & Leon, A. (1995). Update of the NGF saga. *Journal of the Neurological Sciences*, Vol.130, No.2, pp. 119-127, ISSN 0022-510X.

Levi-Montalcini, R. & Hamburger, V. (1951). Selective growth stimulating effects of mouse sarcoma on the sensory and sympathetic nervous system of the chick embryo. *Journal of Experimental Zoology*, Vol.116, No.2, pp. 321-361, ISSN 0022-104X.

Li, L., Kong, L., Fang, X., Jiang, C., Wang, Y., Zhong, Z., Sun, Q., Gu, G., Zheng, D., Meng, R. & Kang, J. (2009). SH2-B beta expression in alveolar macrophages in BAL fluid of asthmatic guinea pigs and its role in NGF-TrkA-mediated asthma. *Respirology*, Vol.14, No.1, pp. 60-68, 1323-7799.

Lomen-Hoerth, C. & Shooter, E.M. (1995). Widespread neurotrophin receptor expression in the immune system and other nonneuronal rat tissues. *Journal of Neurochemistry*, Vol.64, No.4, pp. 1780-1789, ISSN 0022-3042.

Ma, W.Y., Murata, E., Ueda, K., Kuroda, Y., Cao, M.H., Abe, M., Shigemi, K. & Hirose, M. (2010). A synthetic cell-penetrating peptide antagonizing TrkA function suppresses neuropathic pain in mice. *Journal of Pharmacological Sciences*, Vol.114, No.1, pp. 79-84, ISSN 0022-3549.

Martin-Zanca, D., Mitra, G., Long, L.K. & Barbacid, M. (1986). Molecular characterization of the human trk oncogene. *Cold Spring Harbor Symposia on Quantitative Biology*, Vol.51 Pt 2, pp. 983-992, ISSN 0091-7451.

Martin, K.J., Shpiro, N., Traynor, R., Elliott, M. & Arthur, J.S. (2011). Comparison of the specificity of Trk inhibitors in recombinant and neuronal assays. *Neuropharmacology*, Vol.61, No.1-2, pp. 148-155, ISSN 1570-159X.

McNamee, K.E., Burleigh, A., Gompels, L.L., Feldmann, M., Allen, S.J., Williams, R.O., Dawbarn, D., Vincent, T.L. & Inglis, J.J. (2010). Treatment of murine osteoarthritis with TrkAd5 reveals a pivotal role for nerve growth factor in non-inflammatory joint pain. *Pain*, Vol.149, No.2, pp. 386-392, ISSN 0304-3959.

Meakin, S.O. & Shooter, E.M. (1992). The nerve growth factor family of receptors. *Trends in Neurosciences*, Vol.15, No.9, pp. 323-331, ISSN 0166-2236.

Melamed, I., Kelleher, C.A., Franklin, R.A., Brodie, C., Hempstead, B., Kaplan, D. & Gelfand, E.W. (1996). Nerve growth factor signal transduction in human B lymphocytes is mediated by gp140trk. *European Journal of Immunology*, Vol.26, No.9, pp. 1985-1992, ISSN 1521-4141.

Metsis, M. (2001). Genes for neurotrophic factors and their receptors: structure and regulation. *Cellular and Molecular Life Sciences*, Vol.58, No.8, pp. 1014-1020, ISSN 1420-682X.

Meuchel, L.W., Thompson, M.A., Cassivi, S.D., Pabelick, C.M. & Prakash, Y.S. (2011). Neurotrophins induce nitric oxide generation in human pulmonary artery endothelial cells. *Cardiovascular Research*, 2011 May 18, [Epub ahead of print], ISSN 0008-6363.

Micera, A., Vigneti, E., Pickholtz, D., Reich, R., Pappo, O., Bonini, S., Maquart, F.X., Aloe, L. & Levi-Schaffer, F. (2001). Nerve growth factor displays stimulatory effects on human skin and lung fibroblasts, demonstrating a direct role for this factor in tissue repair. *Proceedings of the National Academy of Sciences of the United States of America*, Vol.98, No.11, pp. 6162-6167, ISSN 0027-8424.

Mitra, G. (1991). Mutational analysis of conserved residues in the tyrosine kinase domain of the human trk oncogene. *Oncogene*, Vol.6, No.12, pp. 2237-2241, ISSN 0950-9232.

Nakamura, K., Tan, F., Li, Z. & Thiele, C.J. (2011). NGF activation of TrkA induces vascular endothelial growth factor expression via induction of hypoxia-inducible factor-1alpha. *Molecular and Cellular Neurosciences*, Vol.46, No.2, pp. 498-506, ISSN 1044-7431.

Nassenstein, C., Braun, A., Erpenbeck, V.J., Lommatzsch, M., Schmidt, S., Krug, N., Luttmann, W., Renz, H. & Virchow, J.C., Jr. (2003). The neurotrophins nerve growth factor, brain-derived neurotrophic factor, neurotrophin-3, and neurotrophin-4 are survival and activation factors for eosinophils in patients with allergic bronchial asthma. *Journal of Experimental Medicine*, Vol.198, No.3, pp. 455-467, ISSN 0022-1007.

Nassenstein, C., Dawbarn, D., Pollock, K., Allen, S.J., Erpenbeck, V.J., Spies, E., Krug, N. & Braun, A. (2006). Pulmonary distribution, regulation, and functional role of Trk receptors in a murine model of asthma. *Journal of Allergy and Clinical Immunology*, Vol.118, No.3, pp. 597-605, ISSN 0105-4538.

Ni, X., Li, X., Fang, X., Li, N., Cui, W. & Zhang, B. (2010). NGF/TrkA-mediated Kidins220/ARMS signaling activated in the allergic airway challenge in mice. *Annals of Allergy, Asthma, and Immunology*, Vol.105, No.4, pp. 299-306, ISSN 1081-1206.

Noga, O., Englmann, C., Hanf, G., Grutzkau, A., Guhl, S. & Kunkel, G. (2002). Activation of the specific neurotrophin receptors TrkA, TrkB and TrkC influences the function of eosinophils. *Clinical and Experimental Allergy*, Vol.32, No.9, pp. 1348-1354, ISSN 0954-7894.

Obermeier, A., Halfter, H., Wiesmuller, K.H., Jung, G., Schlessinger, J. & Ullrich, A. (1993). Tyrosine 785 is a major determinant of Trk-substrate interaction. *EMBO Journal*, Vol.12, No.3, pp. 933-941, ISSN 0261-4189.

Olgart, C. & Frossard, N. (2001). Human lung fibroblasts secrete nerve growth factor: effect of inflammatory cytokines and glucocorticoids. *European Respiratory Journal*, Vol.18, No.1, pp. 115-121, ISSN 0903-1936.

Olgart Hoglund, C., de Blay, F., Oster, J.P., Duvernelle, C., Kassel, O., Pauli, G. & Frossard, N. (2002). Nerve growth factor levels and localisation in human asthmatic bronchi. *European Respiratory Journal*, Vol.20, No.5, pp. 1110-1116, ISSN 0903-1936.

Othumpangat, S., Gibson, L.F., Samsell, L. & Piedimonte, G. (2009). NGF is an essential survival factor for bronchial epithelial cells during respiratory syncytial virus infection. *PLoS ONE*, Vol.4, No.7, pp. e6444, ISSN 1932-6203.

Otten, U., Scully, J.L., Ehrhard, P.B. & Gadient, R.A. (1994). Neurotrophins: signals between the nervous and immune systems. *Progress in Brain Research*, Vol.103, pp. 293-305, ISSN 0079-6123.

Patapoutian, A. & Reichardt, L.F. (2001). Trk receptors: mediators of neurotrophin action. *Current Opinion in Neurobiology*, Vol.11, No.3, pp. 272-280, ISSN 0959-4388.

Path, G., Braun, A., Meents, N., Kerzel, S., Quarcoo, D., Raap, U., Hoyle, G.W., Nockher, W.A. & Renz, H. (2002). Augmentation of allergic early-phase reaction by nerve growth factor. *American Journal of Respiratory and Critical Care Medicine*, Vol.166, No.6, pp. 818-826, ISSN 073-449X.

Philippidou, P., Valdez, G., Akmentin, W., Bowers, W.J., Federoff, H.J. & Halegoua, S. (2011). Trk retrograde signaling requires persistent, Pincher-directed endosomes. *Proceedings of the National Academy of Sciences of the United States of America*, Vol.108, No.2, pp. 852-857, ISSN 0027-8424.

Pons, F., Freund, V., Kuissu, H., Mathieu, E., Olgart, C. & Frossard, N. (2001). Nerve growth factor secretion by human lung epithelial A549 cells in pro- and anti-inflammatory conditions. *European Journal of Pharmacology*, Vol.428, No.3, pp. 365-369, ISSN 0014-2999.

Prakash, Y., Thompson, M.A., Meuchel, L., Pabelick, C.M., Mantilla, C.B., Zaidi, S. & Martin, R.J. (2010). Neurotrophins in lung health and disease. *Expert Review of Respiratory Medicine*, Vol.4, No.3, pp. 395-411, ISSN 1747-6348.

Quarcoo, D., Schulte-Herbruggen, O., Lommatzsch, M., Schierhorn, K., Hoyle, G.W., Renz, H. & Braun, A. (2004). Nerve growth factor induces increased airway inflammation via a neuropeptide-dependent mechanism in a transgenic animal model of allergic airway inflammation. *Clinical and Experimental Allergy*, Vol.34, No.7, pp. 1146-1151, ISSN 0954-7894.

Rahbek, U.L., Dissing, S., Thomassen, C., Hansen, A.J. & Tritsaris, K. (2005). Nerve growth factor activates aorta endothelial cells causing PI3K/Akt- and ERK-dependent migration. *Pflugers Archiv (European Journal of Physiology)*, Vol.450, No.5, pp. 355-361, ISSN 0031-6768.

Rajagopal, R., Chen, Z.Y., Lee, F.S. & Chao, M.V. (2004). Transactivation of Trk neurotrophin receptors by G-protein-coupled receptor ligands occurs on intracellular membranes. *Journal of Neuroscience*, Vol.24, No.30, pp. 6650-6658, ISSN 0270-6474.

Ricci, A., Bronzetti, E., Mannino, F., Felici, L., Terzano, C. & Mariotta, S. (2004a). Elevated neurotrophin and neurotrophin receptor expression in spontaneously hypertensive rat lungs. *Growth Factors*, Vol.22, No.3, pp. 195-205, ISSN 0897-7194.

Ricci, A., Felici, L., Mariotta, S., Mannino, F., Schmid, G., Terzano, C., Cardillo, G., Amenta, F. & Bronzetti, E. (2004b). Neurotrophin and neurotrophin receptor protein expression in the human lung. *American Journal of Respiratory Cell and Molecular Biology*, Vol.30, No.1, pp. 12-19, ISSN 1044-1549.

Ricci, A., Greco, S., Amenta, F., Bronzetti, E., Felici, L., Rossodivita, I., Sabbatini, M. & Mariotta, S. (2000a). Neurotrophins and neurotrophin receptors in human pulmonary arteries. *Journal of Vascular Research*, Vol.37, No.5, pp. 355-363, ISSN 1018-1172.

Ricci, A., Greco, S., Mariotta, S., Felici, L., Amenta, F. & Bronzetti, E. (2000b). Neurotrophin and neurotrophin receptor expression in alveolar macrophages: an immunocytochemical study. *Growth Factors*, Vol.18, No.3, pp. 193-202, ISSN 0897-7194.

Ryden, M. & Ibanez, C.F. (1996). Binding of neurotrophin-3 to p75LNGFR, TrkA, and TrkB mediated by a single functional epitope distinct from that recognized by trkC. *Journal of Biological Chemistry*, Vol.271, No.10, pp. 5623-5627, ISSN 0021-9258.

Sawada, J., Itakura, A., Tanaka, A., Furusaka, T. & Matsuda, H. (2000). Nerve growth factor functions as a chemoattractant for mast cells through both mitogen-activated protein kinase and phosphatidylinositol 3-kinase signaling pathways. *Blood*, Vol.95, No.6, pp. 2052-2058, ISSN 0006-4971.

Saxena, S., Howe, C.L., Cosgaya, J.M., Steiner, P., Hirling, H., Chan, J.R., Weis, J. & Kruttgen, A. (2005). Differential endocytic sorting of p75NTR and TrkA in response to NGF: a role for late endosomes in TrkA trafficking. *Molecular and Cellular Neurosciences*, Vol.28, No.3, pp. 571-587, ISSN 1044-7431.

Segal, R.A. & Greenberg, M.E. (1996). Intracellular signaling pathways activated by neurotrophic factors. *Annual Review of Neuroscience*, Vol.19, pp. 463-489, ISSN 0743-4634.

Sherer, T.B., Neff, P.S., Hankins, G.R. & Tuttle, J.B. (1998). Mechanisms of increased NGF production in vascular smooth muscle of the spontaneously hypertensive rat. *Experimental Cell Research*, Vol.241, No.1, pp. 186-193, ISSN 0014-4827.

Sin, A.Z., Roche, E.M., Togias, A., Lichtenstein, L.M. & Schroeder, J.T. (2001). Nerve growth factor or IL-3 induces more IL-13 production from basophils of allergic subjects than from basophils of nonallergic subjects. *Journal of Allergy and Clinical Immunology*, Vol.108, No.3, pp. 387-393, ISSN 0105-4538.

Skaper, S.D. (2008). The biology of neurotrophins, signalling pathways, and functional peptide mimetics of neurotrophins and their receptors. *CNS and Neurological Disorders Drug Targets*, Vol.7, No.1, pp. 46-62, ISSN 1871-5273.

Solomon, A., Aloe, L., Pe'er, J., Frucht-Pery, J., Bonini, S., Bonini, S. & Levi-Schaffer, F. (1998). Nerve growth factor is preformed in and activates human peripheral blood eosinophils. *Journal of Allergy and Clinical Immunology*, Vol.102, No.3, pp. 454-460, ISSN 0105-4538.

Stephens, R.M., Loeb, D.M., Copeland, T.D., Pawson, T., Greene, L.A. & Kaplan, D.R. (1994). Trk receptors use redundant signal transduction pathways involving SHC and PLC-gamma 1 to mediate NGF responses. *Neuron*, Vol.12, No.3, pp. 691-705, ISSN 0896-6273.

Susaki, Y., Shimizu, S., Katakura, K., Watanabe, N., Kawamoto, K., Matsumoto, M., Tsudzuki, M., Furusaka, T., Kitamura, Y. & Matsuda, H. (1996). Functional properties of murine macrophages promoted by nerve growth factor. *Blood*, Vol.88, No.12, pp. 4630-4637, ISSN 0006-4971.

Tacconelli, A., Farina, A.R., Cappabianca, L., Gulino, A. & Mackay, A.R. (2005). TrkAIII. A novel hypoxia-regulated alternative TrkA splice variant of potential physiological and pathological importance. *Cell Cycle*, Vol.4, No.1, pp. 8-9, ISSN 1538-4101.

Takahashi, H., Uno, S., Watanabe, Y., Arakawa, K. & Nakagawa, S. (2000). Expression of nerve growth factor-induced type 1 plasminogen activator inhibitor (PAI-1) mRNA is inhibited by genistein and wortmannin. *Neuroreport*, Vol.11, No.5, pp. 1111-1115, ISSN 0959-4965.

Takahashi, Y., Shimokawa, N., Esmaeili-Mahani, S., Morita, A., Masuda, H., Iwasaki, T., Tamura, J., Haglund, K. & Koibuchi, N. (2011). Ligand-induced downregulation of TrkA is partly regulated through ubiquitination by Cbl. *FEBS Letters*, Vol.585, No.12, pp. 1741-1747, ISSN 0014-5793.

Tam, S.Y., Tsai, M., Yamaguchi, M., Yano, K., Butterfield, J.H. & Galli, S.J. (1997). Expression of functional TrkA receptor tyrosine kinase in the HMC-1 human mast cell line and in human mast cells. *Blood*, Vol.90, No.5, pp. 1807-1820, ISSN 0006-4971.

Torcia, M., Bracci-Laudiero, L., Lucibello, M., Nencioni, L., Labardi, D., Rubartelli, A., Cozzolino, F., Aloe, L. & Garaci, E. (1996). Nerve growth factor is an autocrine survival factor for memory B lymphocytes. *Cell*, Vol.85, No.3, pp. 345-356, ISSN 0092-8674.

Ueda, K., Hirose, M., Murata, E., Takatori, M., Ueda, M., Ikeda, H. & Shigemi, K. (2010). Local administration of a synthetic cell-penetrating peptide antagonizing TrkA function suppresses inflammatory pain in rats. *Journal of Pharmacological Sciences*, Vol.112, No.4, pp. 438-443, ISSN 0022-3549.

Watson, J.J., Allen, S.J. & Dawbarn, D. (2008). Targeting nerve growth factor in pain: what is the therapeutic potential? *BioDrugs*, Vol.22, No.6, pp. 349-359, ISSN 1173-8804.

Weier, H.U., Rhein, A.P., Shadravan, F., Collins, C. & Polikoff, D. (1995). Rapid physical mapping of the human trk protooncogene (NTRK1) to human chromosome 1q21-q22 by P1 clone selection, fluorescence in situ hybridization (FISH), and computer-assisted microscopy. *Genomics*, Vol.26, No.2, pp. 390-393, ISSN 0888-7543.

Wiese, S., Digby, M.R., Gunnersen, J.M., Gotz, R., Pei, G., Holtmann, B., Lowenthal, J. & Sendtner, M. (1999). The anti-apoptotic protein ITA is essential for NGF-mediated survival of embryonic chick neurons. *Nature Neuroscience*, Vol.2, No.11, pp. 978-983, ISSN 1097-6256.

Wiesmann, C. & de Vos, A.M. (2001). Nerve growth factor: structure and function. *Cellular and Molecular Life Sciences*, Vol.58, No.5-6, pp. 748-759, ISSN 1420-682X.

Wilfong, E.R. & Dey, R.D. (2004). Nerve growth factor and substance P regulation in nasal sensory neurons after toluene diisocyanate exposure. *American Journal of Respiratory Cell and Molecular Biology*, Vol.30, No.6, pp. 793-800, ISSN 1044-1549.

Wilfong, E.R. & Dey, R.D. (2005). The release of nerve growth factor from the nasal mucosa following toluene diisocyanate. *Journal of Toxicology and Environmental Health. Part A*, Vol.68, No.15, pp. 1337-1348, ISSN 1528-7394.

Wooten, M.W., Zhou, G., Seibenhener, M.L. & Coleman, E.S. (1994). A role for zeta protein kinase C in nerve growth factor-induced differentiation of PC12 cells. *Cell Growth and Differentiation*, Vol.5, No.4, pp. 395-403, ISSN 1044-9523.

Wu, Z.X. & Dey, R.D. (2006). Nerve growth factor-enhanced airway responsiveness involves substance P in ferret intrinsic airway neurons. *American Journal of Physiology. Lung Cellular and Molecular Physiology*, Vol.291, No.1, pp. L111-118, ISSN 1040-0605.

Xu, M., Remillard, C.V., Sachs, B.D., Makino, A., Platoshyn, O., Yao, W., Dillmann, W.H., Akassoglou, K. & Yuan, J.X. (2008). p75 neurotrophin receptor regulates agonist-induced pulmonary vasoconstriction. *American Journal of Physiology. Heart and Circulatory Physiology*, Vol.295, No.4, pp. H1529-1538, ISSN 0363-6135.

Yamaguchi, Y., Katoh, H., Yasui, H., Mori, K. & Negishi, M. (2001). RhoA inhibits the nerve growth factor-induced Rac1 activation through Rho-associated kinase-dependent pathway. *Journal of Biological Chemistry*, Vol.276, No.22, pp. 18977-18983, ISSN 0021-9258.

York, R.D., Molliver, D.C., Grewal, S.S., Stenberg, P.E., McCleskey, E.W. & Stork, P.J. (2000). Role of phosphoinositide 3-kinase and endocytosis in nerve growth factor-induced extracellular signal-regulated kinase activation via Ras and Rap1. *Molecular and Cellular Biology*, Vol.20, No.21, pp. 8069-8083, ISSN 0270-7306.

Zweifel, L.S., Kuruvilla, R. & Ginty, D.D. (2005). Functions and mechanisms of retrograde neurotrophin signalling. *Nature Reviews. Neuroscience*, Vol.6, No.8, pp. 615-625, ISSN 1471-0048.

Part 6

The Value of the Cytokinome Profile

6

The Value of the Cytokinome Profile

Susan Costantini[1], Ankush Sharma[2]
and Giovanni Colonna[2,3]
[1]"Pascale Foundation" National Cancer Institute - Cancer Research Center, Mercogliano (AV)
[2]Doctorate in Computational Biology - CRISCEB (Second University of Naples), Naples
[3]Department of Biochemistry and Biophysics (Second University of Naples), Naples
Italy

1. Introduction

Many scientific articles describe the pathogenesis of diseases that afflict the modern man (cancer, diabetes, obesity, degenerative diseases, etc.) as a slow common inflammatory process that is the basis of all these diseases. Therefore, we commonly speak of chronic inflammatory diseases (Allavena et al., 2008). The basis of this statement are the numerous experimental observations which show that these diseases are driven, from the earliest moments, by exchange between cells of tissues and organs of molecules that operate as messengers. These molecules, carrying biological messages of great importance, inform and lead a complex system of different cell types on what happens and towards which physiological and metabolic changes they are being carried. The chemical nature of these signaling molecules is diverse, but a group of them, the cytokines, is among the most important and studied inter-cellular messengers (Germano et al., 2008). We know the biological meaning of the signal of many of them, thus we can generally divide these molecules into two major classes: pro-inflammatory cytokines and anti-inflammatory cytokines. They are small proteins, quite numerous, more than about 100, expressed in very low amounts (pico and nano molar) and often short-lived, to cover specific information needs (Macarthur et al., 2004).

The cells recognize these signals through appropriate receptors placed on their external membranes. However their study had some limitations due to the fact that (i) only those more abundant were studied, even if with very sensitive assays based on use of antibodies and fluorescence (ELISA); (ii) the receptors show pleiotropy, i.e. they have good affinity for various cytokines and hence the message can be brought by different cytokines; (iii) the biological significance of the message is known only for some of them, for example, it is not known which is the biological meaning carried out by the under-represented cytokines (the less concentrated ones at phenotypic level) and if the different messages are recognized by the receptor as only redundant or with diverse biological content (Colvin et al., 2004; Costantini et al., 2009; Trotta et al., 2009).

Recently, specific protein chips of considerable and improved sensitivity are being developed. They allow the simultaneous determination of different cytokines based on a fluorescence/laser/antibodies technology which uses microparticle beads (multiplex technology) that allows the analysis of tiny samples (few dozens of microliter) of serum, plasma, or cell cultures supernatant. Each bead set is coated with capture antibody specific for one analyte. The result is the most accurate, sensitive, and reproducible cytokine assay available. An important point of this technology is the ability to appreciate quantitatively also the presence of the under-represented cytokines (Capone et al., 2010; Costantini et al., 2010a). The pattern of these cytokines, being part of the new global or holistic logic, which is used today in the "omics" approach to the study of biological phenomena, can be indicated as "cytokinome" (Costantini et al., 2010b).

The fact is that the cytokines form an informative network, for some ways very similar to the Internet, that capillary connects, as knots to the network, cellular systems also different. The study of this network is important for understanding the evolution of the pathogenesis of many chronic inflammatory diseases. However, there are many questions that must still find the answer. In the case of chronic inflammatory diseases, which development in the time the whole pattern of cytokines shows? Their evolution in time begins in the same way and is common for all the diseases or is pathology correlated and addressed by different types or classes of cytokines? Which one is the cytokinome development during the disease? Answers to these and other questions are essential not only to be able to describe the cytokinome dynamics during the progression of chronic inflammatory diseases but, above all, to try to predict in large advance the prognosis of the disease. If this will be possible, we will be able to intervene with great advance in the early stages of the disease with much more chance of healing or of extending the duration and the expectations of life.

Therefore, the review will focus on:

- Role of the cytokines in chronic inflammatory diseases and cancers
- Challenge and significance of the cytokinome profile
- Hepatocarcinoma as an example of chronic inflammatory disease
- Metabolic pathway analysis of significant genes in hepatoma cells
- Evaluation of cytokines in HCC patients with HCV-related cirrhosis
- Evaluation of cytokines in patients with chronic HCV or with HCV-related cirrhosis
- The need of cytokinome data mining system for a predictive medicine for chronic inflammatory diseases
- The need for structural studies of cytokine/receptor complex: the example of CXCL9, CXCL10 and CXCL11 chemokines and their membrane receptor CXCR3

2. Role of the cytokines in chronic inflammatory diseases and cancers

Inflammation is a physiologic process in response to acute tissue damage resulting from physical injury, ischemic injury, infection, exposure to toxins, chemical irritation, and/or wounding or other types of trauma (Lu et al., 2006; Philip et al., 2004); it is a protective attempt by the organism to remove the injurious stimuli as well as initiate the healing process for the tissue. At the very early stage of inflammation, the phagocytic cells are mainly involved: neutrophils are the first cells to migrate to the inflammatory sites under the regulation of molecules produced by rapidly responding macrophages and mast cells prestationed in tissues (Coussens & Werb, 2002). As the inflammation progresses, various types of leukocytes, lymphocytes, and other inflammatory cells are activated and attracted to the inflamed site by a signaling network involving a great number of growth factors, cytokines, and chemokines (Coussens & Werb, 2002). All cells recruited to the inflammatory site contribute to tissue breakdown and are beneficial by strengthening and maintaining the defense against infection (Coussens & Werb, 2002). The resolution of inflammation also requires a rapid programmed clearance of inflammatory cells: neighboring macrophages, dendritic cells, and backup phagocytes do this job by inducing apoptosis and conducting phagocytosis (Savill et al., 2002).

However, inflammation may become chronic either because an inflammatory stimulus persists or because of dysregulation in the control mechanisms that normally turn the process off. Recently, it has been suggested that inflammation associated with cancer is similar to that seen with chronic inflammation, which includes the production of growth and angiogenic factors that stimulate tissue repair, factors that can also promote cancer-cell survival, implantation, and growth (Philip et al., 2004; Macarthur et al., 2004; Balkwill and Mantovani, 2001). Interestingly, inflammation functions at all three stages of tumor development: initiation, progression and metastasis.

Since many cancers arise from sites of infection, chronic irritation, and inflammation, it is now clear that the tumor microenvironment, which is largely orchestrated by inflammatory cells and cytokines (Fig. 1), is an indispensable participant in the neoplastic process altering not only the metabolic needs of the tissue, but also fostering DNA and protein damage, proliferation, survival, mutagenesis, migration and metastasis of malignant cells (Allavena et al., 2008). Indeed all tumors in the presence of stromal and infiltrating inflammatory cells are facilitated and helped to maintain these metastatic processes. Leukocytes, lymphocytes and other inflammatory cells are activated in this process and attracted to the inflamed site. Inflammation contributes to initiation by inducing the release of a variety of pro-inflammatory cytokines and chemokines and inflammatory enzymes as cyclo-oxygenases that alert the vasculature to release inflammatory cells and factors into the tissue milieu, thereby causing oxidative damage, DNA mutations, and other changes in the microenvironment, making it more conducive to cell transformation, increased survival and proliferation (Germano et al., 2008). We must not forget that many cytokines and chemokines are inducible by hypoxia which is a major physiological difference (Mancino et al., 2008). An important aspect of the tumor microenvironment is the cytokine mediated communication between the tumor and cells. Cytokines and chemokines have many activities that permit cell–cell communication locally at the tissue, with the outcome determined by cytokine concentration milieu and cell type (Germano et al., 2008). Current thinking is that activated immune cells provide both anti- and protumorigenic signals, thus representing targets to be harnessed or attacked for therapeutic advantage depending upon environmental and/or cellular context. Because the control of cytokine production is highly complex and multifactorial, the effects of cytokines are mediated through multiple regulatory networks. The intricate complexity of both cytokine networks clearly conceals the role that a single cytokine may play in the pathogenesis of the disease. It is therefore informative to investigate the immunopathogenesis of a disease process by analyzing multiple cytokines. In this way it is possible to provide a better understanding of the role of cellular, humoral and chemotactic immunity at a critical time in some cancer diseases and also in the treatment course of a correlated infection (Costantini et al., 2009).

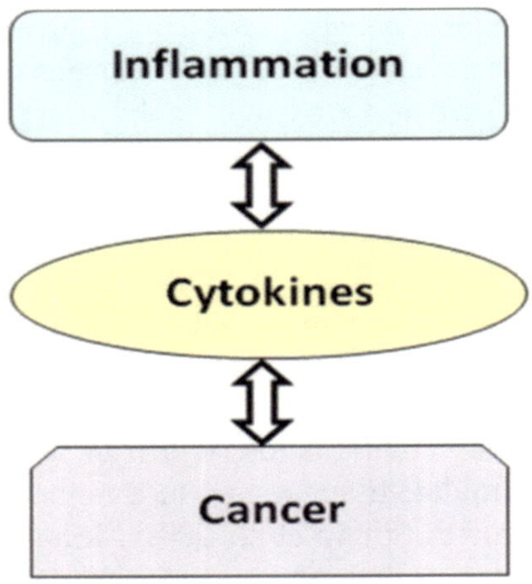

Fig. 1. Relationship between inflammation, cytokines and cancer

3. Challenge and significance of the cytokinome profile

In order to understand the whole universe of human cytokines, the socalled cytokinome, according the "omics" system of definition, it needs to evaluate these proteins and analyse their complex network of interactions by which they regulate their own synthesis or that of their receptors, and antagonize or synergize with each other in many and often redundant ways (Costantini et al., 2010b).

A major effort is the achievement of an efficient database that can collect together correct ontologies, algorithms and tools of analyses, structural and "omics" data of cytokines and their receptors, metabolic pathways, and the whole interactome. Another intriguing problem related to the cytokine family and their receptors is the pleiotropy existing in the cytokine system, where one cytokine is able to activate various receptors and many different cytokines activate the same receptor. When the frame of the whole cytokine network will be known, we will have the possibility to create best and more efficient drugs against the cancer, most probably able to interact with the receptors rather than directly with the cytokine molecules because of their pleiotropic effect. Another element of complexity in the cytokine network is introduced also by the fact that some genes encoding cytokines can give rise to variant forms of cytokines (isoforms) by means of alternative splicing, yielding molecules with slight structural differences but biologically significant changes of activities. This explains why it is always useful to analyze the gene expression profile correlated to the cytokines. In fact, previous studies have identified important mutations in some cancers, but they were primarily focused on a limited set of genes and, thus, provided a constrained view of the mutational spectrum.

However, a correct and comprehensive understanding of cytokine functions can be obtained from simultaneous and coherent measurements of the serum concentrations of cytokines. This point raises the inherent difficulty of a simultaneous measurement of the cytokine concentrations to obtain correct internal ratios among the various molecules present in the same biological fluid due to the often large difference in concentrations spanning several magnitude orders. At present, it is possible to effectively characterize the serum levels of cytokines using a broad-spectrum bead based multiplex immunoassay.

In this complex interactions network, Systems Biology and/or Biologically Integrated Approaches are powerful tools to analyze as a whole, the enormous amount of data coming from the so-called "omics" disciplines (genomics, transcriptomics, proteomics) by computational methods and algorithms, in order to create an information body that allows us to have a comprehensive and integrated vision of the biological phenomenon under investigation. In fact, until the last century, the approach of biological science was to break down the object of study in its elementary parts and to study all the singular units in order to explain the life processes. This was a typical analytical and reductionist procedure, which allowed the understanding of almost all properties of molecular parts of living organisms, such as genes, proteins, metabolites, and was focused on the study of each single component of the system under consideration but was not able to predict the behavior of the systems as a whole. A system can be defined as a number of interacting elements existing within a boundary that is surrounded by an environment. Therefore, a complex system is able to create new properties from the interactions between its components, and also to interact and to respond with the external inputs. When the interactions between the parties are determined by the dynamical processes inducing the emerging properties like adaptability, self-organization and the ability to respond under disturbance, the system becomes complex. In this way these non linear interactions allow a number of possible several states and new emergent behaviors are not predictable from the simple sum of the component parts. These principles were applied to study the living organisms, the stock markets, the ecosystems and the flock of birds. In biology it's necessary to study the living organism as a whole, and the laws of regarding the organizational forces of systems, which yet are not well known, but are essential to solve and to understand the collective phenomena and the framework for the functionality of the systems (Costantini et al., 2008).
Therefore, all the data related to the cytokine evaluations can be analyzed and modeled computationally by using graphs or networks connecting the various data groups (related to gene and protein expression obtained by microarrays and by multiplex biometric ELISA-based immunoassay) in terms of dynamic probabilistic maps of metabolic and/or physiological activities and/or pathogenetic pathways. Hence, the definition and evaluation of a human cytokinome is an important future tool to analyze the interaction network of cytokines both in healthy individuals and in patients affected from a cancer. Using these computational models it will be easier and immediate to understand and investigate how the regression of a chronic inflammation process, by acting on the cellular populations of cytokines, can block the progression of the cancer and how this knowledge can be an useful prognostic and diagnostic tool for clinicians.

4. Hepatocellular carcinoma as an example of chronic inflammatory disease

Hepatocellular carcinoma (HCC) accounts for >5% of all human cancers and for 80% - 90% of primary liver cancer. It is a major health problem worldwide being the fifth most common malignancy in men and the eighth in women; the third most common cause of cancer-related death in the world. Moreover early diagnosis is uncommom and medical treatments are inadeguate (Altekruse et al., 2009).
Yearly 550,000 people worldwide die for HCC, with a 2:1 ratio for men versus women. Its incidence is increasing dramatically, with marked variations among geographic areas (Jemal et al., 2007), racial and ethnic groups, environmental risk factors. The estimated annual number of HCC cases exceeds 700,000, with a mean annual incidence of 3-4% (Jemal et al.,

2007). Most HCC cases (>80%) occur in either sub-Saharan Africa or in Eastern Asia (China alone accounts for more than 50% of the world's cases) (Jemal et al., 2007). In the United States (US) HCC incidence is lower than other countries (0.3/100000) even if there has been a significant and alarming increase in the incidence of HCC in the US, from 1.3 in the late 70s' to 3 in the late 90s', due to HCV infection. In 2008, 21370 new cases of HCC and intrahepatic bile duct cancer were estimated with 18410 deaths (Jemal et al., 2007). In Europe, Oceania and America, chronic hepatitis C and alcoholic cirrhosis are the main risk factors for HCC. The main risk factor for HCC development in patients with hepatitis C is the presence of cirrhosis. Among patients with hepatitis C and cirrhosis, the annual incidence rate of HCC ranges between 1-8%, being higher in Japan (4-8%) intermediate in Italy (2-4%) and lower in USA (1.4%) (Fassio, 2010). Analysis of mortality from HCC in Europe confirmed large variability, with high rates in France (6.79/100000) and Italy (6.72/100000) due to hepatitis C virus (HCV) during the 1960s and 1970s (Bosetti et al., 2008). Southern Italy has the highest rates of HCC in Europe (Fusco et al., 2008).

HCC is unique among cancers occurring mostly in patients with a known risk factor: ninety percent of HCCs develop in the context of chronic liver inflammation and cirrhosis (Altekruse et al., 2009). Hepatitis B (HBV) and C (HCV) viruses are the major cause of liver disease worldwide. Fortunately, the hepatitis B virus vaccine has resulted in a substantial decline in the number of new cases of acute hepatitis B among children, adolescents, and adults in western countries since the mid-1980s. This success is not duplicable for HCV where active or passive vaccination is not available yet. Therefore, the present and next future HCC history will be mainly related to HCV infection. The incidence of HCV infection is hard to quantify since it is often asymptomatic. The World Health Organization estimates that 3% of the world's population - more than 170 million people - are chronically infected (3-4 million new infections every year). Therefore, a tremendous number of people are currently at elevated risk for HCC and its early diagnosis (when surgical intervention is possible) may significantly affect the patients prognosis (Ryder, 2003).

However it is possible also a direct carcinogenesis by hepatitis viruses, without a cirrhotic step (Nash et al., 2010). In particular, it was reported that patients without cirrhosis were younger, survived longer than patients with cirrhosis ($P < 0.0001$) and had a better 5-year survival experience (Chiesa et al., 2000).

In contrast to HBV, HCV does not integrate into the host genome and does not contain a reverse transcriptase. In particular, in the infected subjects both viruses trigger an immune-mediated inflammatory response (hepatitis) that either clears the infection or slowly destroys the liver (Bowen & Walker, 2005).

Effective HCV immunity is limited by the high variability of virion genome; HCV virions turn over rapidly (with a half-life of about 3 h), and up to about 1012 complete viruses are produced per day in an infected person (Ueno et al., 2009). About 80% of newly infected patients develop chronic infection; an estimated 10% to 20% will develop cirrhosis and 1-5% proceeds to end-stage liver cancer over a period of 20 to 30 years (Fig. 2). In the case of HCV, HCC is invariably observed as a complication of cirrhosis, whereas in the case of HBV HCC is often found in non-cirrhotic liver. Therefore, the hepatic fibrosis dramatically increase the incidence of HCC (Castello et al., 2010a).

Many studies were conducted in the last years in regard to anti-HCV immune response. In fact, much attention has recently focused on regulatory T cells (Tregs) being able to secrete inhibitory cytokines such as IL-10 or TGF-β, even if their contribution is yet unclear (Castello et al., 2010b). Increased Treg cells were found in peripheral blood of HCV-infected patients (Boettler et al., 2005) as well as in the tumor microenvironment of HCC patients (Ormandi et al., 2005). The frequency of naturally arising CD4+CD$^{25high+}$ Tregs in the periphery of HCV-infected patients was reported to be higher than that in patients who resolved the infection or uninfected controls (Cabrera et al., 2004). TH1 cytokines are generally up-regulated in patients with HCC, resulting in higher levels of pro-inflammatory cytokines, as IL-1α, IL-15, IL-18, TNF-α, TNF- αRs, TNF-αRI, TNF- αRII, and IL-6 in comparison with healthy individuals (Huang et al., 1999). However, the intra/peri-tumoral cytokines levels are often different from the serum levels (Budhu & Wang, 2006). Higher serum IL-6 level was an independent risk factor for HCC development in female but not male chronic hepatitis C patients (Nakagawa et al., 2009). IL-10 was highly expressed in HCC tumors and serum, correlating with disease progression (Budhu & Wang, 2006). Budhu and Wang reviewed the association between cytokine abnormalities and HCC patients and found that a dominant TH2-like cytokine profile (IL-4, IL-8, IL-10, and IL-5) and a decrease in the TH1-like cytokines (IL-1α, IL-1β, IL-2, IL-12p35, IL-12p40, IL-15, TNF-α, and IFN-γ was associated with the metastatic phenotype of disease (Budhu & Wang, 2006). Thus, it has been hypothesized that TH1 cytokines are involved in tumor development, whereas TH2 cytokines in tumor progression. Recently the cytokine concentrations have been evaluated in patients with HCC patients with HCV-related cirrhosis (Capone et al., 2010).

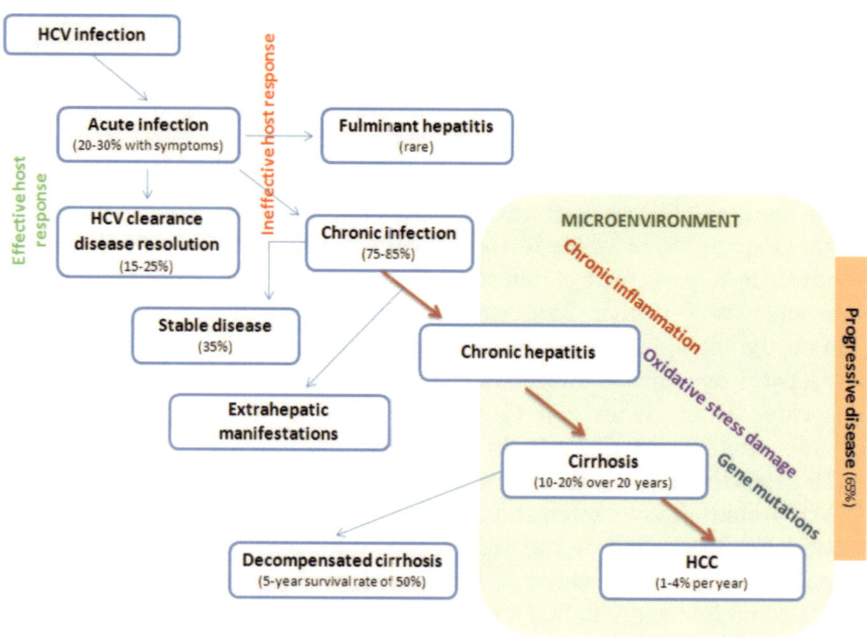

Fig. 2. Evolution from HCV infection to HCC.

5. Metabolic pathway analysis of significant genes in hepatoma cells

The cytokinome study is an important step to our understanding of chronic inflammatory diseases because a global and dynamic knowledge of cellular signaling, at moment only static and mechanistic, will improve our ability to adequately read and understand the meaning in the early time of the information that cells exchange each other. The present technology supports this view from an experimental point of view by DNA and Protein microarrays. These techniques taken together can support a better knowledge of the relationships existing between genome behavior and related phenotypes (cytokines in this case) during the progression of a disease. More difficult is to correlate genomic and phenotypic levels by a logical analysis able to correlate the genes action with their products to extract useful biological information on the disease progression, such as changes in metabolic pathways or activation of new metabolic paths. In general, the knowledge of early metabolic changes during the first stages of an illness is an important moment to develop new more specific drugs by pharmacogenomics as well as to operate a metabolic repair by nutrigenomics. Probably this holistic view of the medicine is perhaps more expensive for the community but it is necessary to efficiently fight the numerous diseases of our time unfortunately founded on chronic inflammation.

The global gene expression has been evaluated in HepG2 cells in comparison to normal human hepatocytes using Illumina microarray. In particular, cRNAs were hybridized to the HumanWG-6 Bead-Chip array which allows to assess the presence of more than 48,000 transcripts (Whole Genome). Our metabolic pathway analysis aims at discovering modifications in and/or activation of new metabolic pathways involved into a perturbation of the hepatoma cell homeostasis. We have used a cluster analysis or "clustering" that is the assignment of a set of data or observations into subsets (called clusters) so that observations in the same cluster are similar. This is a method of analysis used also in bioinformatics to evaluate high-throughput genotyping platforms to build groups of genes with related expression patterns (also known as coexpressed genes). The algorithms we have used are hierarchical algorithms that find successive clusters using previously established clusters and create a hierarchy of clusters which may be represented by a hierarchical clustering dendrogram. The method builds the hierarchy from the individual elements by progressively merging clusters. In particular, hierarchical cluster analysis of genes showed the differential expression of genes in HepG2 cells respect to human hepatocytes used as healthy controls. 2646 genes were significantly down-regulated in HepG2 cells respect to the hepatocytes whereas a further 3586 genes were significantly up-regulated. Moreover, information on the biological functions of the genes that were significantly regulated was obtained by a pathway analysis. Pathways related to these genes were extracted from KEGG (Kyoto Encyclopedia of Genes and Genomes) (Ogata et al 1999), Pathway Interaction Database, and network for CXCL12 in Hepatocellular carcinoma is derived from the HCCnet (Hepatocellular carcinoma network database) (Bing et al, 2010), which contains around 37811 protein-protein interactions from 13 individual datasets having 894 HCC samples containing 30.5%, 44.7 % and 18.7% of HCV infected, HBV infected and unknown factors respectively. Indeed a network of transcription factors that are extracted from microarray data and interact with EGFR gene is constructed by Cytoscape.

Amongst the significantly up-regulated and down-regulated genes several chemokines and some transcription factors (CCL20, CCR6, CX3CL1, Grb2, p53, VCAN, C-MYC, CXCL12, SDC4 and Cyclin D1) were found. CCR6, being the receptor for the chemokine CCL20, is expressed on inactivated memory T-cells, on some dendritic cells and also on Th17 cells. Some studies suggest the involvement of the CCL20/CCR6 system in the carcinogenesis and progression of human HCC (Rubie et al., 2006). CCR6 is implicated in the Chemokine signaling pathway and cytokine–cytokine receptor interaction as obtained from Kegg

(Kyoto encyclopedia of genes) (Ogata et al 1999). In particular, CCL20 interacts with VCAN gene (Fig. 3) which encodes for the Versican protein that plays a role in angiogenesis, inflammation. This protein prevents the growth of cancerous tumors and regulates the activity of several growth factors, which control a diverse range of processes important for cell growth. Moreover elevated levels of Versican have been reported in most malignancies, including brain tumors, melanomas, lymphomas and breast cancers, prostate, colon, lung, pancreas, endometrium, and ovary (Miranda et al., 2011; Kusumoto et al., 2010). CCR6 and CCL20 are known to interact with Versican in the HCC network. This protein was found to be upregulated in HCC patients correlated to Hepatitis B Virus and was indicated as a possible candidate for mediating tumor progression and proliferation in liver and more importantly visual impairment (Paraneoplastic syndrome) associated with HCC patients correlated to HBV.

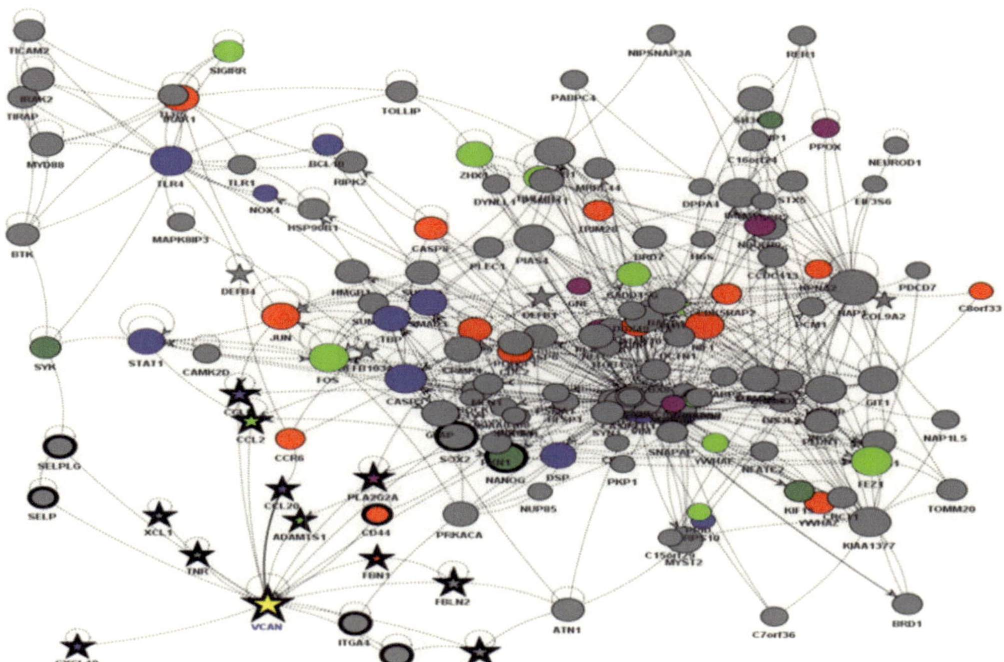

Fig. 3. VCAN Network where the genes are shown by circle and proteins by stars. Different colors: red, up-regulated one; light green, down-regulated one; blue, bidirection-regulated one; grey, not high confident HCC-related one; dark green, genes with selected function info; purple, genes with selected pathway info.

The CXCR4/CXCL12 axis is up-regulated in HCC and participates in HCC cell proliferation. Upon interaction with SDC4 (Syndecan 4), being a heparan sulfate proteoglycans, these proteins function as key regulators of cell signaling via their interactions with multiple growth and angiogenic factors, and promote an aggressive tumor phenotype (Sanderson et al, 2010). CXCL12/SDC4 makes a complex with O Phospho L Tyrosine and upon complex formation it can be hypothesized that it provides stability to p53 protein avoiding cancerous sitations as shown in various cancer cell lines like cervical cancer and lung cancer Renal and

Lung cancer (Sanderson et al, 2010). CXCL12 is found to trans-activating Epidermal growth factor receptor (EGFR) (Porcile,C et al ,2005), that is considered as an important signaling hub where different proliferative and survival signals converge. It is highly evident that EGFR has most important roles to play for controlling signaling cascades from extracellular regions. In particular, the interaction network of EGFR with transcription factors can provide much needed insights to multi factor governing HCC. There were found numerous up- and down- regulated transcription factors interacting with EGFR from microarray data (Fig. 4) and they can produce actions in invasion and metastatis state of the cells and induce simulateounously many biological processes to prevent metastatis, invasion and damage to liver cells.

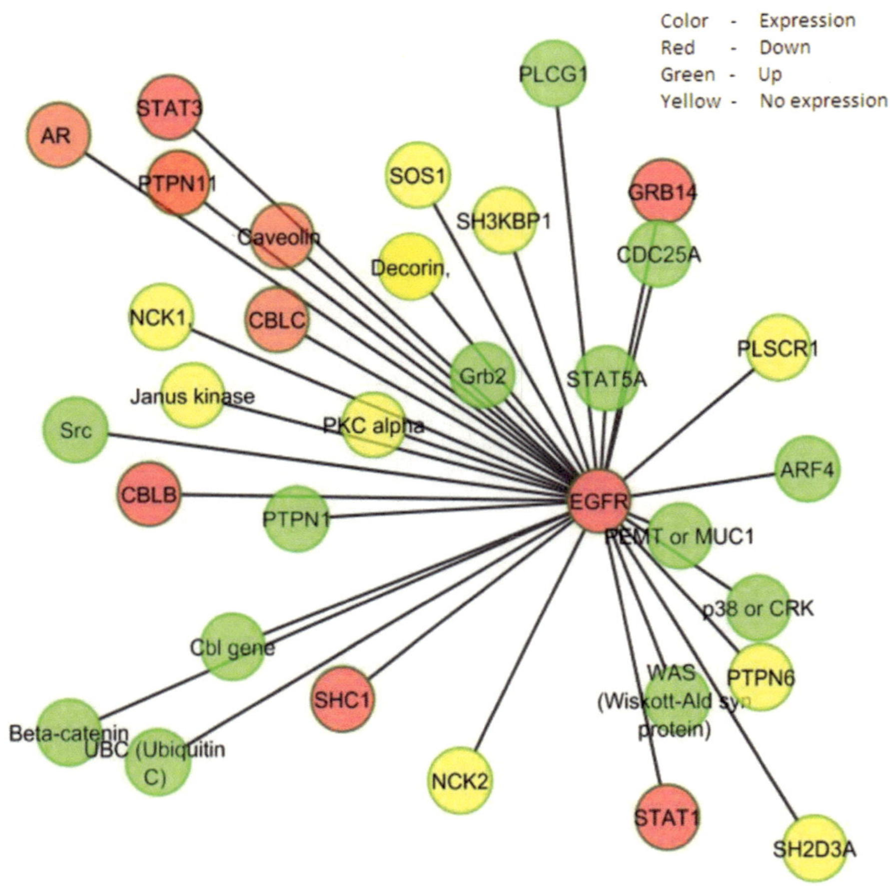

Fig. 4. Interactions of EGFR with de-regulated genes of our microarray data. The down-expressed genes are reported in red, those up-regulated in green and in yellow those no expressed.

Moreover, between the important factors that are governing HCC there is also CX3CL1 (Fractalkine), being a chemokine with both chemoattractant and cell-adhesive functions. Under specific inflammatory conditions, it could regulate the attractions of CX3CR1 bearing cells to tumor site either providing antitumor responses or either pathogenic angiogenesis (Deleterious effects) (Turner et al, 2010). When CX3CL1 is expressed in the tumor, it appears to recruit cytotoxic T cells and NK cells to the tumor site and its expression level is found to correlate with the density of Tumor Infiltrating Lymphocytes (TILs) in some cancers (Ohta et al ,2005).

In addition to these chemokines, Grb2 is also one of the most important upregulated proteins in HCC that was found to be functioning in number of pathways involved in cancer. In particular, Grb2 recruits SOS (exchange protein) for the activating RAS that operates as a molecular switch between MEK and ERK (MAPK) which in nucleus acts on numerous important transcriptions factors like STAT 3 and the expression of STAT3 regulates genes including BCL-x1, CYCLIN D1 and c-MYC which involve in cell apoptosis and cell cycle progression (Sun et al.,2008). In IL6 mediated signaling events, GRB2 interacts with some proteins like FOS and JUN, that are both down regulated in HCC and importantly transcriptional activity of JUN is attenuated and sometimes antagonized by JUNB. This activation takes place in chemically induced murine liver tumours and HCCs of humans, suggesting oncogenic function for this gene in liver tumors of mammals with HSP70 that exhibits regulatory functions of c-JUN, ERK and the JNK pathway, thus inhibiting cell apoptosis (Lee et al., 2005). Moreover, Grb2 plays a specific role in EGF-stimulated EGFR internalization (e.g. receptor sorting, vesicle budding/pinching or vesicle transport (Yamazaki et al., 2002).

From KEGG, other two pathways are found to be deregulated in HCC metastasis, i.e. P53 and MAPK pathways. TP53 plays an important role on regulation of apoptosis and cell cycle arrest and external environment factors or agents are implicated in the development of HCC in correlation with P53, including nutrition, diabetes, oral infection, oral contraceptive, alcohol consumption and some trace elements such as Selenium (Irmak et al., 2003; Wei et al., 2001). A second pathway, which is deregulated in metastatis, is MAPK pathway that is considered to control the most of the activities related to HCC condition by activating around 90 transcription factors although tyrosine kinase inhibitor Sorafenib is used as potential inhibitor of MAPK pathway by inhibiting RAF in HCC and Renal carcinoma (Cabrera et al., 2011).

6. Evaluation of cytokines in HCC patients with HCV-related cirrhosis

The serum levels of 50 different cytokines, chemokines and growth factors were evaluated in patients affected by HCC with chronic HCV-related hepatitis and liver cirrhosis using multiplex biometric ELISA-based immunoassay (Capone et al., 2010). The HCC patients showed a different secretion profile of these proteins compared to healthy controls. Greater amounts of IL-1α, IL-3, IL-12p40, IL-6, IL-8, IL-10, CCL27, CXCL10, CXCL1, IFN-α2, M-CSF, GM-CSF, CXCL9, β-NGF, SCF, SCGF-β, CXCL12, TNF-β were secreted by the HCC patients. No correlation was observed between serum levels and patients age/gender or between patients with a solitary tumour and those with multiple tumours. In particular, the attention was focused only on the proinflammatory molecules (IL-1α, IL-6, IL-8, IL-12p40, GM-CSF, CCL27, CXCL1, CXCL9, CXCL10, CXCL12, β-NGF) that were found to be significantly increased in HCC patients compared to healthy controls. The significantly increased serum levels of IL-6 and IL-8 found in HCC patients agreed with data reported in other studies (Ataseven et al., 2006; Burger et al., 2006). In particular, IL-8 levels measured in HCC patients were found to be increased, and correlated significantly with large tumor size (> 5 cm) suggesting that IL-8 may be involved in disease progression and might prove to be both a useful marker of tumor invasiveness and an independent prognostic factor for HCC patients (Burger et al., 2006, Capone et al., 2010).

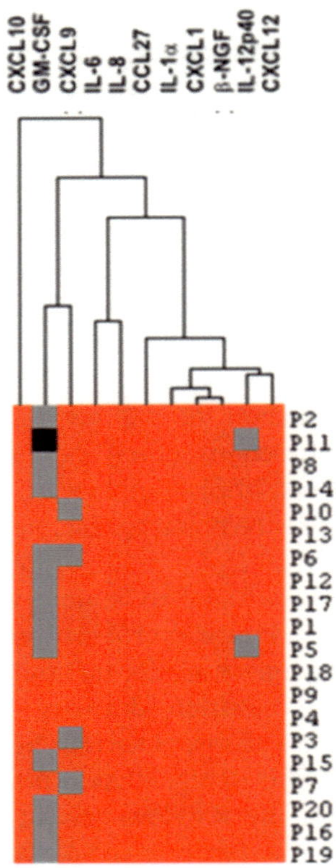

Fig. 5. Protein hierarchy assessed by a computational clustering analysis. More specifically, the length of branches indicates, in inverse proportion, the similarity of protein concentrations, and the scale of protein intensity is indicated by the different colors: over-expressed cytokines, chemokines and growth factors in red, lower values in grey, and values equal to zero in black.

Since IL-8 and IL-6 concentrations correlated significantly with large tumor size (p-value < 0.05 and $R > 0.83$), this confirmed the clinical significance of IL-6 as a prognostic factor of cancer and, in particular, its association with the development of HCC (Łukaszewicz et al., 2007; Wong et al., 2009; Nakagawa et al., 2009). Indeed, CXCL10 levels correlated both with any tumour size and with transaminase levels suggesting that it could be used as marker of liver inflammation status and cancer progression. CXCL12 is known to play a role both in pathogenesis by promoting tumor growth and malignancy, and in the HCC metastatic network by recruiting endothelial cell tumor progenitors (Liu et al., 2008; Burns et al., 2006; Kryczek et al., 2007). Recently, some papers have suggested that β-NGF was involved in cancer growth and metastasis and was detected in diseased liver tissues; in fact this protein has been suggested to be involved in chronic inflammation leading to cancer (Rasi et al., 2007). The correlation evaluation between the concentrations of over-expressed pro-inflammatory molecules measured in HCC patients showed that β-NGF correlated with IL-

1α, IL-12p40, CCL27, CXCL1 and CXCL12. This was confirmed by the related computational clustering analysis which shows that the molecules cluster in two groups, as demonstrated by branches joining them. In particular, β-NGF was grouped with the proteins indicated above (Fig. 5). Therefore, it is possible to suggest that a panel composed of β-NGF and these five proteins may be useful for diagnostic/prognostic purposes.

In conclusion, this approach showed that some pro-inflammatory molecules were significantly up-regulated in these patients, and highlighted the complexity of the cytokine network in this disease. Moreover, this suggests the need to monitor these proteins in order to define a profile that could characterize patients with HCC or to help identify useful markers. In fact, this could lead to better definition of the disease state, and to an increased understanding of the relationships between chronic inflammation and cancer (Capone et al., 2010).

7. Evaluation of cytokines in patients with chronic HCV or with HCV-related cirrhosis

The serum concentrations of a panel of 30 cytokines, chemokines and growth factors were evaluated in patients with chronic inflammation (HC) and liver cirrhosis (LC), and in healthy donors by multiplex biometric ELISA-based assays (Costantini et al., 2010a). The molecules that showed different serum levels in patients respect to healthy controls are reported in Table 1.

	HC vs controls	LC vs controls
IL-1a	0.0196*	0.0077**
IL-1b	<0.0001***	<0.0001***
IL-2R	0.0355*	0.0053**
IL-6	0.0032**	0.0024**
IL-8	0.0004***	0.0001***
CXCL1	0.0076**	0.0034**
CXCL9	0.0004***	0.0002***
CXCL10	0.0015**	0.0003***
CXCL12	0.0364*	0.0443*
MIF	0.04*	0.0033**
b-NGF	0.0008***	0.0002***
HGF		0.0028**

Table 1. P values obtained for all significant molecules in HC and LC patients respect to controls using the nonparametric Mann-Whitney U test.

Greater amounts of IL-1α, IL-1β, IL-2R, IL-6, IL-8, CXCL1, CXCL9, CXCL10, CXCL12, MIF, and β-NGF were secreted by both HC and LC patients.

In particular, in the chronic inflammation and liver cirrhosis patients the same proteins were increased and the only difference was related to HGF being resulted significant and up-regulated only in the patients with liver cirrhosis and not in those with chronic inflammation. In particular, HGF is a multifunctional growth factor that regulates growth and cell motility, exerts mitogenic effects on hepatocytes and epithelial cells and plays diverse roles in organ development, tissue regeneration, and tumor progression (Gentile et al., 2008). Moreover, it is implicated with IL-6, IL-8 and IL-1 in the hepatic stellate cell activation pathway.

However, numerous reports have examined the relationship between HGF and either the facilitation or suppression of HCC occurrence and have suggested that this growth factor could be used as index of cellular growth and of HCC development in liver cirrhosis patients (Yagamamim et al., 2002). In fact, it is interesting that the amount of this molecule was significantly different in liver cirrhosis patients in respect to both healthy controls and chronic inflammation patients and that its concentration in HCC patients was higher than in liver cirrhosis patients. This means that HGF increased in the progression of chronic inflammation leading to liver cirrhosis and cancer and can be used for predicting the occurrence of HCC in chronic HCV-related liver diseases (Costantini et al., 2010a).

7.1 Chronic inflammation versus liver cirrhosis patients

Since IL-1α, IL-1β, IL-2R, IL-6, IL-8, CXCL1, CXCL9, CXCL10, CXCL12, MIF, and β-NGF were increased in both HC and LC patients in respect to healthy control subjects, their mean concentrations were compared by t-test. Fig. 6 shows that the concentrations of all the proteins and, in particular, IL-8, CXCL9 and β -NGF were higher (with $p<0.05$) in patients with liver cirrhosis than in those with chronic inflammation. Afterwards, comparing the serum levels of all cytokines, chemokines and growth factors in HC and LC patients respect to those in HCC patients tested in our recent paper (Capone et al.,2010) is resulted that the mean concentrations of all molecules resulted higher in HCC patients than in those with liver cirrhosis. This indicates that the expression of these pro-inflammatory molecules tends to increase in the chronic inflammation progression leading to liver cirrhosis and HCC and, thus, their evaluation could be used for prognostic studies. The serum levels of statistically significant cytokines, chemokines and growth factors in the HC and LC patients were correlated with clinical data by using the Pearson correlation coefficient. In chronic inflammation patients IL-1α, IL-2R, MIF and β-NGF showed a significant correlation with a positive correlation coefficient between them and with the transaminase values, that were higher in these patients than in healthy controls. Therefore these proteins can be considered as index of immune activation. In particular, these results agreed with literature data reporting that IL-1 and IL-2R participate in the progression from liver injury to fibrosis (Zekri et al., 2010) and that β-NGF is involved in liver cancer growth and metastasis and can be used as an index of chronic infection leading to LC and HCC (Gieling et al., 2009). Indeed, this work suggested for the first time a role of MIF in HCV-related chronic inflammation patients because an increased serum MIF was reported only in HBV patients (Kimura et al., 2006). Moreover, CXCL1, CXCL9, CXCL10 and HFG in liver cirrhosis patients showed a significant correlation and, in details, a positive correlation coefficient between them and a negative correlation coefficient with the albumin values, that were lower in these patients respect to controls. Concerning that HGF resulted the only molecule that was statistically different between HC and LC patients, these data suggested that the four proteins could be useful for diagnostic/prognostic purposes.

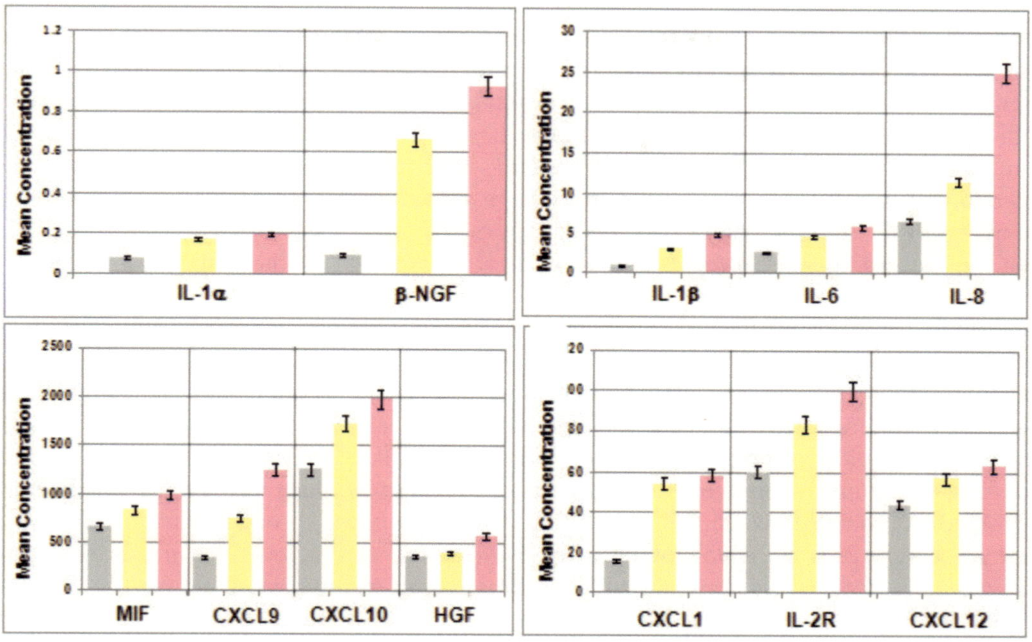

Fig. 6. Mean concentrations of significant cytokines, chemokines and growth factors in healthy control subjects (light grey) and in chronic inflammation (yellow) and liver cirrhosis (pink) patients.

7.2 Chronic inflammation patients with different fibrosis stages

After the classification of their fibrosis stage of chronic inflammation by F Ishak index (Costantini et al., 2010a), the patients were divided in three different subgroups corresponding to F2, F3 and F4 stages and their mean concentrations of significant molecules in three groups compared by t-test. No relevant difference was found between chronic inflammation patients with F3 and F4 fibrosis grade because they corresponded to two already advanced fibrosis stages. Comparing F2 and F4 patients the concentrations of IL-2R, IL-6, IL-8, CXCL9, CXCL10, CXCL12 and MIF were found statistically higher (with $p<0.05$) in chronic inflammation patients with F4 fibrosis grade in respect to F2 fibrosis grade (Costantini et al., 2010a). These data agreed with a recent paper reporting that CXCL9 and CXCL10 were significantly elevated in patients with advanced fibrosis (Zeremski et al. 2009).

In conclusion these results suggested that i) IL-2R, IL-6, IL-8, CXCL9, CXCL10, CXCL12 and MIF could be markers of the progression of chronic hepatitis C leading to liver cirrhosis by increasing fibrosis and ii) HGF, being over-expressed only in liver cirrhosis patients, could be index of fibrosis progression versus liver cirrhosis.

However this work indicated the need of cytokinome data mining system for a predictive medicine, and suggested the utility to integrate all the cytokine data in a network and to make drug design studies on the chemokines resulted significant in the progression from chronic inflammation to HCC.

8. The need of cytokinome data mining system for a predictive medicine

The progressive increase in electronically stored clinical data is opening the possibility of carrying out large-scale studies aimed to discover correlations between new research data and related diseases. For these reasons, many relational databases have implemented data mining techniques (Harrison, 2008) that have been described as the 'extraction of implicit, previously unknown and potentially useful information', such as associations and correlations between data elements from large repositories of data (Lee & Siau, 2001). However, the scientific community needs clinical laboratory databases to collect medical data related to diseases progression and therapy response. In the last years, particular attention has been focused on the protein class comprising cytokines, chemokines and growth factors, because they play a crucial role in promoting angiogenesis, metastasis and subversion of adaptive immunity. Since the control of cytokine production is highly complex and multifactorial, their effects are mediated through multiple regulatory networks. The intricate complexity of these networks clearly conceals the role that a single cytokine may play in the pathogenesis of the disease. Therefore, it is more informative to investigate the immunopathogenesis of a disease process by analyzing a multiple panel of cytokines (Costantini et al., 2009). Utilizing a bead-based broad-spectrum multiplex immunoassay, it is possible not only to evaluate the serum levels of those cytokines ensemble that effectively correlate with the progression of the disease activity but also to define the immunomodulatory effects of a therapy even after months of treatment (Sato et al., 2009; Ozturk et al., 2009; Capone et al., 2010). This indicates that the definition and evaluation of a human cytokinome represents an important future tool to analyze the interaction network of cytokines both in healthy individuals and in patients affected by different diseases. In fact, it will permit one to understand and investigate how the regression of a chronic inflammation process, by acting on the cellular populations of cytokines, can block the progression of a cancer and, therefore, it can be a useful prognostic and diagnostic tool for clinicians.

For these reasons, a portal with user-friendly interfaces, which can be used both by physicians and researchers not only to collect and to correlate clinical data and serum levels of cytokines but also to know quickly what cytokines, chemokines or growth factors are significant in the progression state of a given disease, represents an important and useful tool for clinical prognosis and therapy studies.

Recently it has been developed a software named CDMS (Clinical Data Mining Software) and accessible at the URL: http://www.cro-m.eu/CDMS/ to collect clinical data and serum levels of many cytokines, chemokines and growth factors evaluated on healthy subjects and patients affected by different diseases (i.e. chronic hepatitis C and HCC) using multiplex immunoassays (Evangelista et al., 2010). Moreover, some statistical tools were implemented to correlate significatively clinical and experimental data and to quickly compare standardized cytokinome profile of a patient against a whole data bank that collects cytokinome data from some different diseases. CDMS allows certified users to access some of its services on the basis of their privileges. In detail, physicians and researchers can access the patient administration and statistical analysis sections, and all other authorized figures can access only statistical analysis section. In the patient administration section, there are case histories of patients with information related to their diagnosis, biological analyses as well as clinical data, and evaluations of 50 cytokine concentrations. Moreover, for the same patients, it is possible to insert the cytokine profiles evaluated at different times to compare and evaluate results at different stages of the disease. In the statistical analysis section, the user can select the disease, filter the patients on the basis of gender, age and experiment date and select the most appropriate tool to perform the statistical analysis. In particular, we have implemented: (i) median, mean, variance, standard deviation, min and max values for the selected protein; (ii) t-test value related to the comparison between cytokine concentrations in control group and patients; (iii) Pearson correlation between different cytokines with related graph; (iv) Pearson correlation between each cytokine and some clinical data (i.e. tumor size) with related graph. CDMS represents the first 'user-friendly' tool that can be used by researchers as well as physicians and clinicians to significatively correlate clinical data and cytokine profiles and to identify what cytokines can be significant for the examined disease at a given time. Using its available statistical tools, it has been possible to identify the cyto-chemokines pattern involved in the chronic inflammation processes versus HCC and to verify that IL-8 correlated significantly with large tumor size (>5 cm), and it can be used both as a useful marker of tumor invasiveness and as an independent prognostic factor for HCC patients (Capone et al., 2010; Evangelista et al. 2010). Therefore, this tool can be a useful support to develop a reliable predictive medicine and to improve or discover new predictive relationships among data groups.

9. The need for structural studies of cytokine/receptor complex: The example of CXCL9, CXCL10 and CXCL11 chemokines and their membrane receptor CXCR3

The data obtained on sera of patients with chronic inflammation (HC), liver cirrhosis (LC) and HCC suggested the utility to make drug design studies on three CXCL9, CXCL10 and CXCL11 chemokines for obtaining molecules able to block the progression of fibrotic damage in chronic inflammation patients leading to liver cirrhosis and, then, to HCC (Costantini et al., 2010a).

CXCL9, CXCL10 and CXCL11 are members of a family of small (8–10 kDa) proteins, the chemokines (or chemoattractant cytokines). They play a key role in immune and inflammatory responses by promoting recruitment and activation of different subpopulations of leukocytes, hence they have important proinflammatory and immune modulatory functions (Booth et al., 2002). CXCL9 as well as do CXCL10 and CXCL11 binds and activates the same receptor CXCR3 (chemokine (C-X-C motif) receptor 3) (Booth et al., 2004).

CXCR3 is mainly expressed on activated T and Natural Killer (NK) cells (Zeremski et al., 2007). While CXCL11, CXCL10, and CXCL9 are agonists for CXCR3, they can also act as antagonists for CCR3 (Loetscher et al. 2001). Tumor cells aberrantly express chemokines and/or chemokine receptors, and the interaction of chemokine ligand-receptor pairs is increasingly implicated as a mediator of tumor growth and metastasis. In particular, CXCR3 has now been identified in a variety of malignant cells, including melanoma, breast and prostate carcinomas, neuroblastoma, and a subset of B cell lymphomas (Colvin et al., 2004). CXCL9 and CXCL10 may promote the recruitment of lymphocytes to HCC and released from the HCC cells may induce lymphocyte infiltration. Ruehlmann et al. (2001) suggested that the expression of CXCL9 and CXCL10 might lead to lymphocytic infiltration into HCC, and gene therapy with these CXC chemokines may be effective for patients with HCC. Hrnce, during the past few years, several studies have demonstrated a pathogenenetic role of CXCR3 and its ligands in human inflammatory diseases suggesting the involvement of various segments of their sequences. Therefore, the blockade of CXCR3 interactions with its ligands in vivo has been suggested as a possible therapeutic goal for the treatment of these disorders (Xanthou et al. 2003). Recently the three-dimensional structure of CXCL9 and CXCR3 has been simulated (Trotta et al., 2009). Successively, also the CXCL9/CXCR3 complex (Fig. 7) has been modelled in comparison to CXCL10/CXCR3 and CXCL11/CXCR3 complexes in order to evaluate in details the interaction residues involved in the formation of the complexes and their properties as important structural features to be used for drug design (Trotta et al., 2009).

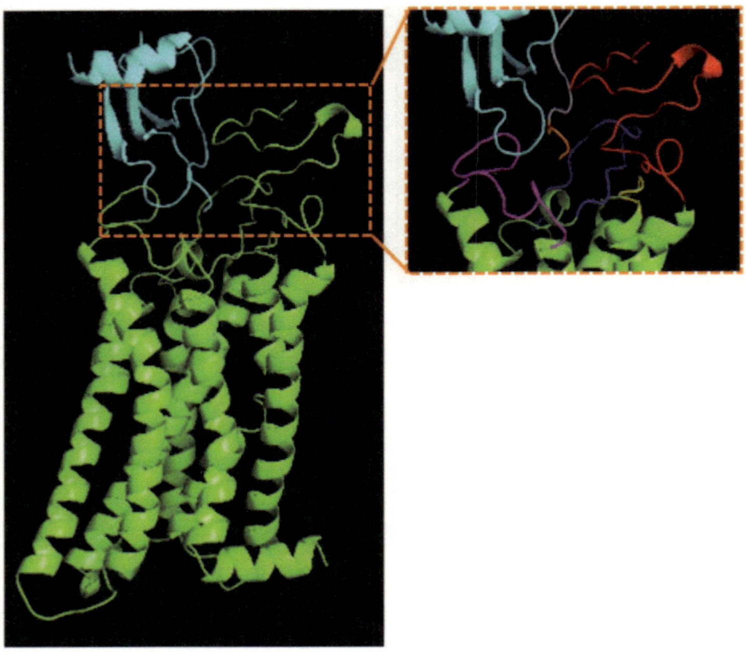

Fig. 7. 3D model of CXCL9/CXCR3 complex where CXCR3 is reported with green ribbon but CXCL9 with cyan ribbon. In details, the loops of the interaction regions are evidenced (i.e. N-terminal, loop1, loop 2 and loop3 of the receptor are shown in red, yellow, blue and magenta, respectively, and N-terminal and N-loop of the chemokine in orange and grey, respectively).

Three chemokines resulted always to interact with their receptor by N-terminal region and N-loop but the receptor by N-terminal region and three extracellular loops according to precedent studies (Xanthou et al. 2003). Moreover the analysis of three complexes showed that the N-loop of all three chemokines was essential for binding the N-terminal region of CXCR3 in agreement to Clark-Lewis et al. (2003) whereas the loop 1 of CXCR3 was essential to bind only CXCL11 and CXCL10 as well as indicated by Xanthou et al. 2003. The analysis of the physical-chemical properties of residues present in these regions in CXCR3 highlighted that: i) N-terminal, loop1 and loop 2 contained some aromatic residues (Phe, Tyr and Trp); ii) N-terminal presented three negatively charged residues (3 Glu), loop2 one (Asp) but loop 3 three (2 Asp and 1 Glu) and iii) both loop 2 and loop 3 had two positively charged residues (2 Arg).These data suggested that the predominant interaction between CXCR3 and its ligands was on electrostatic basis and was favored also from the presence of positively charged residues located in N-terminal region of three chemokines (i.e. three in CXCL9 and CXCL11 and two in CXCL10). Moreover, the presence of aromatic residues stabilized mainly the interaction between CXCR3 and CXCL11, having two Phe residues in N-terminal and might play an important role to favour the stacking interactions with putative drugs and organic compounds.

Therefore the study of the structural basis of the CXCR3 receptor-ligand system through the modeling of three complexes CXCL9/CXCR3, CXCL10/CXCR3, and CXCL11/CXCR3 has evidenced the interaction regions between three chemokines and CXCR3 (Trotta et al., 2009). The related analysis of the physico-chemical properties of residues in these regions suggested that the predominant interaction between CXCR3 and its ligands was on electrostatic basis and favored by the presence of positively charged residues located in the N-terminal region of the three chemokines. The comparison of the three complexes showed that CXCR3 had the highest affinity for CXCL11 in terms of binding energy and higher number of H-bonds, of salt bridges and of interaction residues (Trotta et al., 2009). Since the in silico modelling provided a time- and cost-effective tool for the screening of molecules as well as for designing of novel molecules of desired activity, it was possible to focus the attention on CXCL11. Therefore, in order to develop putative antagonists to CXCR3, a peptide, derived from the N-terminal region of CXCL11, has been synthesized. Preliminary results of this study, taken as a whole, indicated that this peptide may be regarded as a small molecule that, opportunely modified, could represent a good model for an antagonist to CXCR3. Hence, further studies are currently underway to design analogs of this peptide to optimize its physico-chemical properties and to improve the electrostatic and stacking interactions with CXCR3 for novel therapeutic approaches.

10. Conclusion

Over the past several years, there has been a renaissance of research into connection between inflammation and cancer. The inflammation can play a role in tumor suppression by stimulating an antitumor immune response, but more often, under certain conditions, it appears to stimulate tumor development (Mantovani et al., 2008). The intensity and nature of the inflammation could explain this apparent contradiction. In fact, the inflammation may become chronic when the inflammatory stimulus persists. However, it has been suggested that inflammation associated with cancer is similar to that seen with chronic inflammation, which includes the production of growth and angiogenic factors that stimulate tissue repair, factors that can also promote cancer-cell survival, implantation, and growth (Allavena et al., 2008). Thus immune response can promote anticancer effects or carcinogenesis and tumor growth (Mantovani et al., 2008). Cytokines are among molecules that play an important role in the evolution of these processes. In fact, they are proteins that are expressed before and during the inflammatory process and play a key role at the various disease levels so that they can be considered as specific markers of cancer and of its specific evolutive steps (Capone et al., 2010; Costantini et al., 2010a).

The studying model chosen in this chapter is the hepatocellular carcinoma (HCC) that represents a major health problem worldwide being the fifth most common malignancy in men and the eighth in women and the third most common cause of cancer-related death in the world. Indeed its incidence is increasing dramatically, with marked variations among geographic regions, racial and ethnic groups, relatively to the exposure documented environmental risk factors (Castello et al., 2010a, 2010b). In particular, Southern Italy has the

highest rates of HCC in Europe (Fusco et al., 2008). HCC derives from a long clinical history in patients with HCV or HBV infection. In fact, about 80% of newly infected patients develop chronic infection; an estimated 10% to 20% will develop cirrhosis and 1% to 5% advance to end-stage liver cancer (HCC) over a period of 20 to 30 years (Fig. 1).
Recently the serum levels of many cytokines have been evaluated by a broad spectrum bead-based multiplex immunoassay both in patients with chronic HCV or with HCV-related cirrhosis and in patients with HCC patients with HCV-related cirrhosis. These studies have evidenced that some interleukins and chemokines (Fig. 5 and 6) are putative markers of the progression of chronic hepatitis C leading to liver cirrhosis by increasing fibrosis and can be used as templates for designing new drugs able to block the progression of the inflammatory processes (Capone et al., 2010; Costantini et al., 2010a).
However, all the data related to the cytokine evaluations should be modeled computationally by using graphs or networks connecting the various data groups in terms of dynamic probabilistic maps of metabolic and/or physiological activities and/or pathogenetic pathways. In fact only in this way it is possible to define the human cytokinome that can be an useful tool to analyze the interaction network of cytokines both in healthy individuals and in patients affected from HCC (Costantini et al., 2010b). Therefore, CDMS represents the first 'user-friendly' tool that can be used by researchers as well as physicians and clinicians to significatively correlate clinical data and cytokine profiles and to identify what cytokines can be significant for the examined disease at a given time (Evangelista et al., 2010). However further studies will regard the opening of the data sets to other diseases and the implementation of other statistical tools and classification methods to improve or to discover new predictive relationships among data groups.

11. References

Allavena, P.; Sica, A.; Solinas, G.; Porta, C.; Mantovani, A. (2008) The inflammatory microenvironment in tumor progression: the role of tumor-associated macrophages. *Crit. Rev. Oncol. Hematol.*, Vol.66, pp. 1–9, ISSN 1040-8428.

Altekruse, S.F.; McGlynn, K.A.; Reichman, M.E. (2009) Hepatocellular Carcinoma Incidence, Mortality, and Survival Trends in the United States From 1975 to 2005. *J. Clin. Oncol.*, Vol.27, No.9, pp. 1485-91, ISSN 0732-183X.

Ataseven, H.; Bahcecioglu, I.H.; Kuzu, N.; Yalniz, M.; Celebi, S.; Erensoy, A.; Ustundag, B. (2006) The levels of ghrelin, leptin, TNF-alpha, and IL-6 in liver cirrhosis and hepatocellular carcinoma due to HBV and HDV infection. *Mediators Inflamm.*, Vol.2006, pp. 78380, ISSN 0962-9351.

Balkwill, F.; Mantovani, A. (2001) Inflammation and cancer: back to Virchow? *Lancet*, Vol.357, pp. 539-45, ISSN 0140-6736.

Bing, H.; Xiaojie, Q.; Peng, L.; Lishan, W.; Qi, L.; Tieliu, S. (2010) HCCNet: an integrated network database of hepatocellular carcinoma. Cell Research, Vol.20, pp.732-734, ISSN 1001-0602

Boettler, T.; Spangenberg, H.C.; Neumann-Haefelin, C.; Panther, E.; Urbani, S.; Ferrari, C.; Blum, H.E.; von Weizsäcker, F.; Thimme, R. (2005) T cells with a CD4+CD25+ regulatory phenotype suppress in vitro proliferation of virus-specific CD8+ T cells during chronic hepatitis C virus infection. *J. Virol.*, Vol.79, No.12, pp. 7860-7, ISSN 0022-538X.

Booth, V.; Keizer, D.W.; Kamphuis, M.B.; Clark-Lewis, I.; Sykes, B.D. (2002) The CXCR3 binding chemokine IP-10/CXCL10: structure and receptor interactions. *Biochemistry,* Vol.41, pp. 10418-25, ISSN 0006-2960.

Booth, V.; Clark-Lewis, I.; Sykes, B.D. (2004) NMR structure of CXCR3 binding chemokine CXCL11 (ITAC). *Protein Science,* Vol.13, pp. 2022–2028, ISSN 0961-8368.

Bosetti, C.; Levi, F.; Boffetta, P.; Lucchini, F.; Negri, E.; La Vecchia, C. (2008) Trends in mortality from hepatocellular carcinoma in Europe, 1980-2004. *Hepatology,* Vol.48, No.1, pp. 137-45, ISSN 0270-9139.

Bowen, D.G.; Walker, C.M. (2005) Adaptive immune responses in acute and chronic hepatitis C virus infection. *Nature,* Vol.436, No.7053, pp.946-52, ISSN 1537-6591.

Budhu, A.; Wang, X.W. The role of cytokines in hepatocellular carcinoma. *J. Leukoc. Biol.,* Vol.80, No.6, pp. 1197-213, ISSN 0741-5400.

Burger, J.A., Kipps, T.J. (2006) CXCR4: a key receptor in the crosstalk between tumor cells and their microenvironment. *Blood,* Vol.107, pp. 1761-7, ISSN 0006-4971.

Burns, J.M.; Summers, B.C.; Wang, Y.; Melikian, A.; Berahovich, R.; Miao, Z.; Penfold, M.E.; Sunshine, M.J.; Littman, D.R.; Kuo, C.J.; Wei, K.; McMaster, B.E.; Wright, K.; Howard, M.C.; Schall, T.J. (2006) A novel chemokine receptor for SDF-1 and I-TAC involved in cell survival, cell adhesion, and tumor development. *J. Exp. Med.,* Vol.203, pp. 2201-13, ISSN 0022-1007.

Cabrera, R.; Tu, Z.; Xu, Y.; Firpi, R.J.; Rosen, H.R.; Liu, C.; Nelson, D.R. (2004) An immunomodulatory role for CD4+CD25+ regulatory T lymphocytes in hepatitis C virus infection. *Hepatology,* Vol.40, No.5, pp. 1062-71, ISSN 0270-9139.

Cabrera, R.; Pannu, D.S.; Caridi, J.; Firpi, R.J., Soldevila-Pico, C.; Morelli, G.; Clark, V.; Suman, A.; George, T.J.Jr.; Nelson, D.R. (2011) The combination of sorafenib with transarterial chemoembolisation for hepatocellular carcinoma. Aliment. Pharmacol. Ther., 2011 May 23.

Capone, F.; Costantini, S.; Guerriero, E.; Calemma, R.; Napolitano, M.; Scala, S.; Izzo, F.; Castello, G. (2010) Cytokine serum levels in patients with hepatocellular carcinoma. *Eur. Cytok. Net.,* Vol.21, No.2, pp. 99-104.

Castello, G.; Costantini, S.; Scala, S. (2010a) Targeting the inflammation in HCV-associated hepatocellular carcinoma: a role in the prevention and treatment. *J. Trasl. Med.,* Vol.8, pp.109, ISSN 14795876.

Castello, G.; Scala, S.; Palmieri, G.; Curley, S.A., Izzo, F. (2010b) HCV-related hepatocellular carcinoma: From chronic inflammation to cancer. Clin. Immunol., Vol.134, No.3, pp. 237-50, ISSN 1521-7035.

Chiesa, R.; Donato, F.; Tagger, A.; Favret, M.; Ribero, M.L.; Nardi, G.; Gelatti, U.; Bucella, E.; Tomasi, E.; Portolani, N.; Bonetti, M.; Bettini, L.; Pelizzari, G.; Salmi, A.; Savio, A.; Garatti, M.; Callea, F. (2000) Etiology of hepatocellular carcinoma in Italian patients with and without cirrhosis. *Cancer Epidemiology, Biomarkers & Prevention,* Vol. 9, pp. 213-6, ISSN 1538-7755.

Clark-Lewis, I.; Mattioli, I.; Gong, J.H.; Loetscher, P. (2003) Structure-function relationship between the human chemokine receptor CXCR3 and its ligands. *J. Biol. Chem.,* Vol.278, pp. 289-95, ISSN 0021-9258.

Colvin, R.A.; Campanella, G.S.V.; Sun, J.; Luster, A.D. (2004) Intracellular domain of CXCR3 that mediate CXCL9, CXCL10, and CXCL11 function. *J. Biol. Chem.*, Vol.279, pp. 30219-30227, ISSN 0021-9258.

Costantini, S.; Autiero, I.; Colonna, G. (2008) On new challenge for the Bioinformatics. *Bioinformation*, Vol.3, No.5, pp.238-239, ISSN 0973-8894.

Costantini, S.; Capone, F.; Guerriero, E.; Castello, G. (2009) An approach for understanding the inflammation and cancer relationship. *Immunol. Lett.*, Vol.126, pp. 91–92, ISSN 0165-2478.

Costantini, S.; Capone, F.; Guerriero, E.; Maio, P.; Colonna, G.; Castello, G. (2010a) Serum cytokine levels as putative prognostic markers in the progression of chronic HCV hepatitis to cirrhosis. *Eur. Cytokine Netw.*, Vol.21, No.4, pp. 251-6.

Costantini, S.; Castello, G.; Colonna, G. (2010b) Human Cytokinome: a new challenge for systems biology. *Bioinformation*, Vol.5, No.4, pp. 166-167, ISSN 0973-2063.

Coussens, L.M.; Werb, Z. (2002) Inflammation and cancer. *Nature*, Vol.420, pp. 860-7, ISSN 0028-0836.

De Benedetti, V.M.; Welsh, J.A.; Yu, M.C.; Bennett, W.P. (1996) p53 mutations in hepatocellular carcinoma related to oral contraceptive use. Carcinogenesis, Vol.17, pp. 145-149, ISSN 0143-3334.

Evangelista, D.; Colonna, G.; Miele, M.; Cutugno, F.; Castello, G.; Desantis, S.; Costantini, S., (2010) CDMS (Clinical Data Mining Software): a cytokinome data mining system for a predictive medicine of chronic inflammatory diseases. *PEDS*, Vol.123, No.12, pp. 899-902, ISSN 1741-0126.

Fassio, E. (2010) Hepatitis C and hepatocellular carcinoma. *Ann. Hepatol.* Vol.9, pp. 119-22, ISSN 1665-2681.

Fusco, M.; Girardi, E.; Piselli, P.; Palombino, R.; Polesel, J.; Maione, C.; Scognamiglio, P.; Pisanti, F.A.; Solmone, M.; Di Cicco, P.; Ippolito, G.; Franceschi, S.; Serraino, D. (2008) Epidemiology of viral hepatitis infections in an area of southern Italy with high incidence rates of liver cancer. *Eur. J. Cancer.*, Vol.44, No.6, pp. 847-53, ISSN 0959-8049.

Gentile, A.; Trusolino, L.; Comoglio, P.M. (2008) The Met tyrosine kinase receptor in development and cancer. *Cancer Metastasis Reviews*, Vol.27, pp. 85-94, ISSN 0167-7659.

Germano, G.; Allavena, P.; Mantovani, A. (2008) Cytokines as a key component of cancer related inflammation. *Cytokine*, Vol.43, No.3, pp. 374–9, ISSN 0008-5472.

Gieling, R.G.; Wallace, K.; Han, Y.P. (2009) Interleukin-1 participates in the progression from liver injury to fibrosis. *Am. J. Physiol. Gastrointest. Liver Physiol.*, Vol.296, pp. G1324-G1331, ISSN 0193-1857.

Harrison, J.H. (2008) Introduction to the mining of clinical data. *Clin. Lab. Med.*, Vol.28, pp. 1–7, ISSN 0272-2712.

Huang, Y.S.; Hwang, S.J.; Chan, C.Y.; Wu, J.C.; Chao, Y.; Chang, F.Y.; Lee, S.D. (1999) Serum levels of cytokines in hepatitis C-related liver disease: a longitudinal study. *Zhonghua Yi Xue Za Zhi (Taipei)*, Vol.62, No.6, pp. 327-33, ISSN 0578-1337.

Irmak, M.B.; Ince, G.; Ozturk, M.; Cetin-Atalay, R. (2003) Acquired tolerance of hepatocellular carcinoma cells to selenium deficiency: a selective survival mechanism? Cancer Res., Vol.63, pp. 6707-6715, ISSN 0008-5472.

Jemal, A.; Siegel, R.; Ward, E.; Murray, T.; Xu, J.; Thun, M.J. (2007) Cancer Statistics 2007. *CA Cancer J. Clin.*, Vol.57, No.1, pp. 43-66, ISSN 0007-9235.

Kimura, K.; Nagaki, M.; Nishihira, J.; Satake, S.; Kuwata, K.; Moriwaki, H. (2006) Role of Macrophage Migration Inhibitory Factor in Hepatitis B Virus-Specific Cytotoxic-T-Lymphocyte-Induced Liver Injury. *Clinical And Vaccine Immunology*, Vol.13, pp. 415-9, ISSN 1556-6811.

Kryczek, I.; Wei, S.; Keller, E.; Liu, R.; Zou, W. (2007) Stroma-derived factor (SDF-1/CXCL12) and human tumor pathogenesis. *Am. J. Physiol. Cell. Physiol.*, Vol.292, pp. C987-C995, ISSN 0363-6143.

Kusumoto, T.; Kodama, J.; Seki, N.; Nakamura, K.; Hongo, A.; Hiramatsu, Y. (2010) Clinical significance of syndecan-1 and versican expression in human epithelial ovarian cancer. Oncol. Rep., Vol.23 (4), pp. 917–925, ISSN 1021-335X.

Liu, H.; Pan, Z.; Li, A.; Fu, S.; Lei, Y.; Sun, H.; Wu, M.; Zhou, W. (2008) Roles of chemokine receptor 4 (CXCR4) and chemokine ligand 12 (CXCL12) in metastasis of hepatocellular carcinoma cells. *Cell. Mol. Immunol.*, Vol.5, pp. 373-8, ISSN 1672-7681.

Lee, S.; Siau, K. (2001) A review of data mining techniques. *Ind. Manage. Data Syst.*, Vol.100, pp. 41–46, ISSN 0263-5577.

Lee, J.S.; Lee, J.J.; Seo, J.S. (2005) HSP70 deficiency results in activation of c-Jun N-terminal Kinase, extracellular signal-regulated kinase, and caspase-3 in hyperosmolarity-induced apoptosis. J. Biol. Chem., Vol.280, pp. 6634-6641, ISSN 0021-9258.

Loetscher, P.; Pellegrino, A.; Gong, J.H.; Mattioli, I.; Loetscher, M.; Bardi, G.; Baggiolini, M.; Clark-Lewis, I. (2001) The ligands of CXC chemokine receptor 3, I-TAC, MIG, and IP-10, are natural antagonists for CCR3. *The Journal of Biological Chemistry*, Vol.276, pp. 2986–2991, ISSN 0021-9258.

Łukaszewicz, M.; Mroczko, B.; Szmitkowski, M. (2007) Clinical significance of interleukin-6 (IL-6) as a prognostic factor of cancer disease. *Pol. Arch. Med. Wewn.*, Vol.117, pp. 247-51.

Lu, H.; Ouyang, W.; Huang, C. (2006) Inflammation, a key event in cancer development. *Mol. Cancer Res.*, Vol.4, No.4, pp. 221-33, ISSN 1541-7786.

Macarthur, M.; Hold, G.L.; El-Omar, E.M. (2004) Inflammation and cancer. II. Role of chronic inflammation and cytokine polymorphisms in the pathogenesis of gastrointestinal malignancy. *Am. J. Physiol. Gastrointest. Liver Physiol.*, Vol.286, pp. G515-20, ISSN 0193-1857.

Mancino, A.; Schioppa, T.; Larghi, P.; Pasqualini, F.; Nebuloni, M.; Chen, I.H.; Sozzani, S.; Austyn, J.M.; Mantovani, A.; Sica, A. (2008) Divergent effects of hypoxia on dendritic cell functions. *Blood*, Vol.112, pp. 3723–34, ISSN 0006-4971.

Mantovani, A.; Pierotti, M.A. (2008) Cancer and inflammation: a complex relationship. *Cancer Lett.*, Vol.267, pp. 180–1, ISSN 1541-7786.

Miranda, P.W.; Oehler, M.k.; Ricciardelli, C. (2011) Role of Versican, Hyaluronan and CD44 in Ovarian Cancer Metastasis. Int. J. Mol. Sci., Vol.12, pp. 1009-1029, ISSN 1422-0067

Nakagawa, H.; Maeda, S.; Yoshida, H.; Tateishi, R.; Masuzaki, R.; Ohki, T.; Hayakawa, Y.; Kinoshita, H.; Yamakado, M.; Kato, N.; Shiina, S.; Omata, M. (2009) Serum IL-6 levels and the risk for hepatocarcinogenesis in chronic hepatitis C patients: an analysis based on gender differences. *Int. J. Cancer*, Vol.125, pp. 2264-9, ISSN 0020-7136.

Nash, K.L.; Woodall, T.; Brown, A.S.; Davies, S.E.; Alexander, G.J. (2010) Hepatocellular carcinoma in patients with chronic hepatitis C virus infection without cirrhosis. *World J. Gastroenterol.*, Vol.16, No.32, pp. 4061-5, ISSN 1007-9327.

Ogata, H.; Goto, S.; Sato, K.; Fujibuchi, W.; Bono, H.; Kanehisa, M. (2000) KEGG: Kyoto Encyclopedia of Genes and Genomes. NAR, Vol.28, pp. 27-30, ISSN 0305-1048.

Ohta, M.; Tanaka, F.; Yamaguchi, H.; Sadanaga, N.; Inoue, H.; Mori, M. (2005) The high expression of Fractalkine results in a better prognosis for colorectal cancer patients. Int. J. Oncol., Vol.26, pp. 41-47, ISSN 1019-6439

Ormandy, L.A.; Hillemann, T.; Wedemeyer, H.; Manns, M.P.; Greten, T.F.; Korangy, F. (2005) Increased populations of regulatory T cells in peripheral blood of patients with hepatocellular carcinoma. *Cancer Res.*, Vol.65, No.6, pp. 2457-64, ISSN 0008-5472.

Ozturk, B.T.; Bozkurt, B.; Kerimoglu, H.; Okka, M.; Kamis, U.; Gunduz, K. (2009) Effect of serum cytokines and VEGF levels on diabetic retinopathy and macular thickness. *Mol. Vis.*, Vol.15, pp. 1906–1914, ISSN 1090-0535 .

Philip, M., Rowley, D.A.; Schreiber, H. (2004) Inflammation as a tumor promoter in cancer induction. *Semin. Cancer Biol.*, Vol.14, pp. 433-9, ISSN 1522-1059.

Porcile, C.; Bajetto, A.; Barbieri, F.; Barbero, S.; Bonavia, R.; Biglieri, M.; Pirani, P.; Florio, T.; Schettini, G. (2005) Stromal cell-derived factor-1alpha (SDF-1alpha/CXCL12) stimulates ovarian cancer cell growth through the EGF receptor transactivation. Exp. Cell Res., Vol.308, pp.241-253, ISSN 0014-4827.

Rasi, G.; Serafino, A.; Bellis, L.; Lonardo, M.T.; Andreola, F.; Zonfrillo, M.; Vennarecci, G.; Pierimarchi, P.; Sinibaldi Vallebona, P.; Ettorre, G.M.; Santoro, E.; Puoti, C. (2007) Nerve growth factor involvement in liver cirrhosis and hepatocellular carcinoma. *World J. Gastroenterol.*, Vol.13, pp. 4986-95, ISSN 1007-9327.

Rubie, C.; Frick, V. O.; Wagner, M.; Rau, B.; Weber, C.; Kruse, B.; Kempf, K.; Tilton, B.; König, J.; Schilling, M. (2006) Enhanced Expression and Clinical Significance of CC-Chemokine MIP-3α in Hepatocellular Carcinoma. Scandinavian Journal of Immunology, Vol.63, pp. 468–477, ISSN 0300-9475.

Ruehlmann, J.M.; Xiang, R.; Niethammer, A.G.; Ba, Y.; Pertl, U., Dolman, C.S.; Gillies, S.D.; Reisfeld, R.A. (2001) MIG (CXCL9) chemokine gene therapy combines with antibody-cytokine fusion protein to suppress growth and dissemination of murine colon carcinoma. *Cancer Res.*, Vol.61, pp. 8498-503, ISSN 0008-5472.

Ryder, S.D. (2003) British Society of Gastroenterology. Guidelines for the diagnosis and treatment of hepatocellular carcinoma (HCC) in adults. *Gut*, Vol.52, pp. 1-8, ISSN 0003-4819.

Sato, T.; Kusaka, S.; Shimojo, H.; Fujikado, T. (2009) Simultaneous analyses of vitreous levels of 27 cytokines in eyes with retinopathy of prematurity. *Ophthalmology*, Vol.116, pp. 2165–2169, ISSN 0161-6420.

Savill, J.; Dransfield, I.; Gregory, C.; Haslett, C. (2002) A blast from the past: clearance of apoptotic cells regulates immune responses. *Nat. Rev. Immunol.*, Vol. 2, pp. 965-75, ISSN 1474-1733.

Sanderson, R.D.; Yang, Y. (2009) Syndecan-1: a dynamic regulator of the myeloma microenvironment, Clinical and Experiemntal metastasis, Vol.25, pp. 149-159, ISSN 0262-0898.

Staib, F.; Hussain, S.P.; Hofseth, L.J.; Wang, X.W.; Harris, C.C. (2003) TP53 and liver carcinogenesis. Hum. Mutat., Vol.21, pp. 201-216, ISSN 1059-7794.

Sun, X.; Zhang, J.; Wang, L.; Xiang, T. (2008) Growth inhibition of human hepatocellular carcinoma cells by blocking STAT3 activation with decoy- ODN. Cancer lett., Vol.262, pp. 201, ISSN 0304-3835.

Trotta, T.; Costantini, S.; Colonna, G. (2009) Modelling of the membrane receptor CXCR3 and its complexes with CXCL9,CXCL10 and CXCL11 chemokines: Putative target for new drug design. *Molecular Immunology*, Vol.47, pp. 332-339, ISSN 0161-5890.

Turner, S.L.; Mangnall, D.; Bird, N.C.; Blair-Zajdel, M.E.; Rowena, A.D. (2010) Bunning Effects of Pro-Inflammatory Cytokines on the Production of Soluble Fractalkine and ADAM17 by HepG2 Cells. J. Gastrointestin. Liver Dis., Vol.19, pp. 265-71, ISSN 1842-1121.

Ueno, Y.; Sollano, J.D.; Farrell, G.C. (2009) Prevention of hepatocellular carcinoma complicating chronic hepatitis C. *J. Gastroenterol. Hepatol.*, Vol.24, No.4, pp. 531-6, ISSN 0815-9319 .

Wei, Y.; Cao, X.; Ou, Y.; Lu, J.; Xing, C.; Zheng, R. (2001) SeO2 induces apoptosis with down-regulation of Bcl-2 and up-regulation of p53 expression in both immortal human hepatic cell line and hepatoma cell line. Mutat. Res., Vol.490, pp. 113-121, ISSN 1383-5718.

Wong, V.W.; Yu, J.; Cheng, A.S.; Wong, G.L.; Chan, H.Y.; Chu, E.S.; Ng, E.K.; Chan, F.K.; Sung, J.J.; Chan, H.L. (2009) High serum interleukin-6 level predicts future hepatocellular carcinoma development in patients with chronic hepatitis B. *Int. J. Cancer*, Vol.124, pp. 2766-70, ISSN 0020-7136.

Yamagamim, H.; Moriyama, M.; Matsumura, H.; Aoki, H.; Shimizu, T.; Saito, T.; Kaneko, M.; Shioda, A.; Tanaka, N.; Arakawa, Y. (2002) Serum concentrations of human hepatocyte growth factor is a useful indicator for predicting the occurrence of hepatocellular carcinomas in C-viral chronic liver diseases. *Cancer*, Vol.95, pp. 824-34, ISSN 0008-543X.

Yamazaki, T.; Zaal, K.; Hailey, D.; Presley, J.; Lippincott- Schwartz, J.; Samelson, L.E. (2002) Role of Grb2 in EGF-stimulated EGFR internalization. *J. Cell. Sci.*, Vol.115, pp. 1791-802, ISSN 0021-9533.

Zekri, A.R.; Alam El-Din, H.M.; Bahnassy, A.A.; Zayed, N.A.; Mohamed, W.S.; El-Masry, S.H.; Gouda, S.K.; Esmat, G. (2010) Serum levels of soluble Fas, soluble tumor necrosis factor-receptor II, interleukin-2 receptor and interleukin-8 as early predictors of hepatocellular carcinoma in Egyptian patients with hepatitis C virus genotype-4. *Comp. Hepatol.*, Vol.9, pp. 1, ISSN 14765926.

Zeremski, M.; Petrovic, L.M.; Talal A.H. (2007) The role of chemokines as inflammatory mediators in chronic hepatitis C virus infection. *Journal of Viral Hepatitis*, Vol.14, pp. 675–687, ISSN 1352-0504.

Zeremski M, Dimova R, Brown Q, Jacobson IM, Markatou M, Talal AH. Peripheral CXCR3-associated chemokines as biomarkers of fibrosis in chronic hepatitis C virus infection. *Infect. Dis.*, 2009;200:1774-80, ISSN 1537-6613.

Xanthou, G., Williams, T.J., Pease, J.E., 2003. Molecular characterization of the chemokine receptor CXCR3: evidence for the involvement of distinct extracellular domains in a multi-step model of ligand binding and receptor activation. *Eur. J. Immunol.* 33, 2927-36, ISSN 0014-2980.

Part 7

Pancreatic Cancer

7

Periodontal Inflammation as Risk Factor for Pancreatic Diseases

Jelena Milasin[1], Natasa Nikolic Jakoba[2], Dejan Stefanovic[3], Jelena Sopta[4], Ana Pucar[2], Vojislav Lekovic[2] and Barrie E. Kenney[5]

[1]*Institute of Human Genetics, School of Dentistry, University of Belgrade, Belgrade*
[2]*Clinic for Periodontology and Oral Medicine, School of Dentistry, University of Belgrade*
[3]*Clinic for Gastroenterology, School of Medicine, University of Belgrade*
[4]*Institute of Pathology, School of Medicine, University of Belgrade, Belgrade*
[5]*Tarrson Family Endowed Chair in Periodontics, UCLA School of Dentistry, Los Angeles*
[1,2,3,4]*Serbia*
[5]*USA*

1. Introduction

During past decades the relationship between dentistry and internal medicine has been intensely debated. Current evidence suggests that inflammation due to periodontal infections may not be limited to the immediate oral environment but can have systemic effects. Clinical, epidemiological and molecular studies have demonstrated significant association between periodontitis and various diseases, such as coronary heart disease, atherosclerosis, bacterial pneumonia, diabetes mellitus and low birth weight. Individuals with periodontal infections have elevated concentrations of circulating inflammatory markers, disease severity directly correlates with serum concentrations of inflammatory markers, and treatment of periodontal infection can lower markers of systemic inflammatory dysfunction within 2–6 months.

Various hypotheses, including common susceptibility, systemic inflammation, direct bacterial infection and cross-reactivity, or molecular mimicry, between bacterial antigens and self-antigens, have been postulated to explain these relationships. In this scenario, the association of periodontal disease with systemic diseases has set the stage for introducing the concept of periodontal medicine.

At present it is generally agreed on that oral status is connected with systemic health, since poor oral health may occur concomitantly with more serious underlying diseases and/or it may predispose to other systemic diseases. The pioneering approach of periodontal medicine has helped to renew attention on the theory of focal infection and the deepening of the relationship between chronic periodontitis and systemic health.

In recent years, chronic periodontitis has been proposed as a risk factor for pancreatic cancer. Chronic periodontitis might promote pancreatic carcinogenesis, by means of systemic inflammation, or alternatively, through increased production of carcinogens, namely nitrosamines.

The aim of the present study was to investigate pancreatic tissue for the potential presence of periodontopathogenic microorganisms.

2. Periodontal diseases

Periodontal diseases are a group of bacterial inflammatory diseases of the supporting tissues of the teeth (gingiva, periodontal ligament, cementum and alveolar bone). Periodontal diseases include two general conditions based on whether there is attachment or bone loss: gingivitis and periodontitis. Gingivitis is considered a reversible form of the disease, and generally involves inflammation of the gingival tissues without loss of connective tissue attachment. Gingivitis is the most common and prevalent form of periodontal disease among children and adolescents. The incidence and severity increase from childhood to adolescence, reaching a peak prevalence of 80% at 11-13 years of age. The progression from gingivitis to periodontitis is characterized by periodontal pocket development, which favours further plaque accumulation and a shift in its qualitative composition. Thereafter, as the severity of gingivitis decreases, chronic periodontitis measured by attachment loss becomes dominant and continues to increase in severity with age. Periodontitis is a chronic infection involving destruction of tooth-supporting tissues, including the periodontal ligament and alveolar socket support of the teeth. Periodontal disease can affect one tooth or many teeth and, if left untreated, can lead to tooth loss, particularly in adults. It is the most common dental condition in adults, and is also one of the most common chronic inflammatory diseases affecting a majority of the population throughout the world. Some of the clinical signs include bleeding on probing, deep pockets, recession and tooth mobility. Progressive changes from healthy gums to necrotizing periodontitis are given in Figures 1 to 5.

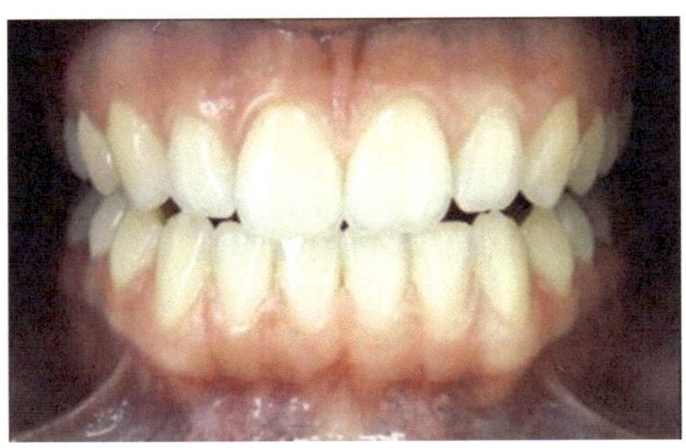

Fig. 1. Healthy gums

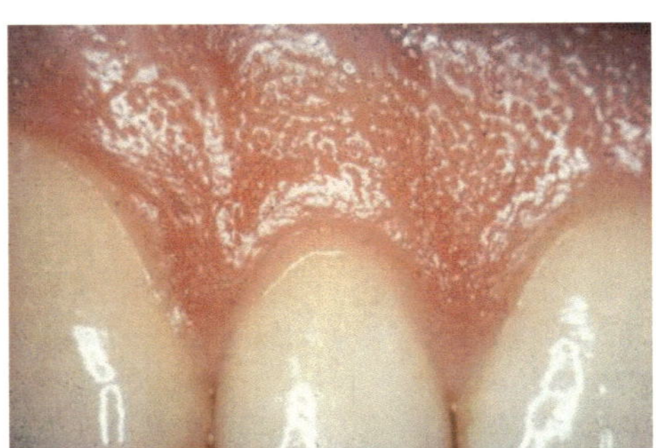

Fig. 2. Gingivitis

2.1 Classification of periodontal diseases

2.1.1 Chronic periodontitis

Chronic periodontitis is the most common form of periodontitis in adults, but can occur at any age. Progression of attachment loss usually occurs slowly, but periods of exacerbation with rapid progression, or periods of remission can occur. The rate of disease progression may be influenced by local (subgingivally placed fillings or crowns, tooth caries…) and/or systemic conditions (diabetes mellitus, pregnancy, puberty, leukemia…) that alter the normal host response to bacterial plaque. The severity of disease can be described as slight, moderate, or severe, based on the level of destruction.

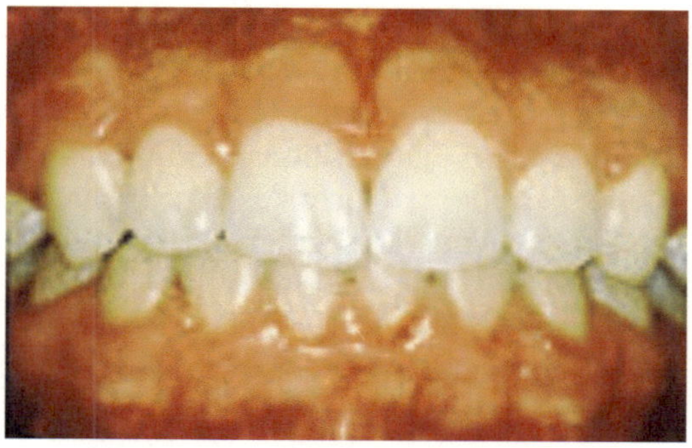

Fig. 3. Gingivitis

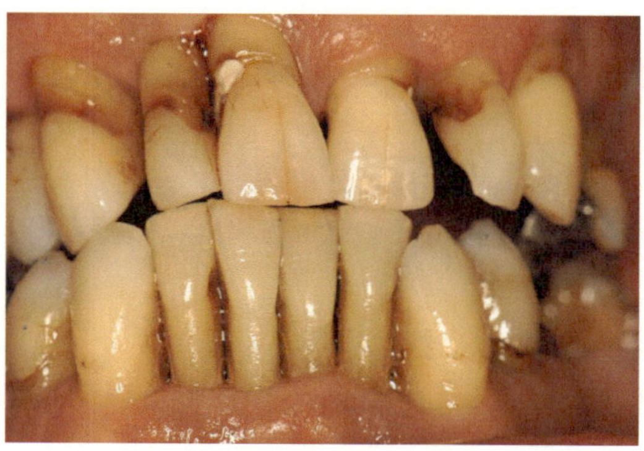

Fig. 4. Periodontitis

2.1.2 Aggressive periodontitis

Aggressive periodontitis (previously Juvenile Periodontitis) is characterized by rapid attachment loss and bone destruction in the absence of significant accumulations of plaque and calculus. (Tonetti&Mombelly, 1999) This form of periodontitis usually affects young individuals, often during puberty, from 10-30 years of age, with genetic predisposition. The bacteria most often associated with aggressive periodontitis is *Aggregatibacter actinomycetemcomitans* (previously *Actinobacillus actinomycetemcomitans*). Aggressive periodontitis can occur as localized or generalized forms. The localized form usually affects first molar and incisor sites. The generalized form usually involves at least three teeth other than first molars and incisors.

2.1.3 Periodontitis as a manifestation of systemic diseases

Periodontitis as a manifestation of systemic diseases may be associated with diabetes, several hematological (acquired, familial, and cyclic neutropenias, leukemias) and genetic disorders (Down's syndrome, certain types of Ehlers-Danlos syndrome, Papillon-Lefevre syndrome, Cohen syndrome and hypophosphatasia). The mechanisms by which all of these disorders affect the health of periodontium are not fully understood, but it is speculated that these diseases can alter host defense mechanisms and upregulate inflammatory responses, resulting in progressive periodontal destruction.

2.1.4 Necrotizing periodontal diseases

Necrotizing periodontal diseases (necrotizing gingivitis, necrotizing periodontitis and necrotizing stomatitis) are the most severe inflammatory periodontal disorders caused by plaque bacteria. These lesions are commonly observed in individuals with systemic conditions such HIV infection, malnutrition and immunosuppression. Clinical characteristics of necrotizing periodontal diseases may include but are not limited to ulcerated and necrotic papillary and marginal gingiva covered by a yellowish and grayish slough or pseudomembrane, blunting and cratering of papillae, bleeding on provocation or spontaneous bleeding, pain, and fetid breath. These diseases may be accompanied by fever, malaise, and lymphadenopathy, although these characteristics are not consistent.

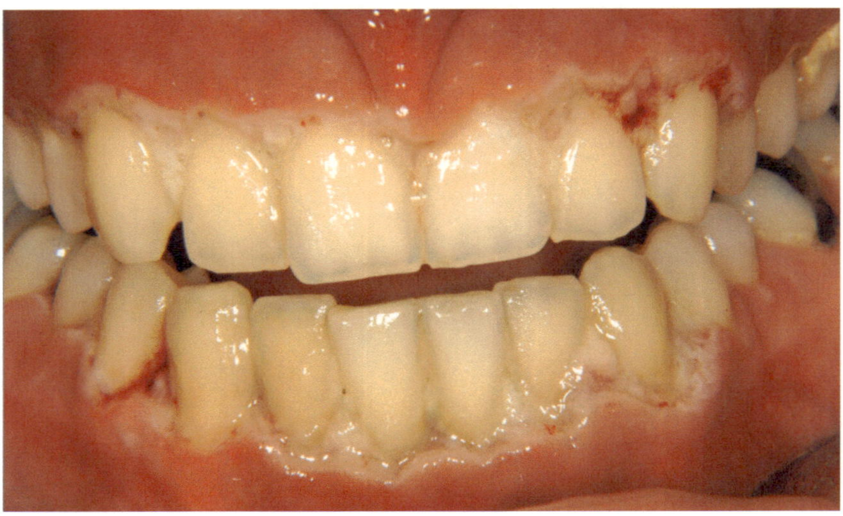

Fig. 5. Necrotizing periodontitis

These diseases appear to have multiple etiologies, microbial and immunological being the two most studied. The primary microbial factor contributing to disease is a shift in the content of the oral microflora, while the primary immunological factor is the destructive host inflammatory response.

2.2 Microbial etiology of periodontal disease

As many as 700 different species of bacteria that colonize the oral cavity can affect the delicate balance of host-bacterial interactions leading to disease. Periodontal infection is initiated by specific invasive oral pathogens that colonize dental plaque biofilms on the tooth root surface. No one knows how many bacterial species, ribotypes, and serotypes coexist in the dental plaque, but the number is very large. With the advent of PCR technologies, many new uncultivable species are being identified.

The onset and progression of periodontal disease is attributed to the presence of elevated levels of a consortium of pathogenic bacteria within the gingival crevice. The plaque is divided into two distinct types based on the relationship of the plaque to the gingival margin, i.e., supragingival plaque and subgingival plaque. The supragingival plaque is dominated by facultative *Streptococcus* and *Actinomyces* species, whereas the subgingival plaque harbors an anaerobic gram-negative flora dominated by uncultivable spirochetal species. It is this gram-negative flora that has been associated with periodontal disease. Since many of its members derive some of their nutrients from the gingival crevicular fluid, a tissue transudate that seeps into the periodontal area, it is possible that their overgrowth is a result of the inflammatory process (Loe et al., 1965).

The disease is a chronic low grade infection involving mainly Gram-negative anaerobic bacteria. There is a clear evidence for the pathogenic role of *Aggregatibacter actinomycetemcomitans, Porphyromonas gingivalis* and *Tannerella forsythia* in periodontal disease development and a reasonably strong evidence exists for the pathogenic role in certain forms of periodontal disease of some other microorganisms such as *Prevotella intermedia, Fusobacterium nucleatum, Campylobacter rectus, Eikenella corrodens* etc (Brajovic et al., 2010; Milicevic et al, 2008). A number of gram-negative rods and spirochetes are putative periodontal pathogens, but these organisms may also be present, although in smaller concentrations, in healthy patients.

Although the plaque is essential for the initiation of periodontal diseases, the majority of the destructive processes associated with these diseases are due to an excessive host response to the bacterial challenge. Periodontal bacteria possess a plethora of virulence factors that, upon interaction with host cells, induce the production of inflammatory mediators at the gingival level.

2.3 Host inflammatory response to bacterial challenge

The fundamental question in regard to periodontal pathology is whether the host is responding to the nonspecific overgrowth of bacteria on the tooth surfaces (inflammatory disease) or to the overgrowth of a limited number of species which produce biologically active molecules that are particularly proinflammatory or antigenic (infection).

There is a distinction between the way the host responds to the supragingival plaque and its response to the subgingival plaque. The response to the supragingival plaque has been thoroughly studied in the experimental gingivitis model described below, whereas the response to the subgingival plaque remains under investigation. Does the host respond to the subgingival plaque as if it were an overgrowth of a bacterial community in which many members produce substances, such as LPS, that are particularly bioactive if they enter the gingival tissue? Or does it respond to a plaque in which certain members produce more biologically active molecules, such as butyric acid (Niederman al., 1997) or hydrogen sulfide (Ratcliff&Johnson, 1999), per cell or possess unique proteases, such as are found in *P. gingivalis* and *Treponema denticola,* which can degrade host molecules, creating a proinflammatory effect (Kuramitsu, 1998)? In either case, although bacteria are involved, it is not the scenario of a typical infection, as the offending bacteria generally remain outside the body, attached to the tooth.

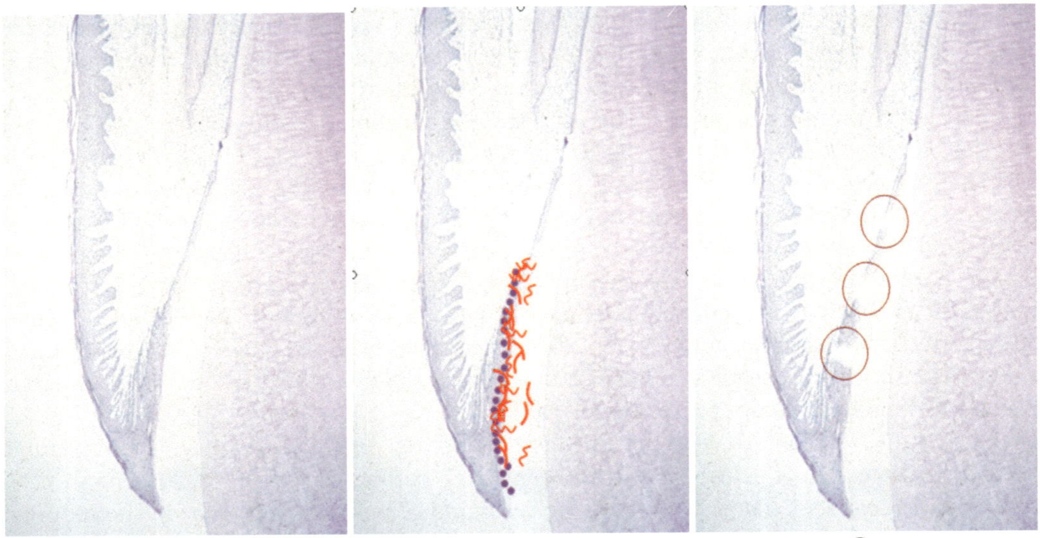

Fig. 6. A) Histology of normal gingiva; B) Accumulation of Gram positive and Gram negative bacteria and bacterial toxins; C) Basement membrane and tissue destruction leading to epithelial ulcerations.

In periodontal disease the inflammatory response causes tissue resistance to bacterial invasion but also provides mechanisms that contribute to tissue damage. Acute inflammatory cells, such as mast cells, macrophages, Langerhans cells, and polymorphonuclear leukocytes, combine their action to form a potent antibacterial defense mechanism. However the initial signs of gingival inflammation (swelling, redness, bleeding on probing) are nothing but the tissue-destructive aspects of the activity of these cells. Neutrophils function to control the bacterial assault by phagocytosis but also secrete matrix metalloproteinases (MMP), which are the agents responsible for collagen loss in the tissues. These latent collagenolytic enzymes can be converted to active forms by proteases and reactive oxygen species in the inflammatory environment, giving rise to elevated levels of interstitial collagenase in the inflammed gingival tissue. The resulting attachment loss deepens the sulcus, or depression, formed where the gingival tissues contact the tooth surface, thereby creating the periodontal pocket. By definition, this loss of attachment converts gingivitis to periodontitis. The depth of the pocket reflects an inflammatory response that causes both the swelling of the gingival tissues at the top of the pocket and the loss of collagen attachment of the tooth to the alveolar bone at the bottom of the pocket. Good oral hygiene can reduce the inflammatory swelling, but the attachment loss and accompanying bone loss is thought to be irreversible. In established periodontal disease, there is also a chronic inflammatory change, with B cells and T cells adding to the antibacterial spectrum. These cells also have capacity to release cytokines, which may induce the synthesis of arachidonate metabolites (especially PGE2), and to stimulate macrophages and osteoclasts to release hydrolases and collagenases, which are responsible for loss of collagen and bone. The interaction of bacterial antigens with peripheral dendritic cells leads to the generation of systemic antibody, whereas interaction with local B cells leads to production of local antibody. Antibody specific to many of the periodontal microorganisms is essential for phagocytosis. Complement components also may contribute to efficient bacterial phagocytosis. The production of interleukin-1β (IL-1β), tumor necrosis factor alpha (TNF-α), and prostaglandin E2 (PGE_2) in response to bacterial lipopolysaccharides (LPS) leads to bone resorption through osteoclast activation, proliferation, and differentiation. Each patient with dental plaque has a complex balance between these protective and damaging scenarios that results either in a slowly progressive loss of attachment (periodontitis) or in a restriction of tissue inflammation to the peripheral tissues (gingivitis).

2.4 Treatment of periodontal disease

Various treatment modalities, such as the traditional debridement procedures (scaling and root planning), surgery (Kwan et al., 1998; Lekovic et al., 1997, 1998a, 1998b, 2001a, 2001b, 2003, 2005; Camargo et al., 1998, 2000, 2002, 2005) and various antimicrobial regimens were introduced for the treatment of periodontal disease.

Traditional treatments reflect the premise that periodontal disease is due to the nonspecific overgrowth of any and all bacteria on the tooth surfaces and that the magnitude of the bacterial overgrowth on the teeth can be controlled by professional cleaning of the teeth at regular intervals. If these accumulations are not removed, various bacterial by-products and their cellular components such as LPS, antigens, or enzymes can provoke an inflammatory response in the gingival tissue. Undisturbed plaques often become calcified, forming dental calculus or tartar, which, if formed below the gingival margin, is often difficult to remove from the root surfaces without some form of surgical access.

This type of periodontal treatment which is considered to be the standard treatment, is based on the premise that if the bacterial overgrowth in dental plaque can be continuously suppressed by mechanical debridement, gingival and periodontal health will be maintained. It is the basis of the "plaque control" programs of organized dentistry and dentifrice manufacturers; as a public health effort, this approach has been very successful.

3. Oral-systemic relationship

In the last decade, the possible association between oral and systemic health has been highlighted in numerous reports. Apart from the seeding infection as a direct consequence of transient bacteraemia, such oral-systemic interactions and outcomes could be due to other, indirect reasons, such as metastatic inflammation as a result of circulating macromolecular complexes and/or metastatic injury due to soluble toxins and bacterial lipopolysaccharide. It has become increasingly clear that the oral cavity can act as the site of origin for dissemination of pathogenic organisms to distant body sites, especially in immunocompromised hosts such as patients suffering from malignancies, diabetes, or rheumatoid arthritis or having corticosteroid or other immunosuppressive treatment. A number of epidemiological studies have suggested that oral infection, especially marginal and apical periodontitis, may be a risk factor for systemic diseases.

3.1 Transient bacteraemia

In common inflammatory conditions such as gingivitis and chronic periodontitis, which are precipitated by the buildup of plaque biofilms, the periodontal vasculature proliferates and dilates, providing an even greater surface area that facilitates the entry of microorganisms into the bloodstream. Often, these bacteraemias are short-lived and transient, with the highest intensity limited to the first 30 min after a trigger episode. On occasions, this may lead to seeding of microorganisms in different target organs, resulting in subclinical, acute, or chronic infections. Yet there are a number of other organs and body sites that may be affected by focal bacteremic spread from the oral cavity. Based on the current evidence, it is likely that bacteria may enter into the bloodstream from oral niches through a number of mechanisms and a variety of portals. First, and most commonly, when there is tissue trauma induced by procedures such as periodontal probing, scaling, instrumentation beyond the root apex, and tooth extractions, a breakage in capillaries and other small blood vessels that are located in the vicinity of the plaque biofilms may lead to spillage of bacteria into the systemic circulation. As stated above, dissemination of oral microorganisms into the bloodstream is common, and less than 1 minute after an oral procedure, organisms from the infected site may have reached the heart, lungs, and peripheral blood capillary system. There are more than 10^{13} microbes on all surfaces of the body, yet the underlying tissues and the bloodstream are usually sterile. In the oral cavity there are several barriers to bacterial penetration from dental plaque into the tissue: a physical barrier composed of the surface epithelium; defensins, which are host-derived peptide antibiotics, in the oral mucosal epithelium; an electrical barrier that reflects the difference between the host cell and the microbial layer; an immunological barrier of antibody-forming cells; and the reticuloendothelial system (phagocyte barrier). Under normal circumstances, these barrier systems work together to inhibit and eliminate penetrating bacteria. When this state of equilibrium is disturbed by an overt breach in the physical system (e.g., trauma), the electrical system (i.e., hypoxia), or immunological barriers (e.g., through neutropenia, AIDS, or immunosuppressant therapy), microorganisms can propagate and cause both acute and chronic infections with increased frequency and severity. With normal oral health and dental care, only small numbers of mostly facultative bacterial species gain access to the bloodstream. However, with poor oral hygiene, the numbers of bacteria colonizing the teeth, especially supragingivally, could increase 2- to 10-fold and thus possibly introduce more bacteria into tissue and the bloodstream, leading to an increase in the prevalence and magnitude of bacteraemia.

Obviously, a higher microbial load would facilitate such dissemination, as it is known that individuals with poor oral hygiene are at a higher risk of developing bacteraemias during oral manipulative procedures. Innate microbial factors may play a role in the latter phenomenon, as only a few species are detected in experimental bacteraemias despite the multitude of diverse bacteria residing within the periodontal biofilm. Species that are commonly found in the bloodstream have virulence attributes that could be linked to vascular invasion. Of particular note are attributes such as endothelial adhesion of *Streptococcus* spp., degradation of intercellular matrices by *Porphyromonas gingivalis*, and impedance of phagocytic activity by *Aggregatibacter actinomycetemcomitans* and *Fusobacterium nucleatum*. As opposed to the more than 700 bacterial species that inhabit the oral cavity, relatively fewer species have been isolated from blood cultures for odontogenic bacteraemias. Phylogenetic studies of the oral microbiome have shown that a large proportion of the oral bacteria comprise the genus *Streptococcus* (Van Dyke et al., 1982.). In a number of controlled clinical trials, streptococci were the predominant organisms isolated, ranging from 40 to 65% of isolates. The highest incidence of bacteraemia results from tooth extractions. Periodontal manipulations are also shown to produce a long-lasting (30 min) bacteraemia. This is probably a reflection of the bacterial load and tissue trauma or associated inflammation at these niches. Other oral procedures are not as significant, at least for individuals with healthy oral cavities. Routine oral hygiene measures such as brushing or flossing are unlikely to cause a significant degree of bacteraemia, but sporadic cleaning after accumulation of a heavy plaque load should be considered a potential risk factor for a bacteremic state.

3.2 Mechanisms linking oral infection to secondary nonoral diseases

Three mechanisms or pathways linking oral infections to secondary systemic effects have been proposed. These are metastatic spread of infection from the oral cavity as a result of transient bacteraemia, metastatic injury from the effects of circulating oral microbial toxins, and metastatic inflammation caused by immunological injury induced by oral microorganisms.

3.2.1 Metastatic infection

As previously discussed, oral infections and dental procedures can cause transient bacteraemia. The microorganisms that gain entrance to the blood and circulate throughout the body are usually eliminated by the reticuloendothelial system within minutes (transient bacteraemia) and as a rule lead to no other clinical symptoms than possibly a slight increase in body temperature. However, if the disseminated microorganisms find favorable conditions, they may settle at a given site and, after a certain time lag, start to multiply.

3.2.2 Metastatic injury

Some gram-positive and gram-negative bacteria have the ability to produce diffusible proteins, or exotoxins, which include cytolytic enzymes and dimeric toxins. The exotoxins have specific pharmacological actions and are considered the most powerful and lethal poisons known (51). Conversely, endotoxins are part of the outer membranes released after cell death. Endotoxin is compositionally a lipopolysaccharide (LPS) that, when introduced into the host, gives rise to a large number of pathological manifestations. LPS is continuously shed from periodontal gram-negative rods during their growth in vivo.

3.2.3 Metastatic inflammation

Soluble antigen may enter the bloodstream, react with circulating specific antibody, and form a macromolecular complex. These immunocomplexes may give rise to a variety of acute and chronic inflammatory reactions at the sites of deposition.

4. Periodontitis affects susceptibility to systemic disease

In a recent review article, Page proposed that periodontitis may affect the host's susceptibility to systemic disease in three ways: by shared risk factors, by subgingival biofilms acting as reservoirs of gram-negative bacteria, and through the periodontium acting as a reservoir of inflammatory mediators.

4.1 Shared risk factors

Factors that place individuals at high risk for periodontitis may also place them at high risk for systemic diseases such as cardiovascular disease. Among the environmental risk factors and indicators shared by periodontitis and systemic diseases, such as cardiovascular disease, are tobacco smoking, stress, aging, race or ethnicity, and male gender. Studies demonstrating genetic factors shared by periodontitis, cardiovascular disease, preterm labor, and osteoporosis have not yet been performed but may be fruitful.

4.2 Subgingival biofilms

Subgingival biofilms constitute an enormous and continuing bacterial load. They present continually renewing reservoirs of LPS and other gram-negative bacteria with ready access to the periodontal tissues and the circulation. Systemic challenge with gram-negative bacteria or LPS induces major vascular responses, including an inflammatory cell infiltrate in the vessel walls, vascular smooth muscle proliferation, vascular fatty degeneration, and intravascular coagulation. LPS upregulates expression of endothelial cell adhesion molecules and secretion of interleukin-1 (IL-1), tumor necrosis factor alpha (TNF-a), and thromboxane, which results in platelet aggregation and adhesion, formation of lipidladen foam cells, and deposits of cholesterol and cholesterol esters.

4.3 Periodontium as cytokine reservoir

The proinflammatory cytokines TNF-a, IL-1b, and gamma interferon as well as prostaglandin E2 (PGE2) reach high tissue concentrations in periodontitis. The periodontium can therefore serve as a renewing reservoir for spillover of these mediators, which can enter the circulation and induce and perpetuate systemic effects. IL-1b favors coagulation and thrombosis and retards fibrinolysis. IL-1, TNF-a, and thromboxane can cause platelet aggregation and adhesion, formation of lipidladen foam cells, and deposition of cholesterol. These same mediators emanating from the diseased periodontium may also account for preterm labor and low-birth-weight infants (Page, 1998).

5. Cardiovascular disease

Cardiovascular disease and periodontal disease are both chronic inflammatory diseases. Numerous cross-sectional and longitudinal epidemiological studies have provided evidence that there is an association between periodontitis and elevated risk for cardiovascular disease. A number of systematic reviews and meta-analyses have described the relationship between periodontal infection and cardiovascular disease, and have suggested that periodontitis may contribute to cardiovascular disease and stroke in susceptible subjects.

It is well accepted that hyperlipidemia is a risk factor for coronary heart disease. Recent studies have shown an association between periodontitis and elevated atherogenic lipid fraction levels and / or decreased anti-atherogenic lipid fraction levels. Most of these were cross-sectional studies, and it is still unclear whether there is a causal relationship between periodontitis and hyperlipidemia. Improvement of serum lipid profiles after periodontal treatment may indicate a causal relationship between periodontitis and hyperlipidemia, and may suggest the possibility of reducing the risk of coronary heart disease by effective periodontal intervention.

C-reactive protein is an important marker for systemic inflammation, and has been consistently found to be elevated in patients with coronary syndromes. Recently, evidence has accumulated demonstrating the association between periodontitis and C-reactive protein. The serum C-reactive protein concentration is increased in systemically healthy subjects with periodontitis. Numerous studies indicate that periodontal intervention therapy may decrease the C-reactive protein-associated cardiovascular disease risk.

Many cytokines play a role in the pathogenesis of both coronary heart disease and periodontitis. These include interleukin-1, interleukin-6, interleukin-8, tumor necrosis factor-a, intercellular adhesion molecule-1 (ICAM-1), P-selectin and E-selectin. Some intervention studies have indicated that periodontal therapy can reduce the levels of these pro-inflammory cytokines, and thus periodontal treatment may lower the cardiovascular disease risk.

Numerous studies of different design and rigor have provided statistical evidence for an association between periodontal disease and cardiovascular disease, raising the possibility that periodontal disease is a risk factor for cardiovascular disease. There are several proposed mechanisms (Fig. 1) by which periodontal disease may trigger pathways leading to cardiovascular disease through direct and indirect effects of oral bacteria. First, evidence indicates that oral bacteria such as *Streptococcus sanguis* and *Porphyromonas gingivalis* induce platelet aggregation, which leads to thrombus formation. These organisms have a collagen-like molecule, the platelet aggregation- associated protein, on their surface. Furthermore, one or more periodontal pathogens have been found in 42% of the atheromas studied in patients with severe periodontal disease (Zambon, 1998). The second factor in this process could be an exaggerated host response to a given microbial or LPS challenge, as reflected in the release of high levels of proinflammatory mediators such as PGE2, TNF-a, and IL-1b. These mediators have been related to interindividual differences in the T-cell repertoire and the secretory capacity of monocytic cells. Typically, peripheral blood monocytes from these individuals with the hyperinflammatory monocyte phenotype secrete 3- to 10-fold-greater amounts of these mediators in response to LPS than those from normal monocyte phenotype individuals. Patients with certain forms of periodontal disease, such as early-onset periodontitis and refractory periodontitis, possess a hyperinflammatory monocyte phenotype. A third mechanism possibly involves the relationship between bacterial and inflammatory products of periodontitis and cardiovascular disease. LPS from periodontal organisms being transferred to the serum as a result of bacteraemias or bacterial invasion may have a direct effect on endothelia so that atherosclerosis is promoted (Pesonen et al., 1981). LPS may also elicit recruitment of inflammatory cells into major blood vessels and stimulate proliferation of vascular smooth muscle, vascular fatty degeneration, intravascular coagulation, and blood platelet function. These changes are the result of the action of various biologic mediators, such as PGs, ILs, and TNF-a on vascular endothelium and smooth muscle. Fibrinogen and WBC count increases noted in periodontitis patients may be a secondary effect of the above mechanisms or a constitutive feature of those at risk for both cardiovascular disease and periodontitis (Kweider et al., 1993).

If so, periodontal disease, because it is both preventable and treatable, becomes a modifiable risk factor for cardiovascular disease. However, if periodontal disease is primarily due to the overgrowth of bacteria in the dental plaque, all individuals would need preventive treatment, since all individuals form dental plaque.

5.1 Atherosclerosis

Atherosclerosis has been defined as a progressive disease process that involves large- to medium-sized muscular and large elastic arteries. The advanced lesion is the atheroma, which consists of elevated focal intimal plaques with a necrotic central core containing lysed cells, cholesterol ester crystals, lipid-laden foam cells, and surface plasma proteins, including fibrin and fibrinogen. In the last few years there were an increasing number of reports dealing with the possible relationship between atherosclerosis and periodontitis, as well as between chronic coronary heart disease and periodontitis (Fien et al., 2005; Ford et al., 2006; Pucar et al., 2007; Spahr et al., 2006). Arteries have been thoroughly explored for the presence of periodontopathogens and a variety of oral microorganisms have been found lodged in arterial walls.

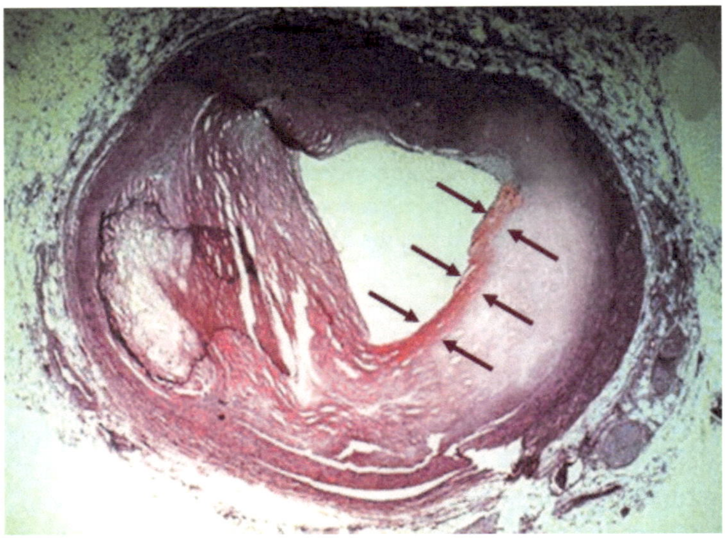

Fig. 7. Coronary artery with stable atheroma. Inflammation and necrosis have replaced the smooth muscle but there is a dense layer of collagen next to lumen (arrows)

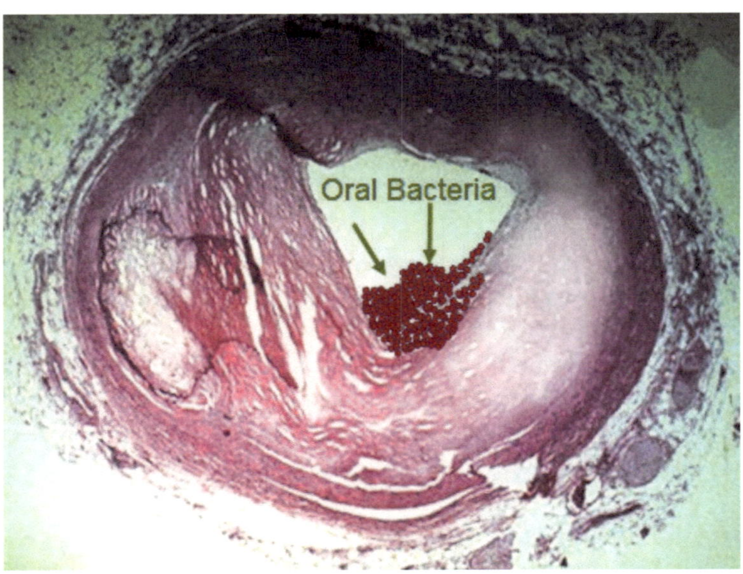

Fig. 8. Circulating oral bacteria have peptides that cause platelet aggregation (arrows)

There are sufficient data to consider that *A.actimomycetamcomitans*, *P. gingivalis* and *P. intermedia* have the ability to invade host cells including epithelium and endothelium evading the neutrophil clearance; in this way periodontal pathogens can penetrate the epithelial barrier of the periodontal tissues and get systemic spreading through the blood stream. By this dynamic, periodontal pathogens can infect directly the vascular endothelium, and atherosclerotic plaques, causing inflammation and plaque instability up to an acute myocardial ischemia. Moreover, periodontal pathogens produce a variety of virulence factors (e.g. adhesions, portliness, haemolysins, membrane vesicles and LPS) that have deleterious effects on vascular system, resulting in platelet aggregation and adhesion, formation of lipid-laden foam cells and deposits of cholesterol, all factors contributing to the formation of atheroma.

Endothelial dysfunction is a fundamental step in the development of atherosclerosis, and can be measured by several methods, including flow-mediated dilatation of the brachial artery. Endothelial dysfunction as determined by measurement of brachial flow-mediated dilatation is considered to be a good predictor of cardiovascular outcomes (Roquer et al., 2009).

Periodontal disease is associated with endothelial dysfunction as measured by brachial flow-mediated dilatation. Endothelial function has been reported to be significantly lower in patients with periodontitis than in control subjects. In addition, endothelial dysfunction in hypertensive patients with periodontitis is more severe compared to hypertensive patients without periodontitis (Higashi et al., 2009). Recently, endothelial function was evaluated in healthy and periodontitis patients with coronary artery disease (Higashi et al., 2008). The results showed that endothelial function was significantly lower in the periodontitis group with coronary artery disease than in the nonperiodontitis group with coronary artery disease. These results suggest that periodontitis is a contributor to endothelial dysfunction, and hence could increase the risk of cardiovascular disease. Based on current evidence, periodontal therapy can improve endothelial dysfunction in periodontitis patients whether they are systemically healthy or have hypertension. This further confirms the causal association between periodontitis and endothelial dysfunction. As endothelial dysfunction is associated with an adverse prognosis for atherosclerosis and cardiovascular disease, periodontal intervention therapy may bring benefits to patients with periodontitis by improving endothelial function, thus reducing the risk of cardiovascular disease. However, this requires further study.

6. Diabetes mellitus

Recent findings indicate that oral health may influence systemic health, and that this may be a bi-directional relationship for some conditions. This is particularly true for the relationship between periodontal disease and diabetes mellitus. The inter-relationship between periodontal disease and diabetes mellitus provides an example of a cyclic association, whereby a systemic disease predisposes the individual to oral infections, and, once the oral infection is established, it exacerbates the systemic disease.

The inflammatory response in the periodontal tissues in response to challenge by dental biofilm is complex and involves networks of cytokines functioning in synergy. The inflammatory response is characterized by localized production of various inflammatory markers and enzymes, such as C-reactive proteins, cytokines (interleukin-1b, interleukin- 6, tumor necrosis factor α), prostanoids (prostaglandin E2) and matrix metalloproteinases.

These increased secretions of inflammatory cytokines contribute to bone loss in periodontitis. The balance between the protective host factors and microbial challenge is greatly influenced by environmental and genetic factors that have an impact on the immuno-inflammatory response of the host. Alterations in immunologically active molecules as a result of diabetes may alter the levels of cytokines in the periodontium, which accelerates progression of the disease. This is the scientific basis for the increased susceptibility to periodontal disease seen in diabetics.

Patients with diabetes exhibited greater periodontal breakdown in response to dental biofilm; however, this depended on the degree of glycemic control (Arrieta-Blanco et al., 2003; Bastard et al., 2006). The highest levels of gingivitis were seen in diabetic patients with poor glycemic control (Mealey, 2006). Clinical and epidemiological studies have reported a higher prevalence and increased severity of periodontal disease in diabetic patients compared with non-diabetic controls (Ciancola et al., 1982; Collin et al., 1998; Safkan-Seppala et at., 1992). Studies have shown that diabetes carries a threefold increased risk of periodontitis compared to non-diabetic individuals (Lo¨e et al., 1978; Sclossman et al., 1990). Alveolar bone loss is enhanced in these individuals, resulting in a more persistent inflammatory response in diabetics. This leads to greater attachment loss and impaired formation of new bone (Liu et al., 2006). In addition, Lo¨e (Lo¨e, 1993) described periodontitis as the 6th complication of diabetes, together with retinopathy, nephropathy, neuropathy, macrovascular diseases and altered wound healing. The complications of diabetes are related to long-term elevation of blood glucose concentrations (hyperglycaemia) that results in the formation of advanced glycation end-products (AGEs). The accumulation of AGEs increases the intensity of the immune-inflammatory response to different pathogens, because inflammatory cells such as monocytes and macrophages have receptors for AGEs with consequent increased production of IL-1β and TNF-α. The AGEs-enriched gingival tissue has greater vascular permeability, greater breakdown of collagen fibers and accelerated destruction of both non-mineralized connective tissue and bone occurs. Diabetes can also cause damage of neutrophil adhesion, chemotaxis and phagocytosis, making patients more susceptible to periodontal destruction. The effects of the hyperglycemic state include the inhibition of osteoblastic proliferation and collagen production. Several studies indicated that diabetes is associated with an increased prevalence, extent and severity of chronic periodontitis. Other studies have suggested that the presence of periodontal infection may be linked to poor metabolic control of diabetes (Southerland et al., 2005). Treatment of periodontal disease can alter glycemic control, and early intervention and treatment of periodontitis may help to prevent the long-term complications of diabetes, thereby having an impact on mortality.

7. Bacterial pneumonia

Pneumonia is an infection of pulmonary parenchyma caused by a wide variety of infectious agents, including bacteria, fungi, parasites, and viruses. Pneumonia can be a life-threatening infection, especially in the old and immunocompromised patient, and is a significant cause of morbidity and mortality in patients of all ages. Most commonly, bacterial pneumonia results from aspiration of oropharyngeal flora into the lower respiratory tract, failure of host defense mechanisms to eliminate them, multiplication of the microorganisms, and subsequent tissue destruction. It is likely that most pathogens first colonize the surfaces of the oral cavity or pharyngeal mucosa before aspiration. These pathogens can colonize from an exogenous source or emerge following overgrowth of the normal oral flora after antibiotic treatment. Common potential respiratory pathogens (PRPs) such as *Streptococcus pneumoniae, Mycoplasma pneumoniae,* and *Haemophilus influenzae* can colonize the oropharynx and be aspirated into the lower airways. Other species thought to comprise the normal oral flora, including *A. actinomycetemcomitans* and anaerobes such as *P. gingivalis* and *Fusobacterium* species, can also be aspirated into the lower airways and cause pneumonia. Pneumonia can result from infection by anaerobic bacteria. Dental plaque would seem to be a logical source of these bacteria, especially in patients with periodontal disease. Such patients harbor a large number of subgingival bacteria, particularly anaerobic species. Among the oral bacterial species implicated in pneumonia are *A. actinomycetemcomitans, Actinomyces israelii, Capnocytophaga* spp., *Eikenella corrodens, Prevotella intermedia,* and *Streptococcus constellatus.* A study has shown that individuals with respiratory disease have significantly higher oral hygiene index scores than subjects without respiratory disease.

8. Low birth weight

Pregnancy can influence gingival health. Changes in hormone levels during pregnancy promote an inflammation termed pregnancy gingivitis. This type of gingivitis may occur without changes in plaque levels. Oral contraceptives may also produce changes in gingival health. Some birth control pill users have a high gingival inflammation level but a low plaque level. Birth control pills may cause changes such as alteration of the microvasculature, gingival permeability, and increased synthesis of estrogen.

Oral infections also seem to increase the risk for or contribute to low birth weight in newborns. Low birth weight, defined as a birth weight of <2,500 g, is a major public health problem in both developed and developing countries. As a remote gram-negative infection, periodontal disease may have the potential to affect pregnancy outcome. During pregnancy, the ratio of anaerobic gram-negative bacterial species to aerobic species increases in dental plaque in the second trimester. The gram-negative bacteria associated with progressive disease can produce a variety of bioactive molecules that can directly affect the host. One microbial component, LPS, can activate macrophages and other cells to synthesize and secrete a wide array of molecules, including the cytokines IL-1b, TNF-a, IL-6, and PGE2 and matrix metalloproteinases. If they escape into the general circulation and cross the placental barrier, they could augment the physiologic levels of PGE2 and TNF-a in the amniotic fluid and induce premature labor.

Human case-control studies have demonstrated that women who have low-birth-weight infants as a consequence of either preterm labor or premature rupture of membranes tend to have more severe periodontal disease than mothers with normal- birth-weight infants. In a recent case-control study, 48 case-control subjects had their gingival crevicular fluid (GCF) levels of PGE2 and IL-1b measured to determine whether mediator levels are related to current pregnancy outcome. In addition, the levels of four periodontal pathogens were measured by using microbespecific DNA probes. The results indicate that GCF PGE2 levels are significantly higher in mothers of preterm low-birthweight infants than in mothers of normal-birth-weight infants (controls). These data suggest a dose-response relationship for increased GCF PGE2 as a marker of current periodontal disease activity and decreasing birth weight. Four organisms associated with mature plaque and progressing periodontitis, *Bacteroides forsythus, P. gingivalis, A. actinomycetemcomitans,* and *Treponema denticola,* are detected at higher levels in mothers of preterm low-birth-weight infants than in controls. These data suggest that biochemical measures of maternal periodontal status and oral microbial burden are associated with preterm birth and low birth weight. 18.2% of preterm low-birth-weight babies may result from periodontal disease— a previously unrecognized and clinically important risk factor for preterm birth and low birth weight. The association between periodontal disease and low birth weight may reflect the patient's altered immune-inflammatory trait that places the patient at risk for both conditions.

Thus, periodontitis may be a marker for preterm delivery susceptibility as well as a potential risk factor. Indeed, the data from animal models suggest that even if periodontal disease is not the primary cause of prematurity, in a subset of patients it may serve as a contributor to the condition. Currently, there is insufficient evidence to link chronic periodontitis to specific adverse pregnancy outcomes.

9. Cancer associated with chronic inflammation

Various sudies confirmed that malignancies may arise from areas of infection and inflammation, simply as part of the normal host response. Indeed, there is a growing body of evidence that many malignancies are initiated by infections (Kuper et al., 2000; Sachter et al., 2002). Persistent infections within the host induce chronic inflammation. Leukocytes and other phagocytic cells induce DNA damage in proliferating cells, through their generation of reactive oxygen and nitrogen species that are produced normally by these cells to fight infection. These species react to form peroxynitrite, a mutagenic agent (Maeda &Akaike, 1998). Hence, repeated tissue damage and regeneration of tissue, in the presence of highly reactive nitrogen and oxygen species released from inflammatory cells, interacts with DNA in proliferating epithelium resulting in permanent genomic alterations such as point mutations, deletions, or chromosomal rearrangements.

More recently, a link between periodontal disease and cancer has been suggested. The scientific rationale behind the proposed association is that inflammation is a major factor in both periodontal disease and cancer.

Oral cancer, gingival squamous cell carcinoma in particular, has been known to mimic advanced periodontal disease in clinical appearance showing similar symptoms of swelling, bleeding, tooth mobility, deep periodontal pockets, and bone destruction. Many cases have been reported of gingival squamous cell carcinoma presenting clinically similar to inflammatory periodontal or periodontal/endodontic lesions. Cases of other types of cancer mistaken for periodontal disease such as metastatic pancreatic cancer and osteogenic sarcoma have also been reported. These examples hint that a similar underlying mechanism may be responsible for both periodontal disease and cancer.

9.1 Cancers and periodontal disease

Several hypotheses are of interest in the potential etiology of a link between, periodontal disease and cancer.

9.1.1 Alteration of the oral flora

It has been suggested that carcinogenic metabolic by-products of periodontal disease might account for the relationship between the two diseases. When considering gastric cancers, it had been argued that the mechanism of increased cancer risk may be an increased production of nitrosamines in situations of poor oral hygiene and that these by-products may function as gastro-intestinal organ specific carcinogens. Nitrosamines have been linked to cancers of the stomach and esophagus. Helicobacter pylori infection also plays a role in stomach cancers (Zarić et al, 2009). Other microorganisms have been studied as well as potential carcinogenic agents. There is also evidence that some strains of candidiasis have been seen at higher frequency in oral cancer patients. Viruses may also play a role. A suggestion has been made that increased periodontal disease may be associated with infection with cytomegalovirus and/or Epstein-Barr Virus 1 with mixed results. EBV of course has been linked to cancer including lymphoma and nasopharyngeal carcinoma.

9.1.2 Increase in systemic circulatory inflammatory markers

The presence of inflammatory cells and mediators such as chemokines, cytokines, and prostaglandins represent indicators associated with tumors. Also, the immune response mounted to a chronic periodontal infection has been proposed as a potential carcinogenic etiologic factor. Also of interest is the relationship between the pro-inflammatory expression of the receptor for advanced glycation end products (RAGE) and esophageal, gastric, colon, biliary, pancreatic, and prostate cancers. RAGE has been shown to play a role in the inflammatory processes of oral infections including periodontal disease. There are several obstacles in accurately determining a relationship between, periodontal disease and cancer.

9.1.3 Confounding factors

Smoking appeared to be the main confounding factor among these studies, especially for cancers strongly linked to tobacco use such as lung cancer. Other potential confounding factors are socio-economic status, diabetes, age, gender and ethnicity, along with genetics.

9.2 Chronic periodontitis as a risk factor for pancreatic cancer

Cancer of the pancreas is a rapidly fatal tumor. Smoking is the only well-documented modifiable risk factors for this cancer, although data suggest that diabetes, obesity and insulin resistance are also risk factors. Alcohol consumption is not an established risk factor for pancreatic cancer, but there is a strong association between alcohol consumption and chronic pancreatitis, and the latter has been associated with a higher risk for pancreatic cancer.

Although viral infections have been strongly associated with cancers, several bacteria can promote or initiate abnormal cell growth by evading the immune system or suppressing apoptosis. Since periodontitis is a chronic oral bacterial infection, few authors have suggested a possible positive association between periodontitis and pancreatic cancer. Chronic periodontitis might promote pancreatic carcinogenesis, by means of systemic inflammation, or alternatively, through increased production of carcinogens, namely nitrosamines. Nitrosamines and gastric acidity have been suggested as factors that have an important role in pancreatic cancer, and tooth loss that occurs through poor dental hygiene may be a marker for more deleterious gastrointestinal flora and, consequently, greater endogenous nitrosation. In fact, endogenous formation of nitrosamines in the oral cavity in

individuals with poor oral hygiene is due to elevated levels of nitrate-reducing oral bacteria, including *H. pylori*. The association between *H. pylori* infection and pancreatic cancer was investigated, but this association could not be confirmed.
A recent study has also suggested positive association between periodontitis and pancreatic cancer risk. Myeloperoxidase and superoxide dismutase help to regulate inflammation and are found to be elevated in periodontitis, and polymorphisms of these genes have been associated with elevated pancreatic cancer risk.

10. Methods

10.1 Patients

Pancreatic tissue specimens were obtained from patients undergoing surgery for ANP (40) and for PC (20) at the Surgical Clinic of the Medical Center of Serbia. The research protocol received institutional evaluation and approval (Ethical Committee of the School of Dentistry, Belgrade). Periodontal evaluation was performed in the hospital, a day before planned surgical procedures, and included assessment of pocket depth (PD in mm) and clinical attachment loss (CAL in mm) at six points of every present tooth (mesio-buccal, mid-buccal, disto-buccal, mesio-lingual, mid-lingual, disto-lingual). The clinical parameters were evaluated with a periodontal probe (XP 23/UNC-15). All measurements were performed by a single periodontist (A.P.). Chronic periodontitis was defined by the presence of at least 4 non-adjacent teeth with sites CAL≥4mm and PD≥5mm (Okuda et al., 2001). All patients that had been taking antibiotics in the previous three months and/or received periodontal treatment were excluded.
12 pancreas specimens obtained during autopsies performed at the Institute of Pathology, School of Medicine, University of Belgrade were also included in the study and used as controls. The cause of death was not related to pancreas.
Immediately after being taken, the specimens were frozen at -20 C until further processing.

10.2 Bacterial DNA detection by PCR

Tissue specimens were treated with proteinase K at 56°C for 30 minutes, followed by 10 minutes of proteinase K inactivation at 95°C and 5 minutes centrifugation in a microfuge to pellet cell debris.
The PCR was performed in volumes of 25 μl containing PCR/Mg++ buffer, 0.2 mM of each dNTP, 0.2 μM of each primer, 0.5 U *Taq* DNA polymerase and 3-5 μl of template DNA containing supernatant.
The amplification was performed in a DNA Thermal Cycler (Hybaid) programmed at 94°C (5 minutes) followed by 35 cycles at 94°C (1 min), annealing temperatures adequate for each primer pair (1 min) and extension at 72°C (1 minute 30 seconds) plus a final extension at 72°C (5 min). The PCR amplified fragments were visualized in an 8% polyacrylamide gel stained with ethidium bromide, on an ultraviolet transilluminator.
Peridontopathogens were detected by means of primer specific PCR. The list of primers, the annealing temperatures as well as the length of the products are given in Table 1. *P. gingivalis* and *A. actinomycetemcomitans* were amplified in the same multiplex PCR reaction, whilst *T. Forshytia* and *P. Intermedia* were coamplified in another multiplex reaction. *E.*

corrodens was amplified separately. Specimens of subgingival dental plaque, positive for those microorganisms were used as positive controls. For the negative control, DNA sample was omitted and replaced by water.

Bacteria	Primer pairs	Annealing. t (C°)	Amplicon Size
Porphyromonas gingivalis	AGA GTT TGA TCC TGG CTC AG CAA TAC TCG TAT CGC CCG TTA TTC	55	460 bp
Aggregatibacter actinomycetemcomitans	AGA GTT TGA TCC TGG CTC AG CAC TTA AAG GTC CGC CTA CGT GC	55	600 bp
Tannerella forsythia	AGA GTT TGA TCC TGG CTC AG GTA GAG CTT ACA CTA TAT CGC AAA CTC CTA	53	840 bp
Prevotella intermedia	AGA GTT TGA TCC TGG CTC AG GTT GCG TGC ACT CAA GTC CGC C	53	660 bp
Eikenella corrodens	CTA ATA CCG CAT ACG TCC TAA G CTA CTA AGC AAT CAA GTT GCC C	53	800 bp

Table 1. Primer sequences, annealing temperatures and size of obtained PCR products used for the detection of tested bacteria

11. Results

All 60 patients included in the study were diagnosed as chronic generalized periodontitis with a mean value of PD 3.12±0.35mm and CAL 2.79±0.82mm.

A total of 72 specimens have been tested for the presence of 5 different periodontopathogens. The result was considered to be positive if a band of expected size was present on the gel. There was no attempt of sequencing the PCR products or quantifying the infectious agents by real-time PCR. 7 out of 40 specimens of acute necrotizing pancreatitis were positive for the presence of: *E. corrodens* (3 cases), *A. actinomycetemcomitans* (1 case), *P. intermedia* (1 case), *T. forsythia* (3 cases, Fig. 9), and *T. forsythia* and *P. intermedia* simultaneously (1 case). In one specimen of pancreatic cancer *P. intermedia* could be detected. Interestingly, two control specimens obtained from cadavers (cause of death was liver cirrhosis) harbored oral microorganisms.

Fig. 9. Polyacrylamide gel electrophoresis showing bands that represent the product of PCR amplification corresponding to *Tannerella forsythia*

Data on tissue specimen origin and PCR findings are summarized in Table 2.

Tissue	no	*Pg*	*Aa*	*Pi*	*Tf*	*Ec*
ANP	40		1	2	2	3
PC	20			1		
NP	12			1	1	

Table 2. The presence of periodontal pathogens in pancreatic tissue. ANP - acute necrotizing pancreatitis, PC - pancreatic cancer, NP - normal pancreatic tissue obtained post-mortem, *Pg – Porphyromonas ginivalis, Aa – Aggregatibacter actinomycetemcomitans, Pi – Prevotella intermedia, Tf - Tannerella forsythia, Ec – Eikenella corroden*

12. Conclusion

To the best of our knowledge, this is the first time that *E. corrodens, A. actinomycetemcomitans, P. intermedia* and *B. forsythia* have been described in ANP. Even though it is for some time obvious that periodontal pathogens can enter the circulation, causing transient bacteraemia, there were no systematic assessments of potential association between oral bacteria and extraoral infections. Although Eikenella species, for instance, have been shown to cause endocarditis and intraabdominal infection, they are considered a very rare etiological agent (Danzinger et al., 1994; Watkin et al., 2002). Interestingly, we found *E. corrodens* in three cases of acute necrotizing pancreatitis. Four other cases of ANP harbored other periodontal pathogens.

Bacterial infections are usual complications in patients with acute pancreatitis but they typically include *Salmonella, Campylobacter, Escherichia coli, Pseudomonas aeruginosa* etc (Garg et al., 2001; Reimund et al., 2008). Generally, acute pancreatitis is not the primary manifestation of these infections. The presence of dental plaque bacteria in our cases of ANP does not exclude the simultaneous occurrence of other pathogens.

Bacterial translocation which can be defined as the passage of intestinal microbes through the mucosa to internal organs is doubtlessly an important cause of pancreas infection. Nonetheless, other infection routes and infection sources should be considered as well, and the presence of periodontal microorganisms in ANP substantiates the hypothesis of alternative paths. Multiple risk factors of bacterial spreading, including surgery, tumour metastasis in the abdomen, compromising local anatomy and circulation, etc., are known to exist. Presumably, from abdominal aorta, where they can be found, oral bacteria are capable of reaching the main arteries supplying pancreas. Their presence in pancreatic tissue could be tentatively explained by compromised local circulation. The finding of bactDNA in two control pancreatic specimens, in which the cause of death was a non-pancreatic disease (cirrhosis), may be due to some contamination during autopsy. Infections in patients with cirrhosis are frequent and varied and their spreading in the peritoneum cannot be ruled out (Frances et al., 2008). In the present study, liver tissue has not been tested for the presence of periodontopathogens.

The finding of only one case positive for *P. intermedia* in the pancreatic cancer group does not support the concept of direct oral bacteria involvement in the pathogenic processes, in the same way as seen in atherosclerosis. On the other hand, pancreatic cancer has been previously related to different bacterial infections. Namely, *Helicobacter* DNA was detected in a very high percentage of pancreatic tumors and surrounding tissue (Nilson et al., 2006; Stolzenberg et at., 2001). As *Helicobacter pylori* is also frequently encountered in the oral cavity of individuals with periodontal disease (Souto et al., 2008, Zarić et al., 2009), its occurrence in the present cases of pancreatic cancer is very probable. A rising body of evidence supports the view on microbially induced and inflammation-driven malignancies (Engels et al., 2008; Lochhead&El-Omar, 2008; Michaud, 2007).

Two large cohort studies looked at a link between pancreatic cancer and history of periodontal disease and found a significant association between the two (Michaud et al., 2007, 2008). According to the authors periodontal disease might be a marker of a susceptible immune system or might directly affect cancer risk. Hujoel found a significant association between pancreatic cancer and periodontitis measured by examination but again had a relatively small number of cases within their cohort. The results published by Michaud on increased incidence of pancreatic cancer among patients with periodontal disease could suggest a possible involvement of periodontopathogens in pancreatic cancer. Our study does not really confirm it, or at least does not point to direct, local contribution of oral microorganisms to the pathogenic process. Their role may be considered in terms of infection and chronic inflammation with systemic effect.

The presence of periodontopathogens in various arteries, however, is an important finding. It means that oral microorganisms have theoretically the possibility to migrate to organs distant from their primary reservoir-the oral cavity, and invade them. Whether it will result in clinical or subclinical pathological changes remains uncertain.

In periodontitis, periodontal pathogens and their products, as well as inflammatory mediators produced in periodontal tissues, might enter the bloodstream and contribute to the global inflammatory burden, causing systemic effects and/or contributing to systemic diseases. Several bacteria can promote or initiate abnormal cell growth by evading the immune system or suppressing apoptosis. Since periodontitis is a chronic oral bacterial infection, few authors have suggested a possible positive association between periodontitis and pancreatic cancer. To our knowledge, this is the first study which demonstrated the presence of periodontal bacteria in pancreatic tissue. Relatively low percentage of positive findings in our study does not represent a reliable proof of a link between periodontopathogens and pancreatic diseases. This might be explained by the fact that destruction of periodontal tissues in our study group was not extensive. Further researches to confirm association between periodontitis and pancreatic diseases are required.

Epidemiological research (cross-sectional and longitudinal studies) can identify relationships but not causation. If some types of periodontal disease merely constitute an oral component of a systemic disorder or have etiological features in common with systemic diseases, periodontal and systemic diseases might frequently occur together without having a cause effect relationship (Slots, 1998). Medical community should be aware of the potential negative effects of periodontal infections on systemic health. First of all, periodontal infections must be recognized and treated, and then a regular oral care must be maintained. Nevertheless, with information accessible at the moment, it seems justified to state that good oral health is important to maintain good general health.

13. Acknowledgments

This work has been financially supported by the grant of the Serbian Ministry of Science (no 175075 and 41008).

14. References

Arrieta-Blanco, J.J.; Bartolome-Villar, B.; Jimenez-Martinez, E.; Saavedra-Vallejo, Arrieta-Blanco, F.J. (2003). Dental problems in patients with diabetes mellitus (II): gingival index and periodontal disease. *Med Oral* , Vol: 8: 233–247.

Bastard, J.P.; Maachi, M.; Lagathu, C.; Kim, M.J.; Caron, M.; Vidal, H.; Capeau, J.; Feve, B. (2006). Recent advances in the relationship between obesity, inflammation, and insulin resistance. *Eur Cytokine Netw*, Vol: 17: 4–12.

Brajović, G.; Stefanović, G.; Ilić, V.; Petrović, S.; Stefanović, N.; Nikolic-Jakoba, N.; Milošević-Jovčić, N. (2010). Association of Fibronectin with Hypogalactosylated Immunoglobulin G (IgG), in Gingival Crevicular Fluid in Periodontitis. *J Periodontol* , Vol: 81:1472-1480.

Camargo, P.M.; Klokkevold, P.R.; Kenney, E.B.; Lekovic, V. (1998). Guided tissue regeneration in Class II furcation involved .maxillary molars: a controlled study of 8 split-mouth cases, *J Periodontol.*, Vol: 69(9):1020-6.

Camargo, P.M.; Lekovic, V.; Weinlaender, M.; Nedic, M.; Vasilic, N.; Wolinsky, L.E.; Kenney, E.B. (2000). A controlled re-entry study on the effectiveness of bovine porous bone mineral used in combination with a collagen membrane of porcine origin in the treatment of intrabony defects in humans. *J Clin Periodontol.*, Vol: (12):889-896.

Camargo, P. M.; Lekovic, V.; Weinlaender, M.; Vasilic, N.; Kenney, E. B. (2002). Platelet-rich plasma and bovine porous bone mineral combined with guided tissue regeneration in the treatment of intrabony defects in humans. *Journal of Periodontal Research*, Vol: 37: 300-306.

Camargo, P. M.; Lekovic, V.; Weinlaender, M.; Vasilic, N.; Madzarevic, M.;Kenney, E. B. (2005). A reentry study on use of bovine porous bone mineral, guided tissue regeneration and platelet-rich plasma in the treatment of intrabony defects in humans. *International Journal of Periodontics and Restorative Dent*, Vol: 25(1):45-59.

Ciancola, L.J.; Park, B.H.; Bruck, E.; Mosovich, L.; Genco, R.J. (1982). Prevalence of periodontal disease in insulin-dependent diabetes mellitus (juvenile diabetes). *J Am Dent Assoc*, Vol: 104: 653–660.

Collin, H.L.; Uusitupa, M.; Niskanen, L.; Kontturi-Na¨rhi, V.; Markkanen, H.; Koivisto, A.M.; Meurman, J.H. (1998). Periodontal finding in elderly patients with non-insulin dependent diabetes mellitus. *J Periodontol*, Vol: 69: 962–966.

Consensus Report Periodontal Diseases: Pathogenesis and Microbial Factors, *Ann. Periodontology* 1 (1996) 926-932.

Danzinger, L.H.; Schoonover, L.L.; Kale, P.; Resnick, D.J. (1994). Eikenella corrodens as an intra-abdominal pathogen. *Am Surg*, Vol: 60(4):296-9.

Engels, E.A. (2008). Inflammation in the development of lung cancer: epidemiological evidence. *Expert Rev Anticancer Ther.* Vol: 8(4):605-15.

Fiehn, N.E.; Larsen, T.; Christiansen, N.; Holmstrup, P.; Schroeder, T.V. (2005). Identification of periodontal pathogens in atherosclerotic vessels. Vol: 76(5):731-6.

Ford, P. J.; Gemmell, E.; Chan, A.; Carter, C.L.; Walker, P.J.; Bird, P.S.; West, M.J.; Cullinan, M.P.; Seymour, G.J. (2006). Inflammation, heat shock proteins and periodontal pathogens in atherosclerosis: an immunohistologic study. Oral *Microbiol Immunol.*, Vol: 21(4):206-11.

Frances, R.; Zapater, P.; Gonzales-Navajas, J.M.; Munoz, C.; Cano, R.; Moreu, R.; Pascual, S.; Bellot, P.; Perez-Mateo, M.; Such, J. (2008). Bacterial DNA in patients with cirrhosis and noninfected ascites mimics the soluble immune response established in patients with spontaneous bacterial peritonitis. *Hepatology*, Vol: 47(3):978-85.

Garg, P.K.; Khanna, S.; Bohidar, N.P.; Kapil, A.; Tandon, R.K. (2001). Incidence, spectrum and antibiotic sensitivity pattern of bacterial infections among patients with acute pancreatitis. *J Gastroenterol Hepatol*, Vol: 6(9):1055-9.

Higashi, Y.; Goto, C.; Jitsuiki, D.; Umemura, T.; Nishioka, K.; Hidaka, T.; Takemoto, H.; Nakamura, S.; Soga, J.; Chayama, K.; Yoshizumi, M., Taguchi, A. (2008). Periodontal infection is associated with endothelial dysfunction in healthy subjects and hypertensive patients. *Hypertension*, Vol: 51: 446–453.

Higashi, Y.; Goto, C.; Hidaka, T.; Soga, J.; Nakamura, S.; Fujii, Y.; Hata, T.; Idei, N.; Fujimura, N.; Chayama, K.; Kihara, Y.; Taguchi, A. (2009). Oral infection-inflammatory pathway, periodontitis, is a risk factor for endothelial dysfunction in patients with coronary artery disease. *Atherosclerosis,* Vol: 206: 604–610.

Hujoel, P.P.; Drangsholt, M.; Spiekerman, C.; Weiss, N,S. (2003). An exploration of the periodontitis -cancer association. *Ann Epidemiol*, Vol: 13 : 312 – 6.

Kinane, D.F. (20010). Causation and pathogenesis of periodontal disease. *Periodontol 2000,* Vol: 25:8-20.

Leković , V.; Klokkevold, P.; Nedić, M.; Kenney, E.B.; Dimitrijević, B.; Đorđević, M. (1997). Histologic and histometric evaluation of two biodegradable membranes following treatment of class II furcation defects. *Journal of Dental Research,*Vol.76:2048.

Lekovic, V.; Klokkevold, P.R.; Kenney, E.B.; Dimitrijevic, B.; Nedic, M.; Weinlaender, M. (1998a). Histologic evaluation of guided tissue regeneration using 4 barrier membranes: a comparative furcation study in dogs.*J Periodontol*, Vol: 69(1):54-61.

Lekovic, V.; Klokkevold, P.R.; Camargo, P.M.; Kenney, E.B.; Nedic, M.; Weinlaender, M. (1998b). Evaluation of periosteal membranes and coronally positioned flaps in the treatment of Class II furcation defects: a comparative clinical study in humans. *J Periodontol.*, Vol: 69(9):1050-5.

Lekovic, V.; Camargo, P.M.; Weinlaender, M.; Kenney, E.B.; Vasilic, N. (2001a). Combination use of bovine porous bone mineral, enamel matrix proteins, and a bioabsorbable membrane in intrabony periodontal defects in humans. *J Periodontol,* Vol: 72(5):583-9.

Lekovic, V.; Camargo, P.M.; Weinlaender, M.; Vasilic, N.; Djordjevic, M.; Kenney, E.B. (2001b). The use of bovine porous bone mineral in combination with enamel matrix proteins or with an autologous fibrinogen/fibronectin system in the treatment of intrabony periodontal defects in humans. *Journal of Periodontology,* Vol: 72: 1157-1163.

Lekovic, V.; Camargo, P.M.; Weinlaender, M.; Vasilic, N.; Madzarevic, M.; Kenney, E.B. (2003). Effectiveness of a combination of platelet-rich plasma, bovine porous bone mineral and guided tissue regeneration in the treatment of mandibular grade II molar furcations in humans. *Journal of Clinical Periodontology*, Vol: 30(8):746-751.

Lekovic, V. & Aleksic Z. (2004). CTG with enamel matrix derivate in papilla augmentation procedure. *Clinical Oral Implants Research*, Vol: 15 (4), 381-392.

Liu, R.; Bal, H.S.; Desta, T.; Krothapalli, N.; Alyyassi, M.; Luan, Q.; Graves, D.T. (2006). Diabetes enhances periodontal bone loss through diminished resorption and diminished bone formation. *J Dent Res*, Vol: 85: 510–514.

Lochhead, P. & El-Omar EM. (2008). Gastric cancer. *Br Med Bull*, Vol: 85:87-100.

Loe, H.; Theilade, E., & Jensen, H.B. (1965). Experimental gingivitis in man. *J. Periodonto*, Vol: 36:177–181.

Lo¨e, H.; Anerud, A.; Boysen, H.; Smith, M. (1978). The natural history of periodontal disease in man. The rate of periodontal destruction before 40 years of age. *J Periodontol*, Vol: 49: 607–620.

Lo¨e, H. (1993). Periodontal disease. The sixth complication of diabetes mellitus. *Diabetes Care*, Vol: 16: 329–334.

Kuper, H.; Adami, H. O. & Trichopoulos, D. (2000).Infections as a major preventable cause of human cancer. *J. Intern. Me*, Vol: 248: 171–183.

Kuramitsu, H. K. (1998). Proteases of *Porphyromonas gingivalis*: what don't they do? *Oral Microbiol. Immunol*, Vol: 13:263–270.

Kwan, S.K.; Lekovic, V.; Camargo, P.M.; Klokkevold, P.R.; Kenney, E.B.; Nedic, M.; Dimitrijevic, B. (1998).The use of autogenous periosteal grafts as barriers for the treatment of intrabony defects in humans. *J Periodontol*, Vol: 69(11):1203-9.

Kweider, M.; Lowe, G. D.; Murray, G.D.; Kinane, D.F.; McGowan A.D. (1993). Dental disease, fibrinogen and white cell count: links with myocardial infarction? *Scott. Med. J*, Vol: 38:73–74.

Maeda, H. & Akaike, T. (1998). Nitric oxide and oxygen radicals in infection, inflammation, and cancer. *Biochemistry*, Vol: 63, 854–865.

Mealey, BL. (2006). Periodontal disease and diabetes. A two-way street. J *Am Dent Assoc*, Vol: 137(Suppl.): 26S–31S.

Michaud, D.S.; Joshipura, K. ; Giovannucci, E. (2007). A prospective study of periodontal disease and pancreatic cancer in US male health professionals. *J Natl Cancer Inst*, Vol: 99:171-175.

Michaud, D.S.; Liu, Y.; Meyer, M.; Giovannucci, E.; Joshipura, K. (2008). Periodontal disease, tooth loss, and cancer risk in male health professionals: a prospective cohort study. *Lancet Oncol*, Vol: 9(6):550-8.

Milicevic, R.; Brajovic, G.; Nikolic-Jakoba, N.; Popovic, B.; Pavlica, D.; Lekovic, V.; B, Milasin, J. (2008). Identification Of Periodontopathogen Microorganisms By PCR Technique. *SRPSKI ARHIV ZA CELOKUPNO LEKARSTVO*, Vol: 136: 476-480.

Niederman, R.; Y. Buyle-Bodin, B. Y.; Lu, Robinson, P.; Naleway, C. (1997). Short-chain carboxylic acid concentration in human gingival crevicular fluid. *J. Dent. Res*, Vol: 76:575–579.

Nilsson, H.O.; Stenram, U. & Ihse I. (2006). Helicobacter species ribosomal DNA in the pancreas, stomach and duodenum of pancreatic cancer patients. *World J Gastroenterol*, Vol: 12:3038-3043.

Okuda, K.; Ishiara, K.; Nakagawa, T.; Hirayama, A.; Inayama, Y., Okuda, K. (2001). Detection of *Treponema denticola* in atherosclerotic lesions. *J Clin Microbiol*, Vol: 39:1114-1117.

Page, R. C. (1998). The pathobiology of periodontal diseases may affect systemic diseases: inversion of a paradigm. *Ann. Periodontol*, Vol: 3:108–120.

Pesonen, E.; Kaprio, E.; Rapola, J.; Soveri, J.; Oksanen, J. (1981). Endothelial cell damage in piglet coronary artery after intravenous administration of *E. coli* endotoxin: a scanning and transmission electron-microscopic study. *Atherosclerosis*, Vol: 40:65–73.

Pucar, A.; Milasin, J.; Lekovic, V.; Vukadinovic, M., Ristic, M., Putnik, S.; Kenny, E.B. (2007). Correlation between atherosclerosis and periodontal putative pathogenic bacterial infections in coronary and internal mammary arteries. *J Periodontol*, Vol: 78(4): 677-82.

Ratcliff, P. A.&Johnson, P.W. (1999). The relationship between oral malodor, gingivitis, and periodontitis. A review. *J. Periodontol*, Vol: 70:485–489.

Reimund, J.M.; Muller, C.D.; Finck, G.; Escalin, G.; Duclos, B.; Baumann, R. (2005). Factors contributing to infectious diarrhea-associated pancreatic enzyme alterations. *Gastroeneterol Clin Biol* , Vol: 29(3):247-53.

Roquer, J.; Segura, T., Serena, J.; Castillo, J. (2009). Endothelial dysfunction, vascular disease and stroke: the ARTICO study. *Cerebrovasc*, Vol: 1: 25–37.

Safkan-Seppala, B.&Ainamo J. (1992). Periodontal conditions in insulin-dependent diabetes mellitus. *J Clin Periodontol*, Vol: 19: 24–29.

Shlossman, M.; Knowler, W.C.; Pettitt, D.J.; Genco, R.J. (1990). Type 2 diabetes mellitus and periodontal disease. *J Am Dent Assoc* , Vol: 121: 532–536.

Slots, J. 1998. Casual or causal relationship between periodontal infection and non-oral disease? *J. Dent. Res.* 77:1764–1765.

Shacter, E. & Weitzman, S. A. (2002). Chronic inflammation and cancer. *Oncology* 16, 217–226.

Southerland, J.H.; Taylor, G.W.; Offenbacher, S. (2005). Diabetes and periodontal infection: making the connection. *Clin Diabetes*, Vol: 23: 171–178.

Souto, R.& Colombo, A.P. (2008). Detection of Helicobacter pylori by polymerase chain reaction in the subgingival biofilm and saliva of non-dyspeptic periodontal patients. *J Periodontol.*, Vol: 79(1):97-103.

Spahr, A.; Klein, E., Khuseyinova, N. et al. (2006). Periodontal infections and coronary heart disease: role of periodontal bacteria and importance of total pathogen burden in the Coronary Event and Periodontal Disease (CORODONT) study. *Arch* Intern, Vol: 1665:554-559.

Stolzenberg-Solomon, R.Z.; Blaser, M.J.; Limburg, P.J. et al. (2001). *Helicobacter pylori* seropositivity as a risk factor for pancreatic cancer. *J Natl Cancer Inst*, Vol: 93:937-941.

Tonetti, M.S.& Mombelly, A. (1999). Early onset periodontitis. *Ann Periodotol*, Vol: 4:39-53.

Van Dyke, T. E.; Bartholomew, E.; Genco, R.J.; Slots, J., Levine, M.J. (1982). Inhibition of neutrophil chemotaxis by soluble bacterial products. *J. Periodontol*, Vol: 53:502–508.

Watkin, R.; Baker, V.; Lang, N.; Ment, J. (2002). Eikenella corrodens infective endocarditis in a previously healthy non-drug user. *Europ J Clin Microbiol Inf Dis*, Vol: 21(12):890-1.

Zambon, J.J. (1996). Periodontal disease: microbial factors. *Ann Periodont*, Vol: 1:879-925.

Zaric, S; Bojic, B; Jankovic, L, et al (2009). Periodontal therapy improves gastric Helicobacter pylori eradication.*J Dent Res*,Vol 88(10):946-50.

Part 8

Role of Polyunsaturated Fatty Acids in Inflammatory Disease

8

Polyunsaturated Fatty Acids and Inflammatory Diseases

Antonio Ferrante and Charles Hii
Department of Immunopathology
SA Pathology at Women's and Children's Hospital
Discipline of Paediatrics, University of Adelaide,
School of Pharmacy and Medical Science
University of South Australia
Australia

1. Introduction

Polyunsaturated fatty acids and their metabolites are crucial to the physiologic and pathophysiologic processes in inflammation. The balance between *n-6* and *n-3* polyunsaturated fatty acids in body tissues is a key to regulating the inflammatory reaction and preventing exacerbated inflammation in inflammatory disorders. Altering fatty acid type and their composition in phospholipids through diet supplements for beneficial outcomes in disease has been of major interest to the community. The sources of polysaturated fatty acid include de novo synthesis, essential fatty acids obtained from the diet, elongation and desaturation to obtain fatty acids of longer chain length by tissues.

The types of fatty acids being esterified in membrane phospholipids provide a characteristic fatty acid composition of the phospholipids which can dictate the characteristics of the inflammatory response depending on the types of metabolites of polyunsaturated fatty acids formed through the lipoxygenase (LOX) and cyclooxygenase (COX) pathways, either promoting or inhibiting the inflammatory process, by controlling intracellular signalling pathways, such as PKC, MAP kinases, PI3 kinase etc

While focusing on the use of n-3 polyunsaturated fatty acids in treating rheumatoid arthritis, cardiovascular diseases and asthma, it is highlighted that such treatments are at a 'cross road' because of poor understanding of the field of lipidomics and in supplementation approaches in those with various illnesses, including inflammatory diseases.

2. Sources of arachidonic acid and other fatty acids

Fatty acids in the body can be obtained by *de novo* synthesis in tissues, through the diet or from the hydrolysis of membrane phospholipids. Human beings can synthesize fatty acids up to 16:0 (palmitate) *de novo* from acetyl coenzyme, by a series of cycles of sequential condensation, reduction, dehydration and reduction. The chain is elongated by two carbon atoms per cycle. 16:0 is then elongated to 18:0 (stearate) and desaturated to yield 18:1*n-9* (oleate). Alternatively, 16:0 is desaturated to 16:1*n-9* (palmitoleate) and elongated to 18:1*n-9*. A variety of longer chain fatty acids can be derived from 18:1*n-9* by a combination of elongation and desaturation reactions. However, mammalian cells are unable to perform these reactions because they do not express the enzymes, Δ12 and Δ15 desaturases to introduce double bonds at carbon atoms beyond C-9. Consequently, mammalian cells cannot synthesise 18:2*n-6* (linoleic) and 18:3*n-3* (α-linolenate). These fatty acids, required by the animal but cannot be synthesised endogenously, are therefore considered as essential fatty acids and are obtained from the diet. The essential fatty acids serve as starting points for the synthesis of longer chain fatty acids such as 20:4*n-6* (arachidonic acid, AA) and the *n-3* fatty acids 20:5*n-3* (eicosapentaenoic acid, EPA) and 22:6*n-3* (docosahexaenoic acid, DHA) by elongation and desaturation through the action of elongases and desaturases (e.g Δ6, Δ5 and Δ4). AA is derived from 18:2*n-6* while EPA and DHA are derived from 18:3*n-3*.

Dietary fatty acids can be obtained from animal meats, fish, green vegetables, and from oils derived from the above. They mainly occur as triacylglycerols. Essential fatty acids are found in abundance in green leafy vegetables and the seeds of most plants. The *n-3* fatty acids EPA and DHA are abundant in marine oils and fish rich diets are another source of these fatty acids. Grain-fed animals are rich in AA (Simopoulos, 1991).

3. Transport and uptake of fatty acids

Following absorption by the intestine, the fatty acids are transported to tissues where they may be utilized immediately or stored. At least four types of vehicles have been shown to be involved in their transportation: (i) chylomicrons, where dietary triacylglycerol is carried in protein-coated lipid droplets and transported to the whole body from the intestine; (ii) ketone bodies (acetoacetate and β-hydroxybutyrate) and (iii) very low density lipoprotein (VLDL), which are responsible for transporting fatty acids, processed by or synthesised in the liver, to either adipose tissue for storage, or to various tissues to be used for cell structure and metabolism and (iv) as non-esterified fatty acid. Triacylglycerol in the blood is enzymatically hydrolysed by lipases, such as lipoprotein lipases, on the surface of endothelial cells. The released free fatty acids become bound to serum fatty acid binding protein eg. albumin, type IV fatty acid transporter, which carries the released fatty acids in the blood stream to appropriate tissue sites. The free fatty acids in the extracellular fluid continuously exchange with the intracellular fatty acids which are released by the action of phospholipase A_2. This process is called intracellular fatty acid turnover (McGarry, 1993).

How fatty acids are taken up by cells remains unclear. It has been proposed that fatty acids firstly become dissociated from albumin and then bind to a fatty acid transporter protein in the plasma membrane or a flip flop mechanism. A fatty acid translocase (FAT) with homology to CD36 has also been reported to be involved in the transport of long chain fatty acids (Bonen et al, 2002). There is evidence that fatty acids can also enter cells by a flip flop mechanism (Kamp et al, 2003). These two modes of fatty acid uptake need not be mutually exclusive. Once inside the cell, fatty acids are transported to various intracellular sites by the cytosolic fatty acid binding protein (FABP, 14-15 kDa) where they interact with appropriate proteins/structures to evoke cellular responses (Spector, 1992; Poirrier et al, 1996). The precise mechanism by which fatty acids are taken up by neutrophils is still poorly defined. However, it has been demonstrated that the ability of a fatty acid to partition into the neutrophil plasma membrane is not sufficient to evoke superoxide production (Steinbeck et al, 1991). Similarly, the observation that saturated fatty acids (lacking biological actions) have a greater ability to partition into the plasma membrane of cytotoxic T lymphocyte than *cis* unsaturated fatty acids, is inconsistent with their biological activity being totally caused by membrane partitioning of a fatty acid (Anel et al, 1993).

4. Arachidonic acid and its metabolites are central to the development of inflammatory reactions

AA is an important promoter of physiologic processes of body tissue and organs. AA and its metabolites can act as an intercellular signalling molecule as well as intracellular secondary signalling molecule (Ferrante et al. 2005). The role of this fatty acid and its products in autoimmune and allergic inflammation has also been abundantly described and appreciated, such that AA and pathways involved in its metabolism have been the targets of medications. The resolution of inflammation initiated through the release of AA from cellular membrane phospholipids is important and where its generation persists, this reaction evolves into a chronic and debilitating condition. The main pathways for its metabolism have been the lipoxygenase (LOX) and cyclooxygenase (COX) enzymes.

AA and its metabolites can be generated at several cellular points. Apart from production at local tissues, be these immune cells or barrier cells such as endothelial cells, epithelial cells etc, the infiltrating cells, particular leukocytes, provide a rich source of these mediators of inflammation. Thus it is not surprising that the lipids influence several key functions of leukocytes which include, chemotaxis, oxygen radical generation, granule enzyme release and cytokine production (Ferrante et al, 2005).

AA may control inflammation through several activities. AA per se has been shown to cause cellular activation independently of its metabolism via the LOX and COX pathways (Ferrante et al, 2005). The generation of several metabolites such as LTB4 and PGE2 gives the system a potent inflammatory potential.

5. Release of AA from the cellular phospholipid pools and the generation of eicosanoids

Cellular activation leads to the activation of Phospholipase A_2 (PLA_2) and the release of AA from the sn-2 position of the phospholipids (Balsinde et al, 2002). This activation can be brought about by many different types of agonists acting usually via a cell surface receptor. This includes intercellular signalling molecules such as cytokines which are involved in inflammatory responses in both the context of physiologic and pathophysiologic states.

Amongst the various structurally different forms of the PLA_2 is the cytosolic ($cPLA_2\alpha$, Group IVA), believed to play an important role in eicosanoids production (Kita et al, 2006; Ghosh et al, 2006). Submicromolar concentrations of Ca^{++} promotes the translocation of $cPLA_2\alpha$ from the cytosol to the perinuclear membrane where it becomes activated by MAP kinases (Lin et al, 1993; Nemenoff et al, 1993). There it causes preferential hydrolysis of AA-containing phospholipids, releasing AA to become available to downstream enzymes including LOX and COX, important in production of leukotrienes and prostaglandins (Fig 1). Its importance has been concluded from studies showing that mice deficient in $cPLA_2\alpha$ were not susceptible to allergy induced brocho-constriction, airway hyper-responsiveness, as well as adult respiratory distress syndrome (Wu et al, 2010). Mice deficient in cPLA2α were also protected from experimental autoimmune encephalomyelitis (Marusic et al, 1995).

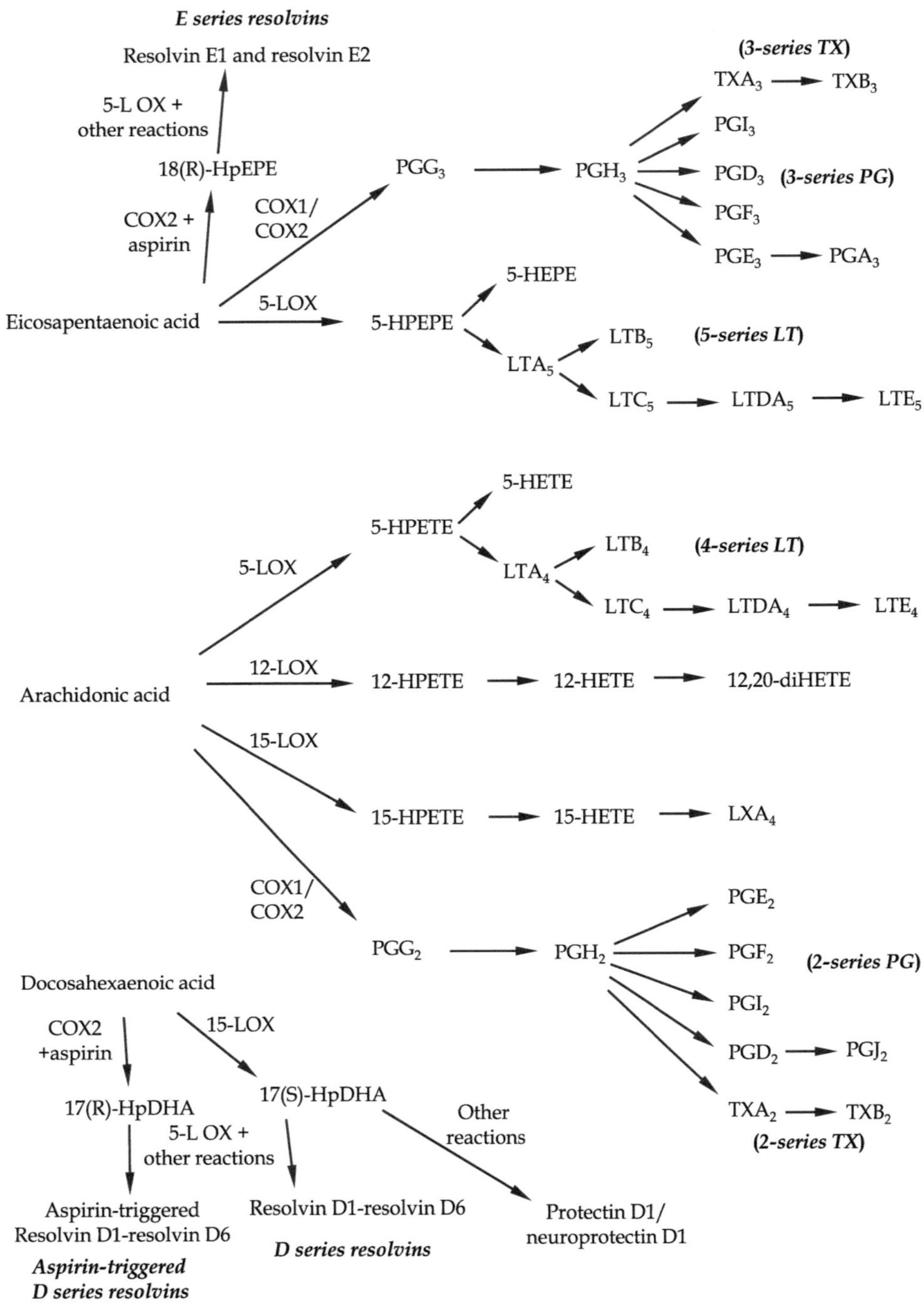

Fig. 1. Outline of the metabolism of arachidonic acid, eicosapentaenoic acid and docosahexaenoic acid by the lipoxygenases and cyclooxygenases. LOX, lipoxygenase; COX, cyclooxygenase; HPETE, hydroperoxyeicosatetraenoic acid; HPEPE, hydroperoxypentaenoic acid; HETE, hydroxyeicosatetraenoic acid; HEPE, hydroxypentaenoic acid; LT, leukotrienes; TX, thromboxane; PG, prostaglandin; LX, lipoxin; HpDHA, hydroperoxyDHA.

Cell activation leads to the generation of AA-derived eicosanoids (Fig 1). The main ones are divided into three groups, leukotrienes (LTs), prostaglandins (PGs) and lipoxins (LXs). Their biological properties give rise to a regulatory network of inflammation, having both an effect on cells of the immune system, macrophages, T cells, neutrophils as well as non-immune cells such as endothelial cells. While the metabolism of AA via the LOX and COX pathways is considered to be inflammatory, it is also evident that some products may exhibit anti-inflammatory properties.

It is clear from several studies that different eicosanoids are generated at different times of an acute inflammatory response (Serhan, 2005; Serhan et al, 2008). Hence, prostaglandins and leukotrienes are rapidly generated, whereas the lipoxins, also produced from AA, are generated later with the onset of the resolution phase. During acute inflammation, activation of cPLA2 results in the conversion of the released AA by 5-LOX and COX to leukotrienes such as LTB4, a potent neutrophil activator and chemoattractant, and proinflammatory prostaglandins which control local blood flow, vascular dilation and permeability changes needed for leukocyte adhesion, diapedesis, and recruitment. The prostaglandins initiate a number of responses relevant in inflammation (i.e., vasoconstriction, vascular permeability changes, pain, vasodilation and edema). However, the production of prostaglandins such as PGE2 and PGD2 which possess proinflammatory properties, also signals the end of the inflammatory response by activating the transcriptional regulation of 15-LOX in neutrophils that initiates an eicosanoid class switch from a proinflammatory profile to a resolving profile, including the generation of EPA- and DHA-derived resolvins and/or protectins. In murine models, resolution of acute inflammation is accompanied by the appearance in exudates of EPA and DHA, which follows the appearance of non-esterified AA. Indeed, leukotrienes (potent chemoattractants) are deactivated and the transcriptional regulation of enzymes required for LX and resolvin production is activated. (Serhan, 2005; Serhan et al, 2008). The combined actions of 5-LOX, 12-LOX and 15-LOX lead to the generation of lipoxins such as LTA_4, resolvins and/or protectins. These mediators have anti-inflammatory and pro-resolving activities.

6. Biological properties of eicosanoids

The cellular actions of the LTB_4 and cysteinyl leukotrienes (cysLTs), LTC_4, LTD_4 and LTE_4, occur through their binding to specific G protein-coupled receptors found on responsive tissues e.g., smooth muscle and inflammatory cells of the immune system e.g., neutrophils. The distribution of receptors for LTs on various cell types are summarised in Table 1 (Okunishi et al, 2011). Two receptors for cysLTs have been well characterised, CysLt1 and CysLt2. LTD_4 has high affinity and LTE_4 has low affinity for these receptors. But other receptors are being recognised for CysLTs which includes a specific receptor for LTE_4 (Maekawa et al, 2008).

LTB_4 has two receptors, a high affinity, BLT1 and lower affinity, BLT2 (Yokomizo et al, 2000). Notably BLT1 is expressed predominantly on leukocytes (Table 1). The biological role of BLT2 requires further studies. LTB_4 is recognised for its potent chemoattractant properties for neutrophils. It also activates other neutrophil responses such as respiratory burst (oxygen radical production) and degranulation. As indicated by the expression of BLT1 on other leukocytes, apart from neutrophils (Table 1), LTB_4 activates also macrophages, eosinophils, T cells and dendritic cells (DCs).

Cell-type	BLT1	CysLT1	CysLT2
Macrophages	+	±#	±
Dendritic cells	+	+	?
B cells	?	+	?
CD4 + T cells	+	+	?
CD8 + T cells	+	?#	?
Neutrophils	+	+	+
Eosinophils	+	+	+
Basophils	+	+	+
Mast Cells	+	+	+
Airway smooth muscle cells	+	+	?
Endothelial cells	+	+	+

Table 1. Leukotriene receptor expression. (+), positive; (±), negligible; (?), not determined; (#) up-regulation upon cell activation (adapted from Okunishi et al, 2011)

The action of PGs is through the rhodopsin-like 7-transmembrane-spanning G protein-coupled receptors. These prostanoid receptors subfamily consists of 8 members EP1/EP2/EP3/EP4 bind PGE_2, DP/CRTH2 bind PGD_2, FP binds $PGF_2\alpha$, IP binds PGI_2, TP binds TXA_2 (Table 2). The CRTH2 receptor is expressed on Th2 lymphocytes and a member of the fMLF receptor superfamily (Ricciotti and FitzGerald, 2011).

7. Eicosanoids and inflammation

7.1 Leukotrienes

Inflammation, whether physiologic or pathophysiologic, is manifested by the accumulation of leukocytes and plasma leakage into the tissue site. The leukotrienes form a major family of the inflammatory mediators generated which significantly contributes to the process. LTB_4 through its chemotactic properties for several cell types including neutrophils and T cells, causes infiltration and accumulation of leukocytes at inflammatory foci. LTB_4 increases vascular permeability of post capillary venules. The ability of LTs to activate DCs has indicated a role in antigen presentation and T cell sensitisation. Relevant to this action is the finding that LTs are produced through the innate immune response, where the various pattern recognition receptors (e.g., Toll-like receptors, TLRs) are expressed on different cell types (Alvarez et al, 2010). Thus LTs may play important roles in the adaptive immune response at an early phase.

Prostaglandin Class	Receptor subtype	Type of cells/tissues
PGE_2	EP1, EP2, EP3, EP4	Brain, kidneys, VSMCs, platelets
PGD_2	DP, CRTH2	Mast cells, brain, airways, Th2 lymphocytes
PGF_{2a}	FPA, FPB	Uterus, airways, VSMCs, eyes
PGI_2	IP-IP, IP-TP_a	Endothelium, VSMCs, platelets, kidney, brain
TxA_2	TP_a, TP_b	Platelets, VSMCs, macrophages, kidney

Table 2. Expression of prostanoid receptors (adapted from Ricciotti and FitzGerald, 2011). VSMC ; vascular smooth muscle cells

The role of LTs has been established as a key mediator in several inflammatory diseases, both in experimental and clinical settings. This includes asthma and allergic rhinitis (Dahlen,

2006; Peter-Golden & Henderson, 2007). Their importance extends to the pathophysiology of atherosclerosis and progression of cancer.

7.2 Prostaglandins

PGE_2 is involved in all the signs of inflammation; redness, swelling and pain (Ricciotti & Fitzgerald, 2011), through its effects on arterial dilation, increased permeability of the microvasculature, peripheral sensory nervous and central sites within the spinal cord and brain. PGE_2 acts via one of its receptors, EP1 to EP4. Using KO mice deficient in these receptors, it has been appreciated that they play important roles in hyperalgesia (PGE_2-EP1), paw swelling in collagen-induced arthritis (EP2, EP4), Carrageenan-induced paw oedema/pleurisy (EP2, EP3), IL-6 production and joint destruction in RA and anti-inflammatory effects of PGE_2 as seen in allergic inflammation.

The regulation of various cell types by PGE_2 occurs through the expression of different EP receptors. PGE_2 exerts an anti-inflammatory effect on functions of neutrophils, macrophages and natural killer cells, the cell-types which underpin the innate immune response (Harris et al. 2002). PGE_2 also exerts regulatory actions on macrophages, DCs, T and B cells which may manifest itself as either inflammatory or anti-inflammatory actions. Examples are regulation of DC cytokine profiles and Th1 or Th2 lymphocyte development (Egan et al, 2004). Engagement of EP4 by PGE_2 in DCs and T cells promotes differentiation to Th1 and also Th17 lymphocytes (Yao et al, 2009). Other ways that PGE_2 regulates the immune response is through its role in the development of DCs with a migratory phenotyping to promote homing to drain lymph nodes (Kabashima et al, 2003; Legler et al, 2006), as well as upregulating the expression of co-stimulatory molecules on these cells (Krause et al, 2009). In an anti-inflammatory manner, PGE_2 suppresses Th1 cell development, B cell function and IgE-driven inflammatory response (Roper et al, 1995; Harris et al, 2002).

PGI_2 has potent vasodilator actions and is known to be important in regulation of cardiovascular homeostasis. The eicosanoid is an inhibitor of platelet aggregation, leukocyte adhesion and vascular smooth muscle cell proliferation (Gryglewski, 2008; Kawabe et al, 2010). Mice deficient in receptors for PGI_2 show an abrogation of the ability of PGI_2 to potentiate the bradykinin-induced microvascular permeability and a substantially reduced carrageenan-induced paw oedema (Murata et al, 1997). Other actions of PGI_2 involving the IP receptors is an allergic inflammation where it may suppress the Th2-mediated lung inflammation (Jaffar et al, 2002).

PGD2 has inflammatory and homeostatic properties. Thus while in the brain it regulates sleep and various other central nervous activities, it has inflammatory function particularly in atropic conditions. The eicosanoid promotes broncho- constriction and airways neutrophil infiltration, typical of allergic asthma (Hardy et al, 1984; Emery et al, 1980; Fujitani et al, 2002). The DP1 and DP2/CRTH2 receptors bind PGD2 with similar high affinity and both are responsible for the pro-inflammatory responses. Effects caused by PGD2 are dictated by the differential expression of these receptors in tissues such as the expression of DP1 receptors in bronchial epithelium is believed to promote the production of cytokines and chemokines which recruit eosinophils and lymphocytes in airway inflammation and hyperreactivity associated with asthma (Kabashima & Narumiya, 2003). Using mice deficient in DP1 receptors the role of PGD2 and the receptor in airway hyperreactivity and Th2-mediated lung inflammation has been documented in animal models (Matsuoka et al. 2000). The use of DP1 antagonists in animal models supports a role for the receptor in antigen-induced microvascular permeability and ovalbumin (OVA)-induced airway hyperreactivity. Reports have also suggested that the DP2/CRTH2 receptors contribute to inflammatory reactions by controlling cell traffic and the effect of function of leukocytes in which it is expressed, Th2 cells, mast cells and eosinophils. An increase in its expression has been shown to be associated with some forms of atopic dermatitis. However inflammation in other contexts may be inhibited by PGD2-DP1 receptor where inhibition of DC migration affects T cell proliferation and cytokine production (Hammad et al, 2003).

TXA_2 is highly unstable and its activity is mediated mainly through the TP receptor. Studies regarding the role of this receptor in physiologic and pathophysiologic responses show that its involved in platelet adhesion and aggregation, activation of endothelial inflammatory response and contraction/proliferation of smooth muscle cells (Nakahata, 2008).

8. Arachidonic acid and metabolites in inflammatory disorders

AA and its metabolites have been shown to play major roles in the pathogenesis of several inflammatory conditions (Table 3). Three inflammatory conditions, asthma, rheumatoid arthritis and atherosclerosis, will be used to demonstrate the interest and the importance of AA and its metabolites in such diseases/conditions.

8.1 Asthma

Arachidonic acid and eicosanoids have been long recognised to play a key role in asthma pathophysiology. The hallmark of this condition is airway inflammation and hyperresponsiveness. The importance of the enzyme responsible for releasing AA from membrane phospholipids, PLA_2 has been established using pharmacological inhibitors and more recently genetically modified mice. Bronchoalveolar lavage fluid of asthmatics contains increased amounts of secretory phospholipase A_2 ($sPLA_2$) and increased activity compared to controls (Triggiani et al, 2009; Chilton et al, 1996; Bowton et al, 1997). Particular interest has centred on group X $sPLA_2$ as this was responsible for most of the activity (Hallstrand et al., 2011). Levels of this $sPLA_2$ correlated with eicosanoid release, severity of asthma and airway inflammation (Hallstrand et al., 2011). Further studies have suggested that group X $sPLA_2$ functions in asthma pathogenesis through the release of cysLTs which are involved in airway inflammation and hyperresponsiveness. Mice genetically deficient in group X $sPLA_2$ showed a marked reduction of asthma induced with OVA, manifested as decreased interstitial oedema, and the accumulation of eosinophils and T cells into the lung (Henderson et al, 2007). The Th2 cytokine levels were also decreased in the deficient mice as were the eicosanoids, PGE_2, PGD_2, LTB_4, and cysLTs (LTC_4, LTD_4, LTE_4) (Henderson et al, 2007). Using knock-in mice with human group X sPLA2, it was demonstrated that this could restore the airway inflammation (Henderson et al., 2011). The important role of the high affinity LTB_4 receptor BLT1 also supports the role of LTs in pathogenesis of asthma (Watanabe et al, 2009).

8.2 Rheumatoid arthritis

AA derived eicosanoids have been shown to play a major role in the pathogenesis of RA. In a murine model of arthritis, a role for cPLA2α was examined using the inhibitor, pyrroxyphine (Tai et al, 2010). There was an increase in $cPLA_2\alpha$ activity which correlated with arthritis severity. Both bone destruction and incidence of arthritis was reduced by the inhibitor. Such effects correlated also with an inhibition of the production of eicosanoids and COX-2 induction.

The importance of eicosanoids in inflammatory arthritis can also be seen from studies with mice which were deficient in either the BLT1 receptor or the low affinity BLT2 receptor. In the collagen-induce arthritis model, BLT1 was found to mediate the disease. Thus, BLT1$^{-/-}$ mice were completely protected and so were the BLT1$^{-/-}$/BLT2$^{-/-}$ double knockout mice (Shao et al, 2006). Because the BLT1$^{-/-}$ mice were completely protected, the authors were not able to determine the contribution of BLT2. This was addressed by Mathis et al (2010) who reported that BLT2$^{-/-}$ mice showed reduced incidence and severity of disease in an autoantibody-induced arthritis model. Note that while the BLT2 receptor is a low affinity receptor for LTB_4, it is in fact a high affinity receptor for the COX-1 derived 12(S)-hydroxyheptadeca-5Z, 8E, 10E-trienoic acid. BTL2 is considered a model target for treating this inflammatory condition.

Prostaglandins levels are elevated in synovial fluid and synovial membranes of RA patients and are believed to play a role in fluid extravasations and pain in synovial tissue, as well as articular cartilage erosion. COX-2 is present in high and COX-1 in smaller amounts in RA synovial tissue. Selective COX-2 inhibitors (e.g. celecoxib, valdecoxib and rofecoxib) have been used to treat inflammation in RA patients, although some (e.g. valdecoxib and rofecoxib) have been withdrawn owing to increased risk of heart attack and stroke in users (James et al, 2007). The presence of the metabolites of AA in RA patients' synovial fluid has been outlined (Grignani et al, 1996). When compared with patients with artherosis (degenerative joint disease), the levels of LTB_4, LTC_4 and 6-keto-PGF1 were significantly higher in RA patients.

8.3 Cardiovascular disease and atheroosclerosis

The 5-LOX/LT pathway has been implicated in the development of cardiovascular disease (CVD) based on studies of human genetic variation (polymorphisms in the genes that code for 5-LOX or its activating protein, 5-LO-activating protein (FLAP)) and in animals, leading to the hypothesis that this pathway promotes atherosclerosis, abdominal aortic aneurysm, and myocardial infarction/reperfusion injury. Much of this is based on the known effects of LTs on leucocyte chemotaxis, vascular inflammation and enhanced permeability, and subsequent tissue/matrix degeneration. Data from a series of studies that involved genetic or pharmacological inhibition of either LT biosynthesis (5-LOX, FLAP, LTA_4 hydrolase, LTC_4 synthase) or the LT receptors, have painted a complex picture of 5-LOX/LT participation in cardiovascular disease, which is further complicated by marked differences between mice and humans (reviewed by Poeckel and Funk, 2010). Added to this is another layer of complexity imposed by the cytokine network specific to a particular pathological condition which impacts on the expression level and hence, the contribution of 5-LOX to the overall disease state. Nevertheless, current data suggest roles for 5-LOX in the early/acute stages of atherosclerosis in mice and humans, but only in the advanced stage of the human pathology. Hence, LTB_4 and CysLT are likely to play critical roles in the early phase of atherosclerosis through their influence on leukocyte recruitment, smooth muscle cell proliferation, migration of endothelial cells (properties of LTB_4) and inflammatory cell recruitment, coronary artery constriction and endothelial cell activation (properties of CysLT). In the advanced phase, LTB_4 may affect plaque stability, and the expression of other components of the 5-LOX pathway such as BLT_1, BLT_2, FLAP, LTA_4 synthase, $CysLT_1$ and $CysLT_2$ are up-regulated (reviewed by Poeckel and Funk, 2010).

The action of LTs in various stages of atherosclerosis development has been reviewed (Back, 2009). The role of LTB4 in the lipid retention and modification stage is seen by the finding that targeting BLT1 receptor decreases the accumulation of lipids and the infiltration of foam cells. The early development of intimal hyperplasia appears also to be influenced by cysLTs and LTB4. Targeting their receptors most likely inhibits intimal hyperplasia with respect to endothelial dysfunction. Cys-LTs have been suggested to play a role in both endothelium relaxation and constriction. The discovery, that endothelial cells express the BLT1 receptor during atherosclerosis (Back et al., 2005) has also implicated LTB4 in causing the changes on the endothelium. The disease progresses into recruitment of leukocytes in the vascular wall and the formation of atherosclerotic plaque. Most likely the macrophages continue to be the centre point of this development, through their ability to produce LTs , such as LTB4 and exacerbate the inflammation at atherosclerotic lesions. This draws in T cells which can stimulate macrophages to generate more LTB4, leading to a vicious cycle, perhaps halted by anti-LT treatments (Back, 2008). Upon rupture of the fibrous cap there is exposure to the blood elements with the consequences of platelet activation and thrombotic occlusion. To date there is only indirect evidence for a role of LTs where it has been shown that 5-LOX is located in areas where matrix metalloproteinases are present and which are responsible for rupture. Plaque in the coronary cerebral arteries will lead to myocardial ischemia and cerebral ischemia, respectively. In myocardial ischemia the role of LTs has been controversial from suggestions of a major, no role and even to possibly protective role (Back, 2009; Adamek et al., 2007). In contrast, in cerebral ischemia, the importance of LTs has been acknowledged. LT synthesis inhibitors and cysLT receptor antagonists limited the damage in animal models.

9. Omega 3 polyunsaturated fatty acids

Supplementation with n-3 fatty acids is of interest because of its potential benefits in treating a range of human diseases and conditions (Table 3). In particular, it is well appreciated that increasing the ratio of *n-3* over *n-6* polyunsaturated fatty acids in membrane phospholipids in patients experiencing inflammation has benefits (Simopoulos, 1991). Thus, fatty acid diet manipulations have been used in treating a wide variety of diseases/conditions including those which have an autoimmune and allergic base. While the mechanisms governing the beneficial effects of certain types of polyunsaturated fatty acids in different types of diseases is likely to vary, it is well appreciated that altering the types of polyunsaturated fatty acids in diets can modify the immune response. This is thought to be the major mechanism by which polyunsaturated fatty acids exert their protective effects in inflammatory and autoimmune disorders (Calder, 2010).

High *n*-3 fatty acid intake for four months significantly increased the general score and sigmoidoscope score of active ulcerative colitis patients compared with a placebo diet (Simopoulos, 1991; Greenfield et al., 1993). The effects were maintained for three months after the fatty acid treatment was discontinued. In a human gingival inflammation model, 28-day treatment with EPA and DHA (1.8g/day) markedly reduced the gingival index in interdental papilla (Campan et al., 1996). Dietary supplementation with fish oil fatty acids in conjunction with conventional treatment (cyclosporin) in psoriasis patients has been shown to improve the skin lesions and decrease the nephrotoxicity of cyclosporin (Simopoulos, 1991). In the treatment of RA, the beneficial effects of fish oil are pronounced and

Conditions
Rheumatoid arthritis
Atherosclerosis
Acute coronary events
Allergic diseases
Asthma
Psoriasis
Inflammatory disease
Multiple sclerosis
Systemic lupus erythematosus
Cystic fibrosis
Type 1 diabetes
Chronic obstructive pulmonary disease

Table 3. Inflammation-based conditions which appear to benefit from n-3 polyunsaturated fatty acid or fish oil supplementation (adapted from Calder et al, 2010)

reproducible in both animal models and in human trials. It has been shown that feeding mice with EPA and DHA, reduces the incidence and severity of type II collagen-induced experimental arthritis (Leslie et al, 1985). Another study demonstrated that n-3 fatty acids given in the form of krill oil or fish oil caused a significant reduction in arthritis score and hind paw swelling in a collagen-induced arthritis model (Ierna et al., 2010). Dietary supplementation with *n-3* polyunsaturated fatty acids in RA patients shows significant relief of joint pain and swelling, and the duration of morning stiffness. This has led to a reduction in requirement for nonsteroidal anti-inflammatory drugs (NSAIDs), with some patients able to discontinue NSAIDs while receiving *n-3* fatty acid supplements (Kremer et al., 1995; Sperling, 1991). A recent clinical study of γ-linolenic acid (GLA, 18:3*n-6*) dietary manipulation in RA patients also showed evidence of the alleviation of disease activity (Zurier et al., 1996). Many recent studies have shown that production of immunological/inflammatory mediators can also be regulated by polyunsaturated fatty acids. Diets rich in *n-3* polyunsaturated fatty acids significantly reduce the production of the pro-inflammatory cytokines, tumour necrosis factor, interleukin-1β and interleukin-2, as well as the lipid mediator, platelet activating factor (Sperling, 1991; Endres, 1989; Williams et al., 1996) and this could account for some of their anti-inflammatory properties. However it has recently been appreciated, through meta analysis, that the use of these fatty acids in the human disease is uncertain (James et al., 2010). These investigators have proposed that fish oil may be of benefit in RA because it may overcome the cardiovascular risk of non-steroidal anti-inflammatory agents.

Supplementation with *n-3* fatty acids also decreases the symptoms of dysmenorrhoea, a prostaglandin-mediated condition in adolescents. After a two month treatment with fish oil, a significant reduction in the Cox Menstrual Symptom Scale was found compared with a placebo diet, probably due to alteration of the prostanoid profile by the high *n-3* fatty acid intake (Harel et al., 1996; Deutch, 1995). Essential fatty acids play an important role in brain and retinal development which mainly occurs during the latter half of pregnancy and the postnatal stage. The growth of fetal brain acquires approximately 21g/wk of DHA during the last trimester of pregnancy. Fatty acids are transported from the maternal circulation across the placenta and fetal blood-brain barrier into the central nervous system. A deficiency of essential fatty acids during pregnancy leads to a reduced level of DHA in the newborn, which is related to a reduction in slow-wave sleep and impaired vision in these infants. Dietary supplementation of *n-3* fatty acids to pregnant women and increasing the amount of DHA in infant formula are beneficial for early neurological development and improve the visual recognition in preterm and term infants (Gibson et al., 1996; Connor et al., 1996; Uauy et al., 1996). It has also been shown that diets rich in *n-3* fatty acids can prevent premature labor and preeclampsia (Olsen & Secher, 1990). Dietary *n-3* fatty acids also reduce the severity and frequency of relapses in patients suffering from multiple sclerosis (Bates, 1990).

Recent work has shown that n-3 fatty acid supplements modify allergic disease development in young children. A systematic review of reports on the effects of *n*-3 fatty acid supplementation during pregnancy and lactation on the risk of developing childhood allergic diseases and asthma, concluded that supplementation during pregnancy but not during lactation decreases childhood asthma and allergy (Klemens et al, 2011; Kremmyda et al, 2009). Thus, fish oil supplements when given to pregnant women with a history of allergic diseases gave rise to significant protection against infant allergy development. This was associated with reduced cord blood IL-13 (Klemens et al, 2011). The difference between supplementation during pregnancy versus in infancy and childhood and the development of eczema, hay fever and asthma has also been highlighted (Calder et al, 2010). Interestingly both the susceptibility and the protection afforded by the n-3 supplements were associated with the levels of protein kinase C (PKC)ζ in cord blood T cells and how those cells mature into Th1 and Th2 cytokine pattern producers. Low PKC ζ expression in the cord blood T cells of an infant increases the risk of development of allergic diseases in childhood (Prescott et al, 2007). In another population study of bronchial inflammation induced by grass pollen allergy challenge showed that the ratio of n-3: n-6 fats were significantly lower for the asthmatics than in healthy subjects (Kitz et al, 2010).

Obese adolescents appear to benefit from n-3 fatty acid supplementation, shown to improve vascular function and cause a reduction in vascular inflammation (Dangardt et al., 2010). Furthermore EPA has been shown to be incorporated into advanced atherosclerotic plaques (Cawood et al, 2010). The higher EPA content in the plaque is associated with reduced plaque inflammation and increased plaque stability (Cawood et al, 2010, Calder & Yaqoob, 2010). There was a reduction in foam cells, T cells and expression of metalloproteinases. In an animal model of atherosclerosis, employing the apoE-deficient mouse, combination of extra virgin oil and fish oil gave rise to protection by a mechanism of anti-thrombotic, anti-hypertriglyceridemic and anti-oxidant (Eilertsen et al., 2011)

The long chain, n-3 polyunsaturated fatty acids, EPA and DHA, are also substrates for the LOX and COX. It is evident that the metabolites of EPA and DHA display several means by which they can contribute to the regulatory network of lipid mediators; by replacing the highly inflammatory products of AA; having anti-inflammatory activity *per se* and displaying inflammation resolving abilities by having cell protection activity. The ability of the LOX and COX systems to generate fatty acid metabolites with substantially lower proinflammatory activity than the AA-derived eicosanoids has provided the basis for classical strategies to manipulate the inflammatory reaction. For example, increasing the ratio of *n*-3 to *n*-6 in membrane phospholipids of leukocytes reduces the production of inflammatory eicosanoids in favour of metabolites with markedly reduced or those which lack proinflammatory activity. Thus diets which contain high levels of the *n-3* fatty acids,

EPA and DHA or their precursors have been used as ways of decreasing inflammatory reactions and relieving the symptoms of these diseases (Simopoulos, 1991).
The EPA metabolised through COX and LOX pathways leads to the generation of 3-series PGs and TXs, and 5-series LTs (Fig 1). These products have some thousand fold less inflammatory activity than the 2-series PGs and 4-series LTs derived from AA. Thus the release of EPA from the sn-2 position of the membrane phospholipids will lead to an increased production of 3-series PGs and 5-series LTs following cell activation. This is believed to be a major mechanism of the beneficial effects of EPA/fish oil supplementation of patients with inflammatory diseases such as RA (James et al., 2010). In another development in the lipid mediator network, more recent work has characterised the generation of another class of inflammation regulators, the aspirin-triggered resolvins. This involves COX-2 aspirin triggered metabolism of EPA and further action of the 5-LOX, leading to the generation of the E-series resolvins, E1 and E2 (Fig 1) (Serhan et al., 2008). These molecules are highly potent in inhibiting neutrophil infiltration and in resolving the inflammatory reaction. Aspirin also triggers the generation of the D - series aspirin-triggered resolvins, RvD1, D2, D3, D4, D5, D6 which are generated from DHA, involving COX-2 and the 5-LOX. DHA metabolism via the 15-LOX and other reactions leads to the release also of these resolvins (Fig 1). DHA can also be oxidised via the 15-LOX to protectin D1. This metabolite inhibits neutrophil and T cell migration, airway inflammation, NF-κB activation, COX-2 induction and TLR macrophage activation. Protectin D1/neuroprotectin D1 is known for its neuroprotective properties (Serhan et al., 2008). It reduces brain ischemia and reperfusion injury, kidney ischemic injury and has anti-fibrotic activity.

10. Concluding remarks

Polyunsaturated fatty acids play critical roles in physiologic and pathophysiologic processes involving the immune system. While these have the ability to alter cellular responses as free fatty acids, most interest is on the properties of the array of metabolic products which they generate. These form a regulatory network which either down- or up-regulates the inflammatory reaction. A major effort continues to be made on the need to achieve an appropriate balance of n-6:n-3 fatty acids in tissues. The levels and ratios of these fatty acids is considered to regulate immune cell function through an effect on cell membrane fluidity, cell membrane structure, the expression of functional cell surface receptors and the types of oxidized products formed. Eicosanoid generation appears to be central to the inflammatory process by influencing the activities of many cell types, T cells, macrophages, neutrophils, eosinophils, DCs, endothelial cells, epithelial cells and smooth muscle cells. The characteristics of the inflammatory response is dependent on the concentrations and types of eicosanoids generated as well as the types of eicosanoid receptors expressed on the cell, which can vary dramatically from cell-type to cell-type. Both exogeneous and endogenous stimuli promote the activation of phospholipase A_2, the release of the polyunsaturated fatty acids from the phopholipids and their metabolism via the LOX and COX pathways. While most of the products formed from AA metabolism are highly proinflammatory, a number of these can also have a dampening effect on the inflammatory response. However, it is evident that the elicitation of a highly pro-inflammatory reaction is offset by the presence of n-3 fatty acids, EPA and DHA. These are metabolised into the low inflammatory, 5-series LTs and 3-series PGs, and anti-inflammatory products, the E-series resolvins/D-series resolvins and neuroprotective lipids, protectins. Because of the diversity of the array of eicosanoids and other fatty acid products generated, there is still much to be discovered on how this network of fatty acid metabolites promote and inhibit the inflammatory response. The time-dependent production of the different types of eicosanoids during various phases of the reaction could explain the types of inflammatory reactions we see, for example resolving and not resolving. The free fatty acids and their metabolic products also govern the synthesis of inflammatory mediators such as cytokines, which are targets for anti-inflammatory medications. Current evidence underscores the importance of phospholipase A2 and eicosanoids in the pathogenesis of inflammatory conditions, including asthma, rheumatoid arthritis and atherosclerosis. In contrast to the view of AA as a promoter of inflammation, n-3 fatty acids are considered as an attractive approach for anti-inflammatory therapy. However, while there is convincing in vitro data and data from animal models of an anti-inflammatory action of n-3 fatty acids in these diseases, results from human studies remain unconvincing or at best only small benefits are achieved. This is likely to reflect still our poor understanding of the actions of these fats when taken as dietary supplements and obviously further and more appropriate clinical trials have been suggested (Fritsche, 2006).

11. Acknowledgement

Our research received funding support from the National Health and Medical Research Council of Australia, the National Heart Foundation of Australia and the Channel 7 Children's Research Foundation of South Australia.

12. References

Adamek, A., Jung, S., Dienesch, C., Laser, M., Ertl, G., Bauersachs, J. & Frantz, S. (2007). Role of 5-lipoxygenases in myocardial ischemia - reperfusion injury in mice. *Eur. J. Pharmacol.* 571(1): 51-54.

Alvarez, Y., Valera, I., Municio, C., Hugo, E., Padrón, F., Blanco, L., Rodríguez, M., Fernández, N. & Crespo, M.S. (2010). Eicosanoids in the innate immune response: TLR and non-TLR routes. *Mediators of Inflammation.* Jun 15, Epub ahead of print.

Anel, A., Richieri, G.V. & Kleinfeld, A.M. (1993) Membrane partition of fatty acids and inhibition of T cell function. *Biochemistry.* 32(2):530-536.

Back, M, (2008). Inflammatory signalling through leukotriene receptors in atherosclerosis. *Curr. Atheroscler. Rep.* 10(3): 244-251.

Back, M. (2009). Leukotriene signalling in atherosclerosis and ischemia. *Cardiovasc. Drugs Ther.* 23(1): 41-48.

Back, M., Bu, D.X., Branstrom, R., Sheikine, Y., Yan, Z.Q. & Hansson, G.K. (2005). Leukotriene B4 signalling through NF-kappaB-dependent BLT1 receptors on vascular smooth muscle cells in atherosclerosis and intimal hyperplasia. *Proc. Natl. Acad Sci. USA* 102(48): 17501-17506.

Balsinde, J., Winstead, M.V. & Dennis, E.A. (2002). Phospholipase A(2) regulation of arachidonic acid mobilization.

Bates, D. (1990) Dietary lipids and multiple sclerosis. *Ups. J. Med. Sci. Suppl.* 48: 173-187.

Bonen, A., Luiken, J.J. &Glatz, JF. (2002). Regulation of fatty acid transport and membrane transporters in health and disease. *Mol. Cell. Biochem.* 239(1-2): 181-192.

Bowton, D.L., Seeds, M.C., Fasano, M.B., Goldsmith, B. & Bass, D.A. (1997) Phospholipase A2 and arachidonate increase in bronchoalveolar lavage fluid after inhaled antigen challenge in asthmatics. *Am. J. Respir. Crit. Care Med.* 155(2): 421-425.

Calder, P.C. (2010). Omega-3 fatty acids and inflammatory processes. *Nutrients*. 2:355-374.

Calder, P.C., Kremmyda, L.S., Vlachava, M., Noakes, P.S. & Miles, E.A. (2010). Is there a role for fatty acids in early life programming of the immune system? *Proc. Nutr. Soc.* 69(3):373-830.

Calder, P.C. & Yaqoob, P. (2010). Omega-3 (n-3) fatty acids, cardiovascular disease and stability of atherosclerotic plaques. *Cell Mol Biol (Noisy-le-grand)*.56(1):28-37.

Campan, P., Planchand, P.O. & Duran D. (1996). Polyunsaturated omega-3 fatty acids in the treatment of experimental human gingivitis. *Bull. Group Int. Rech. Sci. Stomatol. Odontol.* 39(1-2): 25-31.

Cawood, A.L., Ding, R., Napper, F.L., Young, R.H., Williams, J.A., Ward, M.J., Gudmundsen, O., Vige, R., Payne, S.P., Ye, S., Shearman, C.P., Gallagher, P.J., Grimble, R.F. & Calder, P.C. (2010). Eicosapentaenoic acid (EPA) from highly concentrated n-3 fatty acid ethyl esters is incorporated into advanced atherosclerotic plaques and higher plaque EPA is associated with decreased plaque inflammation and increased stability. *Atherosclerosis*. 212(1):252-259.

Chilton, F.H., Averill, F.J., Hubbard, W.C., Fonteh, A.N., Triggiani, M. & Liu, M.C. (1996) Antigen-induced generation of lyso-phospholipids in human airways. *J. Exp. Med.* 183(5): 2235-2245.

Connor, W.E, Lowensohn, R. & Hatcher, L. (1996) Increased docosahexaenoic acid levels in human newborn infants by administration of sardines and fish oil during pregnancy. *Lipids*. Mar 31, Suppl: S183-S187.

Dahlen, S.E. (2006). Treatment of asthma with antileukotrienes: First line or last resort therapy? *Eur. J. Parmacol* . 533(1-3): 40-56.

Dangardt, F., Osika, W., Chen, Y., Nilsson, U., Gan, L.M., Gronowitz, E., Strandvik, B. & Friberg, P. (2010). Omega-3 fatty acid supplementation improves vascular function and reduces inflammation in obese adolescents. *Atherosclerosis*. 212(2):580-585.

Deutch, B. (1995). Menstrual pain in Danish women correlated with low n-3 polyunsaturated fatty acid intake. *Eur. J. Clin. Nutr.* 49(7): 508-516.

Egan, KM., Lawson, JA., Fries, S., Koller, B., Rader, DJ., Smyth, EM. & Fitzgerald, GA. (2004). COX-2-derived prostacyclin confers atheroprotection on female mice. *Science* 306(5703): 1954-1957.

Eilertsen, K.E., Mæhre, H.K., Cludts, K., Olsen, J.O., Hoylaerts, M.F. (2011). Dietary enrichment of apolipoprotein E-deficient mice with extra virgin olive oil in combination with seal oil inhibits atherogenesis. *Lipids Health Dis*. 10:41.

Emery, DL., Djokic, TD., Graf, PD.& Nadel, JA. (1980). Prostaglandin D2 causes accumulation of eosinophils in the lumen of the dog trachea. *J Appl. Physiol* 67(3): 959-962.

Endres, S., Ghorbani, R., Kelley, V.E., Georgilis, K., Lonnemann, G., van der Meer, J.W., Cannon, J.G., Rogers, T.S., Klempner, M.S., Weber, P.C., et al. (1989). The effect of dietary supplementation with n-3 polyunsaturated fatty acids on the synthesis of interleukin-1 and tumor necrosis factor by mononuclear cells. *N. Engl. J. Med.* 320(5): 265-271.

Ferrante, A. & Hii, C. (2006). Progress towards polyunsaturated fatty acid based therapeutics for cardiovascular diseases: turning a millstone into a milestone. *International Atherosclerosis Society Newsletter* September Issue.

Ferrante, A., Hii, C.S. & Costabile (2005). Regulation of neutrophil functions by long chain fatty acids. *in* Gabrilovich, D. (ed.), *The neutrophils; new outlook for the old cell.* Imperial College Press. London. pp169-228.

Fritsche, K. (2006). Fatty acids as modulators of the immune response. *Annu. Rev. Nutr.*26:45-73.

Fujitani, Y., Kanaoka, Y., Aritake, K., Uodome, N., Okazaki-Hatake, K. & Urade, Y. (2002). Pronounced eosinophilic lung inflammation and Th2 cytokine release in human lipocalin-type prostaglandin D synthase transgenic mice. *J. Immunol.* 168(1): 443-449.

Ghosh, M., Tucker, DE., Burchett , SA. & Leslie, CC. (2006) Properties of the Group IV phospholipase A2 family. *Prog Lipid Res.* 45:487-510.

Gibson, R.A., Neumann, M.A. & Makrides, M. (1996). Effect of dietary docosahexaenoic acid on brain composition and neural function in term infants. *Lipids.* Mar 31, Suppl: S177-S181.

Greenfield, S.M., Green, A.T., Teare, J.P., Jenkins, A.P., Punchard, N.A., Ainley, C.C. & Thompson, R.P. (1993). A randomized controlled study of evening primrose oil and fish oil in ulcerative colitis. *Aliment. Pharmacol. Ther.* 7(2): 159-166.

Grignani, G., Zucchella, M., Belai Beyene, N., Brocchieri, A., Saporiti, A. & Chériè Ligniére, E.L. (1996). Levels of different metabolites of arachidonic acid in synovial fluid of patients with arthrosis or rheumatoid arthritis. *Minerva Med.* 87(3):75-79.

Gryglewski, R.J. (2008). Prostacyclin among prostanoids. *Pharmacol. Rep.* 60(1):3-11.

Hallstrand, T.S., Lai, Y., Ni, Z., Oslund, R.C., Henderson, W.R. Jr, Gelb, M.H. & Wenzel, S.E. (2011). Relationship between levels of secreted phospholipase A2 groups IIA and X in the airways and asthma severity. *Clin. Exp. Allergy.* 41(6):801-810.

Hammad, H., de Heer, HJ., Soullie, T., Hoogsteden, HC., Trottein, F. & Lambrecht, BN. (2003). Prostaglandin D2 inhibits airways dendritic cell migration and function in steady state conditions by selective activation of the D prostanoid receptor 1. .*J. Immunol* 171(8): 3936-3940.

Hardy, CC., Robinson, C., Tattersfield, AE.& Holgate, ST. (1984) The bronchoconstrictor effect of inhaled prostaglandin D2 in normal and asthmatic men. *N Engl J.Med.* 311(4): 209-213.

Harel, Z., Biro, F.M., Kottenhahn, R.K. & Rosenthal, S.L. (1996). Supplementation with omega-3 polyunsaturated fatty acids in the management of dysmenorrhea in adolescents. *Am. J. Obstet. Gynecol.* 174(4): 1335-1338.

Harris, S.G., Padilla, J., Kaumas, L., Ray, D. & Phipps, R.P. (2002). Prostaglandins as modulators of immunity. *Trends Immunol.* 23(3): 144-150.

Henderson WR Jr, Chi EY, Bollinger JG, Tien YT, Ye X, Castelli L, Rubtsov YP, Singer AG, Chiang GK, Nevalainen T, Rudensky AY, Gelb MH. (2007). Importance of group X-secreted phospholipase A2 in allergen-induced airway inflammation and remodeling in a mouse asthma model. *J. Exp. Med.* 204(4): 865-877.

Hendersen, W.R. Jr, Oslund, R.C., Bollinger, J.G., Ye, X., Tien, Y.T., Xue, J. & Gelb, M.H. (2011). Blockade of human group X secreted phospholipase A2-induced airway inflammation and hyperresponsiveness in a mouse asthma model by a selective group X secreted phospholipase A2 inhibitor. *J. Biol. Chem.* Jun 7. [Epub ahead of print

Ierna, M., Kerr, A., Scales, H., Berge, K. & Griinari, M. (2010). Supplementation of diet with krill oil protects against experimental rheumatoid arthritis. *BMC Musculoskelet Disord.* 11:136.

Jaffar, Z., Wanks, KS. & Roberts, K. (2002). A key role for prostaglandin I2 in limiting long mucosal Th2, but not Th1, responses to inhaled allergen. *J. Immunol* 169(10) : 5997-6004.

James MJ, Cook-Johnson RJ, Cleland LG. (2007). Selective COX-2 inhibitors, eicosanoid synthesis and clinical outcomes: a case study of system failure. *Lipids.* 42(9):779-785.

James M, Proudman S, Cleland L. (2010). Fish oil and rheumatoid arthritis: past, present and future. *Proc. Nutr. Soc.* 69(3):316-323.

Kabashima, K. & Narumiya, S. (2003) The DP receptor, allergic inflammation and asthma. *Prostaglandins Leukot Essential Fatty Acids.* 69(2-3): 187-194.

Kabashima, K., Sakatal, D., Nagamachi, M., Miyachi, Y., Inaba, K. & Narumiya, S. (2003) Prostaglandin E2-EP4 signalling initiates skin immune responses by promoting migration and maturation of Langerhans cells. *Nat. Med.* 9(6):744-9.

Kamp, F., Guo, W., Souto, R., Pilch, P.F., Corkey, B.E. & Hamilton, J.A. (2003). Rapid flip-flop of oleic acid across the plasma membrane of adipocytes. *J. Biol. Chem.* 278(10): 7988-7995.

Kawabe, J., Ushikubi, F., Hasebe, N. (2010). Prostacyclin in vascular diseases. - Recent insights and future perspectives -. *Circ. J.* 74(5):836-843.

Kita, Y., Ohto, T., Uozumi, N. & Shimizu, T. (2006) Biochemical properties and pathophysiological roles of cytosolic phospholipase A2S. *Biochim. Biophys. Acta.* 1761(11):1317-1322.

Kitz, R., Rose, M.A., Schubert, R., Beermann, C., Kaufmann, A., Böhles, H.J., Schulze, J. & Zielen, S. (2010). Omega-3 polyunsaturated fatty acids and bronchial inflammation in grass pollen allergy after allergen challenge. *Respir. Med.* 104(12):1793-1798.

Klemens, C., Berman, D. & Mozurkewich, E. (2011). The effect of perinatal omega-3 fatty acid supplementation on inflammatory markers and allergic diseases: a systematic review.*BJOG.* 118(8):916-925.

Krause, P., Bruchner. M., Uermosi. C., Singer. E., Groettrup. M.& Legler DF. (2009). Prostaglandin E(2) enhances T-cell proliferation by inducing the costimulatory molecules OX40L, CD70 and 4-1BBL on dendritic cells. *Blood* 113(11): 451-2460.

Kremer, J.M., Lawrence, D.A., Petrillo, G.F., Litts, L.L., Mullaly, P.M., Rynes, R.I., Stocker, R.P., Parhami, N., Greenstein, N.S. & Fuchs, B.R. (1995). Effects of high-dose fish oil on rheumatoid arthritis after stopping nonsteroidal antiinflammatory drugs. Clinical and immune correlates. *Arthritis Rheum.* 38(8): 1107-1114

Kremmyda, L.S., Vlachava, M., Noakes, P.S., Diaper, N.D., Miles, E.A. & Calder, P.C. (2009). Atopy Risk in Infants and Children in Relation to Early Exposure to Fish, Oily Fish, or Long-Chain Omega-3 Fatty Acids: A Systematic Review. *Clin. Rev. Allergy Immunol.* Dec 9. [Epub ahead of print]

Legler, DF., Krause, P., Scandella, E., Singer, E. & Groettrup, M. (2006). Prostaglandin E2 is generally required for human dendritic cell migration and exerts its effect via EP2 and EP4 receptors. *J. Immunol.* 176(2): 966-973.

Leslie, C.A., Gonnerman, W.A., Ullman, M.D., Hayes, K.C., Franzblau, C. & Cathcart, E.S. (1985). Dietary fish oil modulates macrophage fatty acids and decreases arthritis susceptibility in mice. *J. Exp. Med.* 162(4): 1336-1349.

Lin, L.L., Wartmann, M., Lin, A.Y., Knopf, J.L., Seth, A. & Davis, R.J. (1993) cPLA2 is phosphorylated and activated by MAP kinase. *Cell.* 72(2):269-278.

Maekawa, A., Kanaoka, Y., Xing, W. &Austen, K.F. (2008). Functional recognition of a distinct receptor preferential for leukotriene E4 in mice lacking the cysteinyl leukotriene 1 and 2 receptors. *Proc. Natl. Acad. Sci. USA* 105(43): 16695-16700.

Marusic, S., Leach, M.W., Pelker, J.W., Azoitei, M.L., Uozumi, N., Cui, J., Shen, M.W., DeClercq, C.M., Miyashiro, J.S., Carito, B.A., Thakker, P., Simmons, D.L., Leonard, J.P., Shimizu, T., Clark, J.D. (2005) Cytosolic phospholipase A2 alpha-deficient mice are resistant to experimental autoimmune encephalomyelitis. *J. Exp. Med.* 202(6):841-851.

Mathis, S.P., Jala, V.R., Lee, D.M. & Haribabu, B. (2010). Nonredundant role for leukotriene B4 receptors BLT1 and BLT2 in inflammatory arthritis. J. Immunol. 185(5):3049-3056.

Matsuoka, T., Hirata, M., Tanaka, H., Takahashi, Y., Murata, T., Kabashima, K., Sugimoto, Y., Kobayashi, T., Ushikubi, F., Aze, Y., Eguchi, N., Urade, Y., Yoshida, N.m, Kimura, K., Mizoguchi, A., Honda, Y., Nagai, H. & Narumiya, S. (2000). Prostaglandin D2 as a mediator of allergic asthma. *Science* 287(5460): 2013-2017.

McGarry, J.E. (1993) Title of chapter, in Devlin T.M. (ed.), *The textbook of biochemistry with clinical correlations. 3rd edition,* Wiley-Liss, New York, pp 387-422.

Murata, T., Ushikubi, F., Matsuoka, T., Hirata, M., Yamasaki, A., Sugimoto, Y., Ichikawa, A., Aze, Y., Tanaka, T., Yoshida, N., Ueno, A., Oh-ishi, S. & Narumiya, S. (1997). Altered pain perception and inflammatory response in mice lacking prostacyclin receptor . *Nature* 388(6643): 678-682.

Nakahata, N. (2008). Thromboxane A2: physiology/pathophysiologic, cellular signal transduction and pharmacology. *Pharmacol. Ther.* 118(1): 18-35.

Nemenoff, R.A., Winitz, S., Qian, N.X., Van Putten, V., Johnson, G.L., Heasley, L.E. (1993) Phosphorylation and activation of a high molecular weight form of phospholipase A2 by p42 microtubule-associated protein 2 kinase and protein kinase C. *J Biol Chem.* 268(3):1960-1964.

Okunishi, K. & Peters-Goldern, M. (2011). Leukotrienes and Airway Inflammation. *Biochim. Biophys. Acta.* Feb 23. Eprint ahead of print.

Olsen, S.F. & Secher, N.J. (1990). A possible preventive effect of low-dose fish oil on early delivery and pre-eclampsia: indications from a 50-year-old controlled trial. *Br. J. Nutr.* 64(3): 599-609.

Peter-Golden, M. & Henderson, W.R. Jr 2007. Leukotrienes. *N. Engl. J. Med.* 357, 1841-1854.

Poeckel, D. & Funk, C.D. (2010). The 5-lipoxygenase/leukotriene pathway in preclinical models of cardiovascular disease. *Cardiovasc. Res.* 86(2):243-253.

Poirier, H., Degrace, P., Niot, I., Bernard, A. & Besnard, P. (1996). Localization and regulation of the putative membrane fatty-acid transporter (FAT) in the small intestine. Comparison with fatty acid-binding proteins (FABP). *Eur. J. Biochem.* 238(2):368-373.

Prescott, S.L., Irvine, J., Dunstan, J.A., Hii, C. & Ferrante, A. (2007). Protein kinase Czeta: a novel protective neonatal T-cell marker that can be upregulated by allergy prevention strategies. *J. Allergy Clin. Immunol.* 120(1):200-206.

Ricicotti, E. & FitzGerald, G.A. (2011) Prostaglandins and inflammation. *Arterioscler Thromb Vasc Biol* 31(5) 986-1000.

Roper, R.L., Brown, D.M. & Phipps RP. (1995). Prostaglandin E2 promotes B lymphocyte Ig isotype switching to IgE. *J Immunol.* 154(1):162-170.

Serhan, C.N. (2005). Prostaglandins Leukot Essentail Fatty Acids, 73, p139-321.

Serhan, C.N., Yacoubian, S. & Yang, R. (2008). Anti-inflammatory and proresolving lipid mediators. *Annu. Rev. Pathol.;* 3:279-312.

Shao, W.H., Del Prete, A., Bock, C.B. & Haribabu, B. (2006). Targeted disruption of leukotriene B4 receptors BLT1 and BLT2: a critical role for BLT1 in collagen-induced arthritis in mice. *J. Immunol.* 176(10):6254-6261.

Simopoulos, A.P. (1991). Omega-3 fatty acids in health and disease and in growth and development. *Am. J. Clin. Nutr.* 54(3): 438-46.

Spector, A.A. (1992). Fatty acids in Human Biology: Past and Future. *in* Bracco U. and Deckelbaum R.J (ed), *Polyunsaturated fatty acids in human nutrition,* Nestle Nutrition workshop series Vol 28, Raven, New York, pp 1-12.

Sperling, R.I. (1991). Dietary omega-3 fatty acids: effects on lipid mediators of inflammation and rheumatoid arthritis. *Rheum. Dis. Clin. North Am.* 17(2): 373-389.

Steinbeck, M.J., Robinson, J.M. & Karnovsky, M.J. (1991) Activation of the neutrophil NADPH-oxidase by free fatty acids requires the ionized carboxyl group and partitioning into membrane lipid. *J. Leukoc. Biol.* 49(4):360-368.

Tai, N., Kuwabara, K., Kobayashi, M., Yamada, K., Ono, T., Seno, K., Gahara, Y., Ishizaki, J. & Hori, Y. (2010). Cytosolic phospholipase A2 alpha inhibitor, pyrroxyphene, displays anti-arthritic and anti-bone destructive action in a murine arthritis model. Infamm Res 59(1): 53-62.

Triggiani, M., Giannattasio, G., Calabrese, C., Loffredo, S., Granata, F., Fiorello, A., Santini, M., Gelb, M.H. & Marone, G. (2009). Lung mast cells are a source of secreted phospholipases A2. *J. Allergy Clin. Immunol.* 124(3):558-565.

Uauy, R., Peirano, P., Hoffman, D., Mena, P., Birch, D., Birch, E. (1996). Role of essential fatty acids in the function of the developing nervous system. . *Lipids.* Mar 31, Suppl: S167-S176.

Watanabe, S., Yamasaki, A., Hashimoto, K., Shigeoka, Y., Chikumi, H., Hasegawa, Y., Sumikawa, T., Takata, M., Okazaki, R., Watanabe, M., Yokogawa, T., Yamamura, M., Hayabuchi, T., Gerthoffer, W.T., Halayko, A.J. & Shimizu. E. (2009). Expression of functional leukotriene B4 receptors on human airway smooth muscle cells. *J. Allergy Clin. Immunol.* 124(1):59-65.e1-3.

Williams, W.V., Rosenbaum, H. & Zurier, R.B. (1996). Effects of unsaturated fatty acids on expression of early response genes in human T lymphocytes. *Pathobiology.* 64(1): 27-31.

Wu, Y.Z., Abolhassani, M., Ollero, M., Dif, F., Uozumi, N., Lagranderie, M., Shimizu, T., Chignard, M., Touqui, L. (2010). Cytosolic phospholipase A2alpha mediates Pseudomonas aeruginosa LPS-induced airway constriction of CFTR -/- mice. *Respir. Res.* 11:49 .

Yao, C., Sakata, D., Esaki, Y., Matsuoka, T., Kuroiwa, K., Sugimoto, Y. & Narumiya, S. (2009). Prostaglandin E2-EP4 signalling promotes immune inflammation through Th1 cell differentiation and Th17 cell expansion. *Nat. med.* 15(6) : 633-640.

Yokomizo, T., Kato, K., Terawaki, K., Izumi T. & Shimizu, T. (2000). A second leukotriene B(4) receptor, BLT2. A new therapeutic target in inflammation and immunological disorders *J Exp. Med.* 192(3): 421-432.

Zurier, R.B., Rossetti, R.G., Jacobson, E.W., DeMarco, D.M., Liu, N.Y., Temming, J.E., White, B.M. & Laposat, M. (1996). gamma-Linolenic acid treatment of rheumatoid arthritis. A randomized, placebo-controlled trial. *Arthritis Rheum.* 39(11): 1808-1817.

Part 9

Noninvasive Inflammatory Biomarkers

9

A New Era for Assessing Airway Diseases: New Insights in the Asthma Paradigm

J. Bellido-Casado
Institut de Recerca, Pneumology Department, Hospital Santa Creu i Sant Pau Barcelona Spain

1. Introduction

The definition of asthma is constantly being modified and redefined. New knowledge derived from molecular biology and applied immunology is very valuable in interpreting how the airway becomes diseased. At the same time, new biomarkers useful for monitoring patients and detecting inflammatory airway disease are being identified. Currently, patients whose condition is included in the spectrum of inflammatory airway diseases may be reassessed and placed into subgroups so that the biotypes, or endotypes (disease) and phenotypes (patients), form new paradigms to delineate and integrate applied knowledge to this complex and heterogeneously-expressed disease. The definition of asthma and different ways of understanding the disease undergo constant review.

2. Asthma defined as an inflammatory airway disease

The definition of asthma may be established using a set of characteristics that are clinical (recurrent episodes of wheezing and dyspnea), pathophysiological (variability in airflow), or immunological (chronic inflammation) (Global Initiative for Astma [GINA], 2009; British Thoracic Society Scottish Intercollegiate Guidelines Network [BTSSIGN], 2008). They may be found in patients or heterogeneous groups of patients who share these symptoms to a greater or lesser extent. Depending on the emphasis placed on a more specific predominant feature of airway dysfunction, the 'nominalist' view of the concept of asthma is more relevant. On the other hand, if several features are examined together to make the diagnosis, the more 'essentialist' aspect of the specific airway disease stands out [GINA, 2009; BTSSIGN 2008]. Thus, both definitions must be kept in mind when dealing with asthma, and determining an objective system of measurement for the quantifiable aspects that that make up either definition is required [Hargreave & Nair, 2009]. For decades, different methods to quantify and measure the various components of asthma (symptoms, spirometry, maximum peak flow, bronchial provocation) have been used in situations of good health or illness, highlighting the complexity involved in studying, functionally, both the normal and altered airway. Not all the defining characteristics of asthma are present in all patients; moreover, they vary greatly and are often irregular in a single patient. The therapeutic response may also be different depending on the specific pathophysiological characteristics that are predominately found [Lotvall et al., 2011]. Therefore, the classification of asthma severity by daily medication regimen and response to treatment, as well as the different strategies and recommendations for managing patients with difficult to control asthma are essentially needed in clinical practice [Holgate & Polosa, 2006]; otherwise they are limited. New methods based on statistical physics and fluctuation analysis can be a new strategy for assessing and predicting the risk of progression of asthma [Frey & Suki, 2008], but monitoring of airway diseases also requires focus on foundations of the modern biology. Therefore, the application of new technological advancements and the disciplines applied to the study of inflammation, as well as the incorporation of new markers for diagnosis and the monitoring of patients affected by asthma, inspires optimism in the challenge to find a better conceptual understanding of asthma using a dynamic approach that continuously changes and at the same time is more significant than that achieved by mere verification.

In this chapter, specific aspects of the new contributions to the monitoring of asthma and the new research using defined groups of patients to study interrelated heterogeneous aspects of asthma will be described and discussed. These new contributions have modified the approach to grouping and reclassifying characteristics that are clinical, pathophysiological and biological as a whole, and allow for a new definition of asthma in terms of 'phenotypes' and 'endotypes' [Anderson, 2008a; Wenzel, 2006]. Although the addition of these new terms to the definition of asthma may be seen as a conceptual breakthrough, caution must be exercised. For example, new biological knowledge about the pathogenic understanding of inflammatory airway disease (IAD) requires further investigation in many aspects, including how it differs from phenotypes in chronic obstructive pulmonary disease (COPD) [Barnes, 2008], as well as in children [Spycher, 2010]. Hence, a major challenge in the field of respiratory disease today is how to adapt the definition of asthma to new scientific developments. The verification of objective 'biotypes', in terms of the development of asthma and the patients in whom they are observed, is an important conceptual advance, provided better clinical management for each patient is achieved so that the relative uniqueness of each patient with asthma can be better understood, both by the physician and the patients themselves. However, in order to define 'phenotypes' specific to patients or subgroups of patients in addition to the specific pathogenic 'endotypes' that identify them (in other words, how asthma patients become ill), it is necessary to thoroughly identify their defining characteristics. They must therefore be measured and grouped biologically and clinically in a differentiated way, even if certain aspects of the illness are the same [Lotvall et al., 2011; Moore et al., 2010].

Today's objective biological measures and markers used to better understand these biotypes are the central focus of this chapter.

3. Monitoring the airway and monitoring asthma in particular

There are a number of methods available for identifying different aspects related to the natural evolution of IAD. The contribution of each aspect is determined by providing appropriate measures and robust parameters that meet consistent methodological determinants, such as the standardization of the method used, the availability of reference values, the reproducibility of findings, and above all the application of research findings to clinical practice and the global management of patients whose situation is well-defined as well as homogeneous patients or groups of subjects. Not all biological measures studied in recent years have managed to become routinely added as a parameter with clinical value in the management of patients. Furthermore, those used routinely provide specific and limited information only. Therefore, current research being conducted focuses more on the inflammatory aspects of the lung, rather than the classical or clinical function, because it is the central pathogenic mechanism of the disease in the airway [Fabbri et al., 2005]. Severity and control disease assessment requires a multidimensional practical approach including an inflammatory view, as was previously confirmed by some authors [Fitzpatrick et al. 2011a; Haldar et al., 2008].

Technological advancements brought about by modern molecular biology and innovative micron analysis technology applied to the study of inflammation and the pathways of oxidative, lipid, or nitric stress, for example, can allow for a better identification and definition of new parameters, inflammatory profiles, and biomarkers that are more sensitive and specific for predicting the state of progression of IAD, differences in poor outcomes, and the type of anti-inflammatory treatment best suited to manage a particular patient or patient group.

This section briefly discusses the most relevant parameters used in clinical practice for the monitoring of asthma, especially the most recent parameters that contribute greatly to the overall management of patients and other more promising parameters, from the perspective derived by direct measurement and monitoring of inflammatory activity.

3.1 Global systems of measurement for airway disease

From a clinical point of view, patients are typically monitored through the measurement of the symptoms present, questionnaires on the degree of control of the disease [Curtis et al., 1997] or the impact on quality of life related to health [Juniper et al., 2004], pathophysiological parameters such as the degree of bronchial obstruction [FEV_1 or PEF] [Miller, 2005], and variability [Reddel, 2006] or the degree of bronchial hyper-reactivity, both specific and nonspecific [Anderson, 2008b, Cockcroft & Davis 2006; Crapo et al., 2000; Sont et al., 1999; Sterk et al., 1993]. Each of these are more or less direct methods of measuring the clinical impact of inflammatory diseases of the airways, providing complementary information to diagnostic and therapeutic management [Fuhlbrigge, 2004; Gibson & Powell, 2004; Taylor et al., 2008] and, to a lesser degree, clinical interpretation [Frey & Suki, 2008]. They have become absolutely necessary and indispensable for the classification of the patient's and establishment of control disease. In terms of study, testing of the whole response of the total airway implies knowing several pathogenic mechanisms of disease [Bousquet et al., 2000; Leuppi et al., 2001]. Understanding how control of the severity or clinical evolution of the disease is developed retains some specific limitations that result in advantages and disadvantages. For example, the main advantage of studying bronchial hyper-responsiveness to histamine or methacholine challenge is the high negative predictive value of the test [Luks et al., 2010]. On the contrary, its presence and the severity observed indicate functional impairment of the airway. This may be interpretable in either a physiological (dysfunction, with or without an associated inflammatory basal profile) or pathological context (chronic inflammation, injury, mucosal or submucosal remodelling), which may or may not be modified by treatment once established [Hargreave et al., 1981; Rosi et al., 1999; Sont et al., 1999; van Essen-Zandvliet et al., 1994]. Recent advances in the clinical use of substances, such as adenosine or mannitol, provide additional data on the association between bronchial hyper-responsiveness, as measured by these indirect stimuli, and markers of inflammation [Polosa et al., 2000; Rutgers et al., 2000].

Other findings arising from the current radiological spectrum of diseases of the airway also provide useful data to study dynamic airway inflammation, expressed as the degree of trapped air and bronchial wall thickness [Gupta et al., 2010].
It is therefore possible to say that although the parameters and measurements discussed in this section can be applied to both asthma and COPD in order to achieve better clinical management, its meaning and clinical interpretation are often heterogeneous or variable depending on the patient, the therapy administered at the time of measurement, and the spectrum of IADs identified in the subject, both initially and over time [Avital et al., 1995; Dima et al., 2010]. Discrimination of all the spectrum of obstructive airway diseases is the goal to achieve at present time.

3.2 Direct systems of injury and repair measurement in pulmonary biology

The pathology of the airway has a clearly inflammatory pathophysiological basis, although the role this plays, both in the short term and in the long term, in the biological continuum of integrity, dysfunction, injury, and repair continues to undergo constant research. Traditionally, the gold standard in inflammatory activity has been to use various measurements and markers, both inflammatory and those of oxidative stress, obtained invasively by bronchial biopsy and bronchoalveolar lavage [Bergeron et al., 2007; Brasier et al., 2010; Hallstrand et al., 2011]. Although various parameters and histological patterns of inflammation have been identified with these techniques, many of them are shared by the anatomopathological spectrum of IAD. This causes ambiguity, both in the various pathogenic contexts in which pathophysiological interpretation is difficult and, consequently, non-pathognomonic situations in which discrimination regarding asthma or COPD occurs. Only some of these findings have demonstrated applicability to clinical care and a certain ability to differentiate or discriminate between the inflammatory pathogenic states of an underlying pathologic lesion, as in the study of bronchial remodelling [Sont et al., 1999; Sont et al., 2003], or the prevalence of the cellular profile of bronchial infiltration, as in the case of life-threatening asthma [Mauad et al., 2004; Mauad et al., 2008]. Furthermore, both techniques also have some significant limitations when carried out routinely. The first is that only one compartment of the airway is represented unless both procedures are done at the same time. The second limitation is the invasiveness of the procedure. This is an obstacle when routinely performed on the patient, despite the fact that these methods have been standardized and allow for a better visualization of the type of inflammation and anatomical injury caused by IAD in certain patients. They are also useful in studying the pathogenic mechanisms involved, as well as classifying and identifying the stage of disease [Fabbri et al., 2003; Fabbri et al., 2005; Moore et al., 2011], but the requirements of the procedure do not make them suitable for routine monitoring of the patient and are therefore generally reserved today for the systematic study of inflammation in pulmonary biology research.
The new semi-invasive methods, such as induced sputum, or non-invasive methods, such as the measurement of nitric oxide, condensation, or exhaled temperature, provide new and useful data directly from the airway that may be used in the classification of IADs and the management of patients [Popov, 2011]. Some markers derived from blood samples can also be used in assessing inflammatory disease and its systemic impact. These include eosinophil cationic proteins, as well as cationic peroxidase and leucotriens [Koh et al., 2007; Rabinovitch, 2007], but other novel systemic blood biomarkers are also promising [Verrills

et al., 2011]. The most important contributions of non-invasive methods currently used to measure inflammation of the airway and the most promising research being carried out with new applied technologies in molecular biology and immunology are discussed below.

3.2.1 Induced sputum

This semi-invasive technique is used to obtain a representative sample of bronchial secretions in the airway. Some methodological variations in the induction procedure may produce samples from a more central or peripheral compartment of the airway, providing versatility in IAD screening in terms of both central and peripheral orientation. This is characterized as such because the differential inflammatory profile obtained is reproducible and can be correctly interpreted in a clinical context. However, this is not the case in the study of the various markers of inflammation and oxidative stress obtained from the supernatant, which have strict methodological considerations and limitations in the interpretation of results [Nicholas, 2009]. Bearing this in mind, induced sputum has become the gold standard non-invasive method for measuring bronchial cell inflammation and for certain soluble markers that are identifiable and of specific dilution [Bakakos, 2011; Djukanovic 2004]. The standardization of the method and procedure, adequate safeness of the technique, good toleration by the patient, ease of use, and the obtainment of reference values have made it an essential technique in the study of complex patients who require the characterization of the bronchial inflammatory pattern in order to be managed correctly [Djukanovic, 2002]. The current characterization of the endotypes and phenotypes of patients with inflammatory airway disease, based on inflammatory cell patterns [Balzar et al., 2011; Haldar et al., 2008], and the combination of different biomarkers, such as those derived from 'esputoma' [Gray et al., 2008; Nicholas, 2006] and oxidative stress [Louhelainen et al., 2008a; Louhelainen et al., 2008b], 15-lipoxygenase pathway [Chu, et al., 2002], gluthation oxidation [Fitzpatrick et al., 2011b] or genetics and protein identification [Baines et al., 2011; Hastie et al, 2010] make sputum an indisputable protagonist in the new definition of phenotypes, the classification of patients with asthma and COPD [Fabbri et al., 2003; Fatj et al., 2009; Louis et al., 2002; Wang et al., 2011], the therapeutic management of these patients, the prediction of therapeutic response [Green et al., 2002; Jayaram et al., 2006, Caramori et al., 2005], and the evaluation of efficacy in the most recent anti-inflammatory molecules [Haldar et al, 2009; Pavord et al. 2009, van Rensen et al. 2009]. Currently, new techniques in molecular biology may be applied to the study of sputum in order to study the expression shown in the cellular response of certain subtypes of cell lines, as found for example, by studying toll-like cell receptors or local innate immunity measured by flow cytometry [Lay et al, 2011], or those derived from cell cultures [Bettiol et al., 2002], the cellular response to markers of cell migration [Dent et al., 2004], or even those obtained from the analysis of proteomics traces or esputoma [Park & Rim, 2011; Nicholas & Djukanovic, 2009], as well as the genome [Baines et al., 2011; Bisgaard et al., 2011].

3.2.2 The exhaled fraction determined singularly or in combination

The use of exhaled markers capable of reflecting a clinically useful measurement of the inflammation and oxidative stress present in the airway currently involves bronchial nitric oxide (NO) as the main marker [Barnes et al., 2010]. This measurement is reproducible and the method has been standardized [ATS/ERS, 2005]. Because its concentration is dependent on the flow and the source of production, a compartmental model of alveolar or bronchial origin of exhaled nitric oxide has been developed in order to study of the origin of the alteration and the lung injury, situating it at a more central or peripheral level in the airway [Puckett et al., 2010]. This model allows the production variability within the spectrum of IAD and the anti-inflammatory modulation produced by the therapy administered to be studied in depth. While this method is certainly advantageous when carrying out clinical monitoring within a timeframe because of its non-invasivity, it may only be used in certain patients, i.e. those in whom the main source of NO has been identified as a clearly modifiable and dependent element of the course of inflammation with therapeutic anti-inflammatory management, or for the screening of type of activated inflammation [Anderson et al., 2011]. The use of NO in the research of no homogeneously selected patients leads to a clinically confusing interpretation in terms of its identification and therefore must be considered limited or biased under these circumstances [Dweik et al., 2010]. In addition, certain methodological considerations conditioned by the design of NO research studies regarding the cut-off used to make a management decision must be taken into account during diagnosis and treatment, i.e. conditioning the patient management strategy based on the levels of NO [Gibson, 2009; Quaedvlieg et al., 2009; Schleich et al., 2009; Schneider et al., 2009].

Other exhaled markers of the bronchial airway, such as the detection of carbon monoxide and other volatile hydrocarbon compounds, products of lipid peroxidation, have also been studied [Antczak et al., 2011]. However, a definitive standardization of methods for immediate application in a clinical context has not been achieved. Similarly, the measurement of exhaled temperature increase at the start of breathing with regard to the reference point marked during the entire period of measurement of the increase is associated with the presence of active inflammation and airway remodelling [Paredi, 2005]. This also occurs with the measurement of bronchial blood flow, estimated by mass spectrometry using the Fick principle, and the calculation of the dilution of exhaled acetylene [the initial concentration inhaled is known]. Both methods may have their place in the spectrum of non-invasive monitoring of bronchial inflammation if the optimal exhaled flow is standardized methodologically for the purpose of measurement [Paredi & Barnes, 2010].

The identification of different volatile compounds produced by oxidative stress, nitrosative stress, inflammation and metallic elements, and obtained from the exhaled condensate has also been possible through the use of chromatography and mass spectrometry [Corradi et al. 2007; Corradi et al, 2010]. Some of these compounds may be considered biomarkers in clinical practice [Baraldi et al., 2009 Kostikas et al., 2008; Loukides et al, 2011], such as pH determination [Kostikas et al., 2011; Antus et al, 2010]. However, it is necessary to simplify the instrumentation of the procedure for routine use in clinical practice. The standardization of methodology and applicability to clinical practice of other compounds under investigation as potential biomarkers has yet to be sufficiently achieved due, among other things, to certain limitations, such as contamination of condensate compounds of the mouth (especially if concomitant oral inflammation occurs), difficulty in calculating the optimal dilution of the selected parameter, or instability, volatility, and interaction of the mixture of soluble compounds that can take place during this process [Horvàth et al. 2005]. Comparisons with other biomarkers obtained and already standardized are needed to establish the utility of the different compounds of exhaled condensate, especially if

performed one by one [Baraldi et al., 2009]. However, recent specific phenotypes of asthma patients, like aspirin intolerant asthmatics can be identified [Sanak et al, 2011].
Calculating the nasal exhaled fraction may be useful for the study and diagnosis of primary ciliary dyskinesia and is virtually abolished in this disease [Horváth et al., 2003]. On the contrary nasal NO levels are higher in rhinitis [Struben et al., 2006]

3.2.3 The multiple molecular studies of biological lung samples, or systemic samples, significant to pulmonary disease

Since the detection of a single marker of inflammation or oxidative stress does not identify a specific inflammatory disease of the airway as defined today, but rather proves the heterogeneity of inflammatory conditions and diseases of the airway, current research on biological markers focuses on a combination of identifying patterns of proteins and volatile compounds that can be identified by molecular marks or traces they contain. At the molecular level, many omic compounds (proteomic, metabolomic, genomic) may be identified. Within the field of respiratory medicine, these compounds will remain an enigma until the wealth of empirical molecular information is organized and interpreted, free of *a priori* hypotheses, and the subsequent translation to clinical practice can be carried out. Such information would have the great advantage of producing a custom 'fingerprint' of inflammation during a specific time point in the evolution of the disease process in a particular patient. The correct interpretation of molecular information will allow the clinician to identify and predict the patient and disease biotypes (phenotype and endotype), the severity of the inflammatory process in progress, the clinical evolution, the type of treatment to be applied, the response to the therapy administered, and the prognosis for each individual patient [Crameri, 2005; Vijverberg et al., 2011]. The new molecular application technology based on bioinformatics, cluster analysis, and artificial intelligence algorithms that are being developed at present provide all this information for the purpose of prediction and interpretation at a biological level. This is useful in understanding the new biology of systems integration [Perpiñá, 2010; Scott et al., 2007; Thaler & Hanson, 2005]. The following is a description of the research currently being conducted.
First, chromatography and mass spectrometry have been used to identify hundreds of volatile exhaled organic compounds originating from the metabolic pathways involved in pulmonary biology. However, their use as biomarkers with a clinical application is still under study [Freidrich, 2009]. Secondly, the addition of other specific technology for determining the spectrum of metabolites, proteins or organic compounds in different biological samples (cellular, fluid, or gas) in blood, sputum, or bronchoalveolar lavage, and developed on line, such as the application a multiple set of nanosensors (arrays) or the application of high-resolution nuclear magnetic resonance, has achieved rapid progress in identifying potential profiles and patterns of disease-specific biomarkers. For example, different patterns of compounds originating in breathing and exhaled breath evaluated by the so-called *electronic nose* identify molecules of different size, volume and dipole [Lewis, 2004]. These patterns have shown good sensitivity and discrimination capabilities for this combination and may be as helpful as those already described for the identification of certain odours, producing an odoriferous mark or *smellprint*. This would specifically identify the type of inflammation present and could be useful in the differential diagnosis of specific IADs [Dragonieri et al., 2007] in addition to the particular diagnostic and therapeutic strategies for each patient.

4. The future of targeted and individualized biological respiratory therapy

The new concept of biotypes (endotypes and phenotypes) of IAD is transforming the definition of asthma to the point where it will soon be possible to obtain a more accurate simplification of what is understood today as asthma in order to better adapt to patient management and the clinical reality. However, the definition of asthma that currently exists is complex and will remain so, despite continuous modification and rehabilitation, given that although the heterogeneity of the IAD is better understood and the subtypes of the disease and patient subgroups are better classified, the multifactorial and dynamic aspects of the biological responses involved make applying reductionist criteria very difficult. It is therefore necessary to maintain a flexible and mentally versatile attitude that is as dynamic as biology itself. This attitude will facilitate the understanding of respiratory medicine of the future, which in turn will affect therapeutic management. This approach may be considered the cornerstone of individualized therapy for respiratory patients. It will aid in the progressive incorporation of biopharmaceuticals capable of regulating or altering inflammatory pathways, the remodelling process and the smooth muscle response. Both strategies are complementary and briefly commented.

First, the action and biological and immunological mechanisms will modulate the degree of response obtained at the molecular level and will result clinically in a very specific action. Being able to have these modulating biopharmaceuticals will be crucial and improve the quality of life for patients with IAD and asthma [Adock et al., 2008; Casale & Stokes, 2008]. However, the availability of these drugs will lead to a major challenge at the clinical level that they will be reflected in trying to establish well-defined therapeutic indications to ensure safe, efficient, and cost-effective use. Some examples of modulating biopharmaceuticals in the context of eosinophilic inflammation that have been used in patients with poor control and greater severity of symptoms are those that interfere with the biological action of IgE, IL-5 or TNFα. The attainment of adequate control and improvement of outcome in these patients is a sign of success in the development of new molecules, such as the monoclonal antibodies, mepolizumab, etarnercept or omalizumab [Holgate et al, 2011; Pavord et al., 2010; Pelaia et al., 2011]. Other biological modulating drugs acting at the neutrophilic, mast o lymphocite cells or other relevant molecules in the pathways and the inflammatory response, are being tested for the purpose of incorporation into the therapeutic arsenal available for IAD [Chung & Marwick, 2010, Barnes, 2009]. Pharmacogenetics and understanding of innate immunty pathways are promising areas of research to discover determined mechanisms and specific molecules to reverse the altered inflammatory response [Caramori et al., 2004; Kanagaratham et al., 2011; Gupta & Agrawal, 2010; Slager, 2010].

Second, the important thing to considering the therapy of releaving symptoms in the asthma clinic course is the understanding of the mechanical obstruction in the airways and the air-trapping compensatory consequence [Sorkness et al., 2008]. New long-acting smooth muscle relaxant molecules are been incorporated alone or in combination to the inhaler therapy [Cazzola et al., 2011; Chung et al., 2009; Kiyokawa et al., 2011; Postma et al., 2011], but recent knowing of the genetics of airway smooth muscle points out a new strategies to develop asthma targeted molecules [Hai, 2008]. Another specific therapy focus on smooth muscle of the airways, like bronchial thermoplasty, is still under evaluation [Thompson et al., 2011].

5. Conclusion

Inflammatory diseases of the airway, and asthma in particular, are complex and heterogenous, both in terms of the biological expression of inflammation they produce and in terms of the 'biotypes' (endotypes and phenotypes) that can be objectively translated from this condition. New information provided by new technology applied to modern molecular biology and immunology requires the current concept and definition of asthma to be modified and adapted. The attainment of this important progressive scientific knowledge can help to address how and why this condition occurs and may contribute to a better understanding of the classification of each asthma patient, the proper diagnosis of the type of asthma presented, the monitoring approach, the personalized treatment required, and the method to determine prognosis. A wide spectrum of biomarkers is currently being incorporated as clinically useful parameters. What remains is to gradually adapt them to comprehensive of multidimensional approaches and medical procedures, and establish the appropriate indications and clinical applications in respiratory disease.

6. References

[1] Adcock, IM.; Caramori, G. & Chung, KF. (2008). New targets for drug development in asthma. *Lancet*. Vol. 372, No. 9643, (September 2008), pp.1073-1087, ISSN 0140-6736.

[2] American Thoracic Society; & European Respiratory Society. (2005). ATS/ERS recommendations for standardized procedures for the online and offline measurement of exhaled lower respiratory nitric oxide and nasal nitric oxide, 2005. *Am J Respir Crit Care Med*. Vol.171, No 8, (April 2005), pp.912-930, ISSN 1073-449X.

[3] Anderson, GP. (2008a). Endotyping asthma: new insights into key pathogenic mechanisms in a complex, heterogenous disease. *Lancet*. Vol. 372, No. 9643, (September 2008), pp. 1107-1119, ISSN 0140-6736.

[4] Anderson, JT.; Zeng, M.; Li, Q.; Stapley, R.; Moore, DR 2nd.; Chenna, B.; Fineberg, N.; Zmijewski, J.; Eltoum, IE.; Siegal, GP.; Gaggar, A.; Barnes, S.; Velu, SE.; Thannickal, VJ.; Abraham, E.; Patel, RP.; Lancaster, JR Jr.; Chaplin, DD.; Dransfield, MT. & Deshane, JS. (2011). Elevated levels of NO are localized to distal airways in asthma. *Free Radic Biol Med*. Vol. 50, No.11, (Juny 2011), pp.1679-1688, ISSN 0891-5849.

[5] Anderson, SD. (2008b). Provocative challenges to help diagnose and monitor asthma: exercise, methacholine, adenosine, and mannitol. *Curr Opin Pulm Med*. Vol. 14, No. 1, (January 2008), pp. 39-45, ISSN 1070-5287.

[6] Antczak, A.; Ciebiada, M.; Kharitonov, SA.; Gorski, P. & Barnes, PJ. (2011). Inflammatory Markers: Exhaled Nitric Oxide and Carbon Monoxide During the Ovarian Cycle. *Inflammation*. May 18. [Epub ahead of print].

[7] Antus, B.; Barta, I.; Kullmann, T.; Lazar, Z.; Valyon, M.; Horvath, I. & Csiszer, E. (2010). Assessment of exhaled breath condensate pH in exacerbations of asthma and chronic obstructive pulmonary disease: A longitudinal study. *Am J Respir Crit Care Med*. Vol.182, No.12, pp.1492-1497, ISSN 1073-449X.

[8] Avital, A.; Springer, C.; Bar-Yishay, E. & Godfrey, S. (1995). Adenosine, methacholine, and exercise challenges in children with asthma or paediatric chronic obstructive pulmonary disease. *Thorax*. Vol. 50, No.5, (May 1995), pp.511-516, ISSN 0040-6376.

[9] Baines, KJ.; Simpson, JL.; Wood, LG.; Scott, RJ. & Gibson, PG. (2011). Transcriptional phenotypes of asthma defined by gene expression profiling of induced sputum samples. *J Allergy Clin Immunol*. Vol. 127. No.1, (January 2011), pp.153-160, ISSN 0091-6749.

[10] Bakakos, P.; Schleich, F.; Alchanatis, M. & Louis, R. (2011). Induced sputum in asthma: from bench to bedside. *Curr Med Chem*. Vol. 18, No. 10, pp.1415-1422. ISSN 0929-8673.

[11] Balzar, S.; Fajt, ML.; Comhair, SA.; Erzurum, SC.; Bleecker, E.; Busse, WW.; Castro, M.; Gaston, B.; Israel, E.; Schwartz, LB.; Curran-Everett, D.; Moore, CG. & Wenzel, SE. (2011). Mast cell phenotype, location, and activation in severe asthma: data from the severe asthma research program. *Am J Respir Crit Care Med*. Vol.183, Vol.3, pp.299-309, ISSN 1073-449X.

[12] Baraldi, E.; Carraro, S.; Giordano, G.; Reniero, F.; Perilongo, G. & Zacchello, F. (2009). Metabolomics: moving towards personalized medicine. *Ital J Pediatr*. Vol. 35, No.1, (October 2009), p.30, ISSN 1720-8424.

[13] Barnes, PJ. (2008). Immunology of asthma and chronic obstructive pulmonary disease. *Nat Rev Immunol*. Vol. 8, No. 3, (March 2008), pp. 183–192, ISSN 1474-1733.

[14] Barnes, PJ. (2009). Histone deacetylase-2 and airway disease. *Ther Adv Respir Dis*. Vol.3, No.5, (October 2009), pp.235-243, ISSN 1753-4658.

[15] Barnes, PJ.; Dweik, RA.; Gelb, AF.; Gibson, PG.; George, SC.; Grasemann, H.; Pavord, ID.; Ratjen, F.; Silkoff, PE.; Taylor, DR. & Zamel, N. (2010). Exhaled nitric oxide in pulmonary diseases: a comprehensive review. *Chest*. Vol. 138, No. 3, (September 2010), pp.682-692, ISSN 0012-3692.

[16] Bergeron, C.; Tulic, MK. & Hamid, Q. (2007). Tools used to measure airway remodelling in research. *Eur Respir J*. Vol. 29, No.3, (March 2007), pp.596-604, ISSN 0903-1936.

[17] Bettiol, J.; Sele, J.; Henket, M.; Louis, E.; Malaise, M.; Bartsch, P. & Louis, R. (2002). Cytokine production from sputum cells after allergenic challenge in IgE-mediated asthma. *Allergy*. Vol.57, No.12, (December 2002), pp.1145-1150, ISSN 0105-4538.

[18] Bisgaard, H.; Pipper, CB. & Bønnelykke, K. (2011). Endotyping early childhood asthma by quantitative symptom assessment. *J Allergy Clin Immunol*. Vol. 127, No. 5, (May 2011), pp.1155-1164, ISSN 0091-6749.

[19] Bousquet, J.; Jeffery, PK.; Busse, WW.; Johnson, M. & Vignola, AM. (2000). Asthma. From bronchoconstriction to airways inflammation and remodeling. *Am J Respir Crit Care Med*. Vol.161, No.5, (May 2000), pp.1720-1745, ISSN 1073-449X.

[20] Brasier, AR.; Victor, S.; Ju, H.; Busse, WW.; Curran-Everett, D.; Bleecker, E.; Castro, M.; Chung, KF.; Gaston, B.; Israel, E.; Wenzel, SE.; Erzurum, SC.; Jarjour, NN. & Calhoun, WJ. (2010). Predicting intermediate phenotypes in asthma using bronchoalveolar lavage-derived cytokines. *Clin Transl Sci*. Vol. 3, No.4, (August 2010), pp.147-157, ISSN 1752-8054.

[21] British Thoracic Society Scottish Intercollegiate Guidelines Network. (2008) British guideline on the management of Asthma. *Thorax*. Vol.63, No. Suppl. 4, pp. iv1–121, ISSN 0040-6376.

[22] Caramori, G.; Adcock, IM. & Ito, K. (2004). Anti-inflammatory inhibitors of IkappaB kinase in asthma and COPD. *Curr Opin Investig Drugs.* Vol.5, No.11, (November 2004), pp.1141-1147, ISSN 1472-4472.

[23] Caramori, G.; Pandit, A. & Papi, A. (2005). Is there a difference between chronic airway inflammation in chronic severe asthma and chronic obstructive pulmonary disease?. *Curr Opin Allergy Clin Immunol.* Vol. 5, No.1, (February 2005), pp.77-83. ISSN 1528-4050.

[24] Casale, TB, & Stokes, JR. (2008). Immunomodulators for allergic respiratory disorders. *J Allergy Clin Immunol.* Vo.121. No. 2, (February 2008), pp. 288-296, ISSN 0091-6749.

[25] Cazzola, M.; Calzetta, L. & Matera, MG. (2011). β(2) -adrenoceptor agonists: current and future direction. *Br J Pharmacol.* Vol.163, No.1, (May 2011) pp.4-17, ISSN 1476-5381.

[26] Chu, HW.; Balzar, S.; Westcott, JY.; Trudeau, JB.; Sun, Y.; Conrad, DJ. & Wenzel, SE. (2002). Expression and activation of 15-lipoxygenase pathway in severe asthma: relationship to eosinophilic phenotype and collagen deposition. *Clin Exp Allergy.* Vol. 32, No 11, pp.1558-1565, ISSN 1365-2222.

[27] Chung, KF, & Marwick, JA. (2010). Molecular mechanisms of oxidative stress in airways and lungs with reference to asthma and chronic obstructive pulmonary disease. *Ann N Y Acad Sci.* Vol. 1203, (August 2010), pp. 85-91, ISSN 0077-8923.

[28] Chung, KF.; Caramori, G. & Adcock, IM. (2009). Inhaled corticosteroids as combination therapy with beta-adrenergic agonists in airways disease: present and future. *Eur J Clin Pharmacol.* Vol. 65, No.9, (Sepetember 2009), pp.853-871, ISSN 0031-6970.

[29] Cockcroft, DW. & Davis, BE. (2006). Mechanisns of airway hyperresponsiveness. *J Allergy Clin immunol.* Vol. 118, No. 3 (Setember 2006), pp. 551-559, ISSN 0091-6749.

[30] Corradi, M.; Gergelova, P. & Mutti, A. (2010). Use of exhaled breath condensate to investigate occupational lung diseases. *Curr Opin Allergy Clin Immunol.* Vol. 10, No. 2, (April 2010), pp.93-98, ISSN 1528-4050.

[31] Corradi, M.; Zinelli, C. & Caffarelli, C. (2007). Exhaled breath biomarkers in asthmatic children. *Inflamm Allergy Drug Targets.* Vol. 6, No. 3, (Sepetember 2007), pp.150-159, ISSN 1871-5281.

[32] Crameri, R. (2005). The potential of proteomics and peptidomics fro allergy asnd asthma. *Allergy.* Vol. 60, No.10, (October 2005), pp. 1227-1237, ISSN 0105-4538.

[33] Crapo, RO.; Casaburi, R.; Coates, AL.; Enright, PL.; Hankinson, JL.; Irvin, CG.; MacIntyre, NR.; McKay, RT.; Wanger, JS.; Anderson, SD.; Cockcroft, DW.; Fish, JE. & Sterk, PJ. (2000). Guidelines for methacoline and exercise challenge testing-1999. This official statement of the American Thoracic Society was adopted by the ATS Board of Directors, July 1999. *Am J Respir Cri Care Med.* Vol.161, No.1, (January 2000), pp. 309-329, ISSN 1073-449X.

[34] Curtis, JR.; Martin, DP. & Martin, TR. (1997). Patient-assessed Health Outcomes in Chronic Lung Disease. *Am J Respir Crit Care Med.* Vol. 156, No. 4 pt1, (October 1997), pp.1032-1039, ISSN 1073-449X.

[35] Dent, G.; Hadjicharalambous, C.; Yoshikawa, T.; Handy, RL.; Powell, J.; Anderson, IK.; Louis, R.; Davies, DE. & Djukanovic, R. (2004). Contribution of eotaxin-1 to

eosinophil chemotactic activity of moderate and severe asthmatic sputum. *Am J Respir Crit Care Med*. Vol. 169, No.10, (May 2004), pp.1110-1117, ISSN 1073-449X.

[36] Dima, E.; Rovina, N.; Gerassimou, C.; Roussos, C. & Gratziou, C. (2010). Pulmonary function tests, sputum induction, and bronchial provocation tests: diagnostic tools in the challenge of distinguishing asthma and COPD phenotypes in clinical practice. *Int J Chron Obstruct Pulmon Dis*. Vol. 5, (September 2010), pp.287-296, ISSN 1176-9106.

[37] Djukanovi,c R.; Sterk, PJ.; Fahy, JC. & Hargreave, FE. (2002). Standardised methodology of sputum induction and processing. *Eur Respir J*. Vol. 20, No. suppl 37, (September 2002), pp. 1s-55s. ISSN 0903-1936.

[38] Djukanovic, R. & Sterk, PJ. (2004). *An atlas of induced sputum: an aid for research and diagnosis*. The Partenon Publishing Group, ed. ISBN 1842140051. London.

[39] Dragonieri, S.; Schot, R.; Mertens, BJ.; Le Cessie, S.; Gauw, SA.; Spanevello, A.; Resta, O.; Willard, NP.; Vink, TJ.; Rabe, KF.; Bel, EH. & Sterk, PJ. (2007). An electronic nose in the discrimination of patients with asthma and controls. *J Allergy Clin Immunol*. Vol. 120, No.4, (October 2007), pp.856-862, ISSN 0091-6749.

[40] Dweik, RA.; Sorkness, RL.; Wenzel, S.; Hammel, J.; Curran-Everett, D.; Comhair, SA.; Bleecker, E.; Busse, W.; Calhoun, WJ.; Castro, M.; Chung, KF.; Israel, E.; Jarjour, N.; Moore, W.; Peters, S.; Teague, G.; Gaston, B.; Erzurum, SC. & National Heart, Lung, and Blood Institute Severe Asthma Research Program. (2010). Use of exhaled nitric oxide measurement to identify a reactive, at-risk phenotype among patients with asthma. *Am J Respir Crit Care Med*. Vol.181, No.10, (May 2010), pp.1033-1341. ISSN 1073-449X.

[41] Fabbri, L.; Peters, SP.; Pavord, I.; Wenzel, SE.; Lazarus, SC.; Macnee, W.; Lemaire, F. & Abraham, E. (2005). Allergic rhinitis, asthma, airway biology, and chronic obstructive pulmonary disease in AJRCCM in 2004. *Am J Respir Crit Care Med*. Vol.171, No.7, (April 2005), pp.686-698, ISSN 1073-449X.

[42] Fabbri, LM.; Romagnoli, M.; Corbetta, L.; Casoni, G.; Busljetic, K.; Turato, G.; Ligabue, G.; Ciaccia, A.; Saetta, M. & Papi, A. (2003). Differences in airway inflammation in patients with fixed airflow obstruction due to asthma or chronic obstructive pulmonary disease. *Am J Respir Crit Care Med*. Vol.167, No. 3, (Frebruary 2003), pp.418-424, ISSN 1073-449X.

[43] Fajt, ML. & Wenzel, SE. (2009). Asthma phenotypes in adults and clinical implications. *Expert Rev Respir Med*. Vol.3, No. 6, (December 2009), pp.607-625, ISSN 1747-6348.

[44] Fitzpatrick, AM, Teague, WG, Meyers, DA, Peters, SP, Li, X, Li, H, Wenzel, SE, Aujla, S, Castro, M, Bacharier, LB, Gaston, BM, Bleecker, ER, Moore, WC; National Institutes of Health/National Heart, Lung, and Blood Institute Severe Asthma Research Program. Heterogeneity of severe asthma in childhood: confirmation by cluster analysis of children in the National Institutes of Health/National Heart, Lung, and Blood Institute Severe Asthma Research Program. (2011a). *J Allergy Clin Immunol*. Vol.127, No.2, (Febreuary 2011), pp.382-389. ISSN 0091-6749.

[45] Fitzpatrick, AM.; Teague, WG.; Burwell, L.; Brown, MS.; Brown, LA; & NIH/NHLBI Severe Asthma Research Program. (2011b). Glutathione oxidation is associated

with airway macrophage functional impairment in children with severe asthma. *Pediatr Res*. Vol. 69, No.2, (February 2011), pp.154-159. ISSN 0031-3998.

[46] Frey, U. & Suky, B. (2008). Complexity of chronic asthma and chronic obstructive pulmonary disease: implications for risk assessment, and disease progression and control. *Lancet*. Vol. 372, No. 9643, (September 2008), pp.1088-1099, ISSN 0140-6736.

[47] Friedrich, MJ. (2009). Scientists seek to sniff out diseases: electronic "noses" may someday be diagnostic tools. *JAMA*. Vol. 301, No.6, (February 2009), pp.585-586, ISSN 0098-7484.

[48] Fuhlbrigge, AL. (2004). Asthma severity and asthma control: symptoms, pulmonary function, and inflammatory markers. *Curr Opin Pulm Med*. Vol. 10, No. 1, (January 2004), pp. 1-6, ISSN 1070-5287.

[49] Gibson, PG. & Powell, H. (2004) Written actions plans for asthma: an evidence-based review of the key components. *Thorax*. Vol. 59, No. 2, (February 2004), pp. 94-99, ISSN 0040-6376.

[50] Gibson, PG. (2009). Using fractional exhaled nitric oxide to guide asthma therapy: design and methodological issues for AStthma TReatment ALgorithm studies. *Clin Exp Allergy*. Vol.39, No.4, (April 2009), pp.478-490, ISSN 1365-2222.

[51] Global Initiative for Asthma. Global strategy for asthma management and prevention. Available at http//www.ginasthma.org [accessed 8 March 2009].

[52] Gray, RD.; MacGregor, G.; Noble, D.; Imrie, M.; Dewar, M.; Boyd, AC.; Innes, JA.; Porteous, DJ. & Greening, AP. (2008). Sputum proteomics in inflammatory and suppurative respiratory diseases. *Am J Respir Crit Care Med*. Vol. 178, No. 5, (September 2008), pp.444-452, ISSN 1073-449X.

[53] Green, RH.; Brightling, CE.; McKenna, S.; Hargadon, B.; Parker, D.; Bradding, P.; Wardlaw, AJ. & Pavord, ID. (2002). Asthma exacerbations and sputum eosinophil counts: a randomised controlled trial. *Lancet*. Vol. 360, No. 9347, (November 2002), pp.1715-1721, ISSN 0140-6736.

[54] Gupta, GK. & Agrawal, DK. (2010). CpG oligodeoxynucleotides as TLR9 agonists: therapeutic application in allergy and asthma. *BioDrugs*. Vol. 24, No. 4, (August 2010), pp.225-35, ISSN 1173-8804.

[55] Gupta, S.; Siddiqui, S.; Haldar, P.; Entwisle, JJ.; Mawby, D.; Wardlaw, AJ.; Bradding, P.; Pavord, ID.; Green, RH. & Brightling, CE. (2010). Quantitative analysis of high-resolution computed tomography scans in severe asthma subphenotypes. *Thorax*. Vol. 65, No.9, (September 2010), pp.775-781, ISSN 0040-6376.

[56] Hai, CM. Mechanistic systems biology of inflammatory gene expression in airway smooth muscle as tool for asthma drug development. (2008). *Curr Drug Discov Technol*. Vol.5, No.4, (December 2008), pp.279-288, ISSN 1570-1638.

[57] Haldar, P.; Brightling, CE.; Hargadon, B.; Gupta, S.; Monteiro, W.; Sousa, A.; Marshall, RP.; Bradding, P.; Green, RH.; Wardlaw, AJ. & Pavord, ID. (2009). Mepolizumab and exacerbations of refractory eosinophilic asthma. *N Engl J Med*. Vol. 360, No. 10, (March 2009), pp. 973-984. Erratum in: *N Engl J Med* Vol. 364, No.6, (February 2011), p.588, ISSN 1533-4406.

[58] Haldar, P.; Pavord, ID.; Shaw, DE.; Berry, MA.; Thomas, M.; Brightling, CE.; Wardlaw, AJ. & Green, RH. (2008). Cluster analysis and clinical asthma phenotypes. *Am J Respir Crit Care Med*. Vol. 178, No.3, (August 2008), pp.218-224, ISSN 1073-449X.

[59] Hallstrand, TS.; Lai, Y.; Ni, Z.; Oslund, RC.; Henderson, WR Jr.; Gelb, MH. & Wenzel, SE. (2011). Relationship between levels of secreted phospholipase A[2] groups IIA and X in the airways and asthma severity. *Clin Exp Allergy*. Vol. 41, No. 6, (June 2011), pp.801-810, ISSN 1365-2222.

[60] Hargreave, FE. & Nair, P. (2009). The definition and diagnosis of asthma. *Clin Exp Allergy*, Vol. 39, No.11, (November 2009), pp.1652-1658, ISSN 1365-2222.

[61] Hargreave, FE.; Ryan, G.; Thomson, NC.; O'Byrne, PM.; Latimer, K.; Juniper, EF & Dolovich, J. (1981). Bronchial responsiveness to histamine or methacholine in asthma: measurement and clinical significance. *J Allergy Clin Immunol*. Vol. 68, No. 5, (November 1981), pp.347-355, ISSN 0091-6749.

[62] Hastie, AT.; Moore, WC.; Meyers, DA.; Vestal, PL.; Li, H.; Peters, SP.; Bleecker, ER. & National Heart, Lung, and Blood Institute Severe Asthma Research Program. Analyses of asthma severity phenotypes and inflammatory proteins in subjects stratified by sputum granulocytes. (2010). *J Allergy Clin Immunol*. Vol. 125, No. 5, (May 2010), pp:1028-1036, ISSN 0091-6749.

[63] Holgate, ST. & Polosa, R. (2006). The mechanisms, diagnosis, and management of severe asthma in adults. *Lancet*. Vol. 368, No. 9537, (August 2006), pp.780-93, ISSN 0140-6736.

[64] Holgate, ST.; Noonan, M.; Chanez, P.; Busse, W.; Dupont, L.; Pavord, I.; Hakulinen, A.; Paolozzi, L.; Wajdula, J.; Zang, C.; Nelson, H. & Raible, D. (2011). Efficacy and safety of etanercept in moderate-to-severe asthma: a randomised, controlled trial. *Eur Respir J*. Vol. 37, No. 6, (Juny 2011), pp.1352-1359, ISSN 0903-1936.

[65] Horváth, I.; Hunt, J.; Barnes, PJ.; Alving, K.; Antczak, A.; Baraldi, E.; Becher, G.; van Beurden, WJ.; Corradi, M.; Dekhuijzen, R.; Dweik, RA.; Dwyer, T.; Effros, R.; Erzurum, S.; Gaston, B.; Gessner, C.; Greening, A.; Ho, LP.; Hohlfeld, J.; Jöbsis, Q.; Laskowski, D.; Loukides, S.; Marlin, D.; Montuschi, P.; Olin, AC.; Redington, AE.; Reinhold, P.; van Rensen, EL.; Rubinstein, I.; Silkoff, P.; Toren, K.; Vass, G.; Vogelberg, C.; Wirtz, H. & ATS/ERS Task Force on Exhaled Breath Condensate. (2005). Exhaled breath condensate: methodological recommendations and unresolved questions. *Eur Respir J*. Vol.26, No.3, (September 2005), pp. 523-548, ISSN 0903-1936.

[66] Horváth, I.; Loukides, S.; Wodehouse, T.; Csiszér, E.; Cole, PJ.; Kharitonov, SA. & Barnes, PJ. (2003). Comparison of exhaled and nasal nitric oxide and exhaled carbon monoxide levels in bronchiectatic patients with and without primary ciliary dyskinesia. *Thorax*. Vol. 58, No.1, (January 2003), pp.68-72. Erratum in: (2004) *Thorax*. Vol. 59, No.6, p.543, ISSN 0040-6376.

[67] Jayaram, L.; Pizzichini, MM.; Cook, RJ.; Boulet, LP.; Lemière, C.; Pizzichini, E.; Cartier, A.; Hussack, P.; Goldsmith, CH.; Laviolette, M.; Parameswaran, K. & Hargreave, FE. (2006). Determining asthma treatment by monitoring sputum cell counts: effect on exacerbations. *Eur Respir J*. Vol. 27, No.3, (March 2006), pp.483-494, ISSN 0903-1936.

[68] Juniper, EF.; Wisniewski, ME.; Cox, FM.; Emmett, AH.; Nielsen, KE. & O'Byrne, PM. (2004). Relationship between quality of life and clinical status in asthma: a factor analysis. *Eur Respir J*. Vol. 23, No. 2, (February 2004), pp.287-291, ISSN 0903-1936.

[69] Kanagaratham, C.; Camateros, P.; Flaczyk, A. & Radzioch, D. (2011). Polymorphisms in TOLL-like receptor genes and their roles in allergic asthma and atopy. *Recent Pat Inflamm Allergy Drug Discov*. Vol.5, No.1, pp.45-56, ISSN 1872-213X.

[70] Kiyokawa, H.; Matsumoto, H.; Nakaji, H.; Niimi, A, Ito, I.; Ono, K.; Takeda, T.; Oguma, T.; Otsuka, K. & Mishima, M. (2011). Centrilobular Opacities in the Asthmatic Lung Successfully Treated with Inhaled Ciclesonide and Tiotropium: With Assessment of Alveolar Nitric Oxide Levels. *Allergol Int*. February 25. [Epub ahead of print], ISSN 1323-8930.

[71] Koh, G C-H.; Shek, L P-C.; Goh, D Y-T.; Van Bever, H. & Koh, D S-Q. (2007). Eosinophil cationic protein: is it useful in asthma?. A systematic review. *Respir Med*. Vol. 101, No. 4, (April 2007), pp.696-705, ISSN 0954-6111.

[72] Kostikas, K.; Koutsokera, A.; Papiris, S.; Gourgoulianis, KI. & Loukides, S. (2008). Exhaled breath condensate in patients with asthma: implications for application in clinical practice. *Clin Exp Allergy*. Vol. 38, No.4, (April 2008), pp.557-565, ISSN 1365-2222.

[73] Kostikas, K.; Papaioannou, AI.; Tanou, K.; Giouleka, P.; Koutsokera, A.; Minas, M.; Papiris, S.; Gourgoulianis, KI.; Taylor, DR.& Loukides, S. (2011). Exhaled NO and exhaled breath condensate pH in the evaluation of asthma control. *Respir Med*. Vol.105, No.4, (April 2011), pp.526-532, ISSN 0954-6111.

[74] Lay, JC.; Peden, DB. & Alexis, NE. (2011). Flow cytometry of sputum: assessing inflammation and immune response elements in the bronchial airways. *Inhal Toxicol*. Vol. 23, No. 7, (Juny 2011), pp.392-406, ISSN 0895-8378.

[75] Leuppi, JD.; Salome, CM.; Jenkins, CR.; Koskela, H.; Brannan, JD.; Anderson, SD.; Andersson, M.; Chan, HK. & Woolcock, AJ. (2001). Markers of airway inflammation and airway hyperresponsiveness in patients with well-controlled asthma. *Eur Respir J*. Vol.18, (No.3, Sepetember 2001), pp.444-450, ISSN 0903-1936.

[76] Lewis, NS. (2004). Comparisons between mammalian and artificial olfaction based on arrays of carbon black-polymer composite vapor detectors. *Acc Chem Res*. Vol. 37, No.9, (September 2004), pp.663-672, ISSN 1520-4898.

[77] Lötvall, J.; Akdis, CA.; Bacharier, LB.; Bjermer, L.; Casale, TB.; Custovic, A.; Lemanske, RF Jr.; Wardlaw, AJ.; Wenzel, SE. & Greenberger, PA. Asthma endotypes: a new approach to classification of disease entities within the asthma syndrome. (2011). *J Allergy Clin Immunol*. Vol.127, No.2, (February 2011), pp.355-360, ISSN 0091-6749.

[78] Louhelainen, N.; Myllärniemi, M.; Rahman, I. & Kinnula, VL. Airway biomarkers of the oxidant burden in asthma and chronic obstructive pulmonary disease: current and future perspectives. (2008a). *Int J Chron Obstruct Pulmon Dis*. Vol. 3, No. 4, Pp. 585-603, ISSN 1176-9106.

[79] Louhelainen, N.; Rytilä, P.; Obase, Y.; Mäkelä, M.; Haahtela, T.; Kinnula, VL. & Pelkonen, A. (2008b). The value of sputum 8-isoprostane in detecting oxidative stress in mild asthma. *J Asthma*. Vol. 45, No.2, (March 2008), pp.149-154, ISSN 1532-4303.

[80] Louis, RE.; Cataldo, D.; Buckley, MG.; Sele, J.; Henket, M.; Lau, LC.; Bartsch, P.; Walls, AF. & Djukanovic, R. (2002). Evidence of mast-cell activation in a subset of patients with eosinophilic chronic obstructive pulmonary disease. *Eur Respir J*. Vol. 20, No.2, (August 2002), pp.325-331, ISSN 0903-1936.

[81] Loukides S.; Kontogianni K.; Hillas G.& Horvath I. (2011). Exhaled breath condensate in asthma: from bench to bedside. *Curr Med Chem*. Vol.18, No.10, pp.1432-1443, ISSN 1568-0118.

[82] Luks, VP.; Vandemheen, KL. & Aaron, SD. (2010). Confirmation of asthma in an era of overdiagnosis. *Eur Respir J*. Vol.36, No. 2, (August 2010), pp.255-260, ISSN 0903-1936.

[83] Mauad, T.; Ferreira, DS.; Costa, MB.; Araujo, BB.; Silva, LF.; Martins, MA.; Wenzel, SE. & Dolhnikoff, M. (2008). Characterization of autopsy-proven fatal asthma patients in São Paulo, Brazil. *Rev Panam Salud Publica*. Vol. 23, No.6, (June 2008), pp.418-423, 1020-4989.

[84] Mauad, T.; Silva, LF.; Santos, MA.; Grinberg, L.; Bernardi, FD.; Martins, MA.; Saldiva, PH. & Dolhnikoff, M. (2004). Abnormal alveolar attachments with decreased elastic fiber content in distal lung in fatal asthma. *Am J Respir Crit Care Med*. Vol.170, No.8, (October 2004), pp.857-862, ISSN 1073-449X.

[85] Miller, MR.; Hankinson, J.; Brusasco, V.; Burgos, F.; Casaburi, R.; Coates, A.; Crapo, R.; Enright, P.; van der Grinten, CP.; Gustafsson, P.; Jensen, R.; Johnson, DC.; MacIntyre, N.; McKay, R.; Navajas, D.; Pedersen, OF.; Pellegrino, R.; Viegi, G.; Wanger, J. & ATS/ERS Task Force. Series "Standardisation of spirometry. ATS/ERS task force, standardization of lung function testing". (2005). *Eur Respir J*. Vol. 26, No. 2, (August 2005), pp. 319-338, ISSN 0903-1936.

[86] Moore, WC.; Evans, MD.; Bleecker, ER.; Busse, WW.; Calhoun, WJ.; Castro, M.; Fan Chung, K.; Erzurum, SC.; Curran-Everett, D.; Dweik, RA.; Gaston, B.; Hew, M.; Israel, E.; Mayse, ML.; Pascual, RM.; Peters, SP.; Silveira, L.; Wenzel, SE. & Jarjour, NN; for the National Heart, Lung, and Blood Institute's Severe Asthma Research Program. Safety of investigative bronchoscopy in the Severe Asthma Research Program. (2011). *J Allergy Clin Immunol*. Apr 13. [Epub ahead of print].

[87] Moore, WC.; Meyers, DA.; Wenzel, SE.; Teague, WG.; Li, H.; Li, X.; D'Agostino, R Jr.; Castro, M.; Curran-Everett, D.; Fitzpatrick, AM.; Gaston, B.; Jarjour, NN.; Sorkness, R.; Calhoun, WJ.; Chung, KF.; Comhair, SA.; Dweik, RA.; Israel, E.; Peters, SP.; Busse, WW.; Erzurum, SC.; Bleecker, ER. & The National Heart, Lung, and Blood Institute's Severe Asthma Research Program. Identification of asthma phenotypes using cluster analysis in the Severe Asthma Research Program. (2010). *Am J Respir Crit Care Med*. Vol.181, No.4, (February 2010), pp.315-323, ISSN 1073-449X.

[88] Nicholas, B. & Djukanovic, R. (2009). Induced sputum: a window to lung pathology. *Biochem Soc. Trans*. Vol. 37, No Pt4, (August 2009), pp.868-872, ISSN 0300-5127.

[89] Nicholas, B.; Skipp, P.; Mould, R.; Rennard, S.; Davies, DE.; O'Connor, CD. & Djukanović, R. (2006). Shotgun proteomic analysis of human-induced sputum. *Proteomics*. Vol. 6, No.15, (August 2006), pp.4390-4401, ISSN 1615-9853.

[90] Paredi, P. & Barnes, PJ. (2009). The airway vasculature: recent advances and clinical implications. *Thorax*. Vol. 64, No. 5, (May 2009), pp.444-450, ISSN 0040-6376.

[91] Paredi, P.; Kharitonov, SA. & Barnes, PJ. (2005). Correlation of exhaled breath temperature with bronchial blood flow in asthma. *Respir Res*. Vol.6, (February 2005), p.15, ISSN 1465-993X.

[92] Park, CS. & Rhim, T. (2011). Application of proteomics in asthma research. *Expert Rev Proteomics*. Vol. 8, No. 2, (April 2011), pp.221-230, ISSN 1478-9450.

[93] Pavord, ID.; Haldar, P.; Bradding, P. & Wardlaw, AJ. (2010). Mepolizumab in refractory eosinophilic asthma. *Thorax*. Vol. 65, No.4, (April 2010), p. 370, ISSN 0040-6376.

[94] Pavord, ID.; Jeffery, PK.; Qiu, Y.; Zhu, J.; Parker, D.; Carlsheimer, A.; Naya, I. & Barnes, NC. (2009). Airway inflammation in patients with asthma with high-fixed or low-fixed plus as-needed budesonide/formoterol. *J Allergy Clin Immunol*. Vol.123, No. 5, pp.1083-1089, ISSN 0091-6749.

[95] Pelaia, G.; Gallelli, L.; Renda, T.; Romeo, P.; Busceti, MT.; Grembiale, LD.; Maselli, R.; Marisco, SA. & Vatrella, A. (2011). Update on optimal use of omalizumab in management of asthma. *J Asthma and Allergy*. Vol.4, pp.49-59 ISSN 1178-6965.

[96] Perpiñá Tordera, M. (2010). Why do we look at asthma through the keyhole?. *Arch Bronconeumol*. Vol. 46, No. 8, (Augus 2010), pp.433-438, ISSN 0300-2896.

[97] Polosa, R.; Ciamarra, I.; Mangano, G.; Prosperini, G.; Pistorio, MP.; Vancheri, C. & Crimi, N. (2000). Bronchial hyperresponsiveness and airway inflammation markers in nonasthmatics with allergic rhinitis. *Eur Respir J*. Vol.15, No.1, (January 2000), pp.30-35, ISSN 0903-1936.

[98] Popov, TA. Human exhaled breath analysis. (2011). *Ann Allergy Asthma Immunol*. Vol.106, No.6, (June 2011), pp.451-456, ISSN 1081-1206.

[99] Postma, DS.; O'Byrne, PM. & Pedersen, S. (2011). Comparison of the effect of low-dose ciclesonide and fixed-dose fluticasone propionate and salmeterol combination on long-term asthma control. *Chest*. Vol.139, No.2, (February 2011), pp.311-318, ISSN 0012-3692.

[100] Puckett, JL.; Taylor, RW.; Leu, SY.; Guijon, OL.; Aledia, AS.; Galant, SP. & George, SC. (2010). Clinical patterns in asthma based on proximal and distal airway nitric oxide categories. *Respir Res*. Vol. 11, (April 2010), p.47, ISSN 1465-993X.

[101] Quaedvlieg, V.; Sele, J.; Henket, M. & Louis, R. (2009). Association between asthma control and bronchial hyperresponsiveness and airways inflammation: a cross-sectional study in daily practice. *Clin Exp Allergy*. Vol. 39, No. 12, (December 2009), pp.1822-1829, ISSN 1365-2222.

[102] Rabinovitch, N. (2007). Urinary leukotriene E_4. *Immunol Allergy Clin N Am*. Vol. 27. No. 6, (June 2007), pp. 451-464, ISSN 0889-8561.

[103] Reddel, HK. Peak flow monitoring in clinical practice and clinical asthma trials. (2006). *Curr Opin Pulm Med*. Vol. 12, No. 1, (January 2006), pp. 75–81, ISSN 1070-5287.

[104] Rosi, E.; Ronchi, MC.; Grazzini, M.; Duranti, R. & Scano, G. (1999). Sputum analysis, bronchial hyperresponsiveness, and airway function in asthma: results of a factor analtysis. *J Allergy Clin Immunol*. Vol. 103, No. 2 pt1, (February), pp.232-237, ISSN 0091-6749.

[105] Rutgers, SR.; Timens, W.; Tzanakis, N.; Kauffman, HF.; van der Mark, TW.; Koëter, GH. & Postma, DS. (2000). Airway inflammation and hyperresponsiveness to adenosine 5'-monophosphate in chronic obstructive pulmonary disease. *Clin Exp Allergy*. Vol.30, No.5, (May 2000), pp.657-662, ISSN 1365-2222.

[106] Sanak, M.; Gielicz, A.; Bochenek, G.; Kaszuba, M.; Niżankowska-Mogilnicka, E. & Szczeklik, A. (2011). Targeted eicosanoid lipidomics of exhaled breath condensate provide a distinct pattern in the aspirin-intolerant asthma phenotype. *J Allergy Clin Immunol*. Vol. 127, No.5, (May 2011), pp.1141-1147, ISSN 0091-6749.

[107] Schleich, FN.; Seidel, L.; Sele, J.; Manise, M.; Quaedvlieg, V.; Michils, A. & Louis, R. (2010). Exhaled nitric oxide thresholds associated with a sputum eosinophil count ≥3% in a cohort of unselected patients with asthma. *Thorax*. Vol. 65, No.12, (December 2010), pp.1039-1044, ISSN 0040-6376.

[108] Schneider, A.; Tilemann, L.; Schermer, T.; Gindner, L.; Laux, G.; Szecsenyi, J. & Meyer, FJ. (2009). Diagnosing asthma in general practice with portable exhaled nitric oxide measurement--results of a prospective diagnostic study: FENO < or = 16 ppb better than FENO < or =12 ppb to rule out mild and moderate to severe asthma. *Respir Res*. Vol. 10, p.15. Erratum in (2009). *Respir Res*. Vol.10, (March 2009), p. 64, ISSN 1465-993X.

[109] Scott, SM.; James, D. & Ali, Z. (2007). Data analysis for electronic nose systems. *Microchim Acta*. Vol. 156, pp. 183-207, ISSN 0026-3672.

[110] Slager, RE.; Hawkins, GA.; Ampleford, EJ.; Bowden, A.; Stevens, LE.; Morton, MT.; Tomkinson, A.; Wenzel, SE.; Longphre, M.; Bleecker, ER. & Meyers, DA. (2010). IL-4 receptor α polymorphisms are predictors of a pharmacogenetic response to a novel IL-4/IL-13 antagonist. *J Allergy Clin Immunol*. Vol.126, No.4, (October 2010), pp.875-878, ISSN 0091-6749.

[111] Sont, JK.; De Boer, WI.; van Schadewijk, WA.; Grünberg, K.; van Krieken, JH.; Hiemstra, PS.; Sterk, PJ. & Asthma Management Project University of Leiden Study Group. (2003). Fully automated assessment of inflammatory cell counts and cytokine expression in bronchial tissue. *Am J Respir Crit Care Med*. Vol.167, No.11, (June 2003), pp.1496-1503, ISSN 1073-449X.

[112] Sont, JK.; Willems, LN.; Bel, EH.; van Krieken, JH.; Vandenbroucke, JP. & Sterk PJ. (1999). Clinical control and histopathologic outcome of asthma when using airway hyperresponsiveness as an additional guide to long-term treatment. The AMPUL Study Group. *Am J Respir Crit Care Med*. Vol. 159, No. 4 pt 1, (April 1999), pp. 1043–1051, ISSN 1073-449X.

[113] Sorkness, RL.; Bleecker, ER.; Busse, WW.; Calhoun, WJ.; Castro, M.; Chung, KF.; Curran-Everett, D.; Erzurum, SC.; Gaston, BM.; Israel, E.; Jarjour, NN.; Moore, WC.; Peters, SP.; Teague, WG.; Wenzel, SE. & National Heart, Lung, and Blood Institute Severe Asthma Research Program. (2008). Lung function in adults with stable but severe asthma: air trapping and incomplete reversal of obstruction with

bronchodilation. *J Appl Physiol.* Vol.104, No.2, (February 2008), pp.394-403, ISSN 8750-7587.

[114] Spycher, BD.; Silverman, M. & Kuehni, CE. (2010). Phenotypes of childhood asthma: are they real?. *Clin Exp Allergy.* Vol. 40, No.8, (August 2010), pp.1130-1141, ISSN 1365-2222.

[115] Sterk, PJ.; Fabbri, LM.; Quanjer, PH.; Cockcroft, DW.; O'Byrne, PM.; Anderson, SD.; Juniper, EF. & Malo, JL. (1993). Airway responsiveness. Standardized challenge testing with pharmacological, physical and sensitizing stimuli in adults. Report Working Party Standardization of Lung Function Tests, European Community for Steel and Coal. Official Statement of the European Respiratory Society. *Eur Respir J Suppl.* Vol. 16, (March 1993), pp.53-83, ISSN 0106-4347.

[116] Struben, VM.; Wieringa, MH.; Feenstra, L. & de Jongste, JC. (2006). Nasal nitric oxide and nasal allergy. *Allergy.* Vol. 61, No. 6, pp.665-670, ISSN 0105-4538.

[117] Taylor, DR.; Bateman, ED.; Boulet, LP.; Boushey, HA.; Busse, WW.; Casale, TB.; Chanez, P.; Enright, PL.; Gibson, PG.; de Jongste, JC.; Kerstjens, HA.; Lazarus, SC.; Levy, ML.; O'Byrne, PM.; Partridge, MR.; Pavord, ID.; Sears, MR.; Sterk, PJ.; Stoloff, SW.; Szefler, SJ.; Sullivan, SD.; Thomas, MD.; Wenzel, SE. & Reddel, HK. (2008). A new perspective on concepts of asthma severity and control. *Eur Respir J.* Vol. 32, No. 3, (September 2008), pp.545-554, ISSN 0903-1936.

[118] Thaler, ER. & Hanson, CW. (2005). Medical applications of electronic nose technology. *Exert Rev Med Devices.* Vol. 2, No. 5, (September 2005), pp. 559-566, ISSN 1743-4440.

[119] Thomson, NC.; Rubin, AS.; Niven, RM.; Corris, PA.; Siersted, HC.; Olivenstein, R.; Pavord, ID.; McCormack, D.; Laviolette, M.; Shargil,l NS.; Cox, G. & AIR Trial Study Group. (2011). Long-term (5 year) safety of bronchial thermoplasty: Asthma Intervention Research (AIR) trial. *BMC Pulm Med.* Vol.11, (February 2011), p.8, ISSN 1471-2466.

[120] van Essen-Zandvliet, EE.; Hughes, MD.; Waalkens, HJ.; Duiverman, EJ. & Kerrebijn, KF. (1994). Remission of childhood asthma after long-term treatment with an inhaled corticosteroid [budesonide]: can it be achieved? Dutch CNSLD Study Group. *Eur Respir J.* Vol.7, No.1, (January 1994), pp.63-68. ISSN 0903-1936.

[121] van Rensen, EL.; Evertse, CE.; van Schadewijk, WA.; van Wijngaarden, S.; Ayre, G.; Mauad, T.; Hiemstra, PS.; Sterk, PJ. & Rabe, KF. (2009). Eosinophils in bronchial mucosa of asthmatics after allergen challenge: effect of anti-IgE treatment. *Allergy.* Vol. 64, No.1, (January 2009), pp.72-80, ISSN 0105-4538.

[122] Verrills, NM.; Irwin, JA.; He, XY.; Wood, LG.; Powell, H.; Simpson, JL.; McDonald, VM.; Sim, A. & Gibson, PG. Identification of Novel Diagnostic Biomarkers for Asthma and Chronic Obstructive Pulmonary Disease. (2011). *Am J Respir Crit Care Med.* Vol.183, No. 12, (June 2011), pp.1633-1643, ISSN 1073-449X.

[123] Vijverberg, SJ.; Koenderman, L.; Koster, ES.; van der Ent, CK.; Raaijmakers, JA. & Maitland-van der Zee, AH. (2011). Biomarkers of therapy responsiveness in asthma: pitfalls and promises. *Clin Exp Allergy.* Vol. 41, No.5, (May 2011), pp.615-629, ISSN 1365-2222.

[124] Wang, F.; He, XY, Baines, KJ.; Gunawardhana, LP.; Simpson, JL.; Li, F. & Gibson, PG. (2011). Different inflammatory phenotypes in adults and children with acute asthma. *Eur Respir J*. Jan 13. [Epub ahead of print].

[125] Ward, C.; Reid, DW.; Orsida, BE.; Feltis, B.; Feltis, B.; Ryan, VA.; Johns, DP. & Walters, EH. (2005). Inter-relationships between airway inflammation, reticular basement memebrane thikening and bronchial hyper-reactivity to methacholine in asthma: a systematic bronchoalveolar lavage and airway biopsy analysis. *Clin Exp Allergy*. Vol. 35, No.12, (December 2005), pp. 1565-1571, ISSN 1365-2222.

[126] Wenzel, SE. (2006). Asthma: defining of the persistent adult phenotypes. *Lancet*. Vol. 368, No. 9537, (August 2006), pp. 804-813, ISSN 0140-6736.

Part 10

Role of AC0T7

10

Role of ACOT7 in Arachidonic Acid Production and Inflammation

Crystall Swarbrick, Noelia Roman and Jade K. Forwood
Charles Sturt University
Australia

1. Introduction

Acyl-CoA Thioesterases (ACOTs) perform a wide range of cellular functions by catalysing the thiolytic cleavage of activated fatty acyl-CoAs. Substrates of ACOTs include short to long-chain acyl-CoAs as well as a range of methyl-branched, and dicarboxylic bile acid-CoAs (M. C. Hunt & Alexson, 2008). Expression of ACOTs have been detected in both prokaryotes and eukaryotes with expression in higher organisms being detected in cytosol, mitochondria, peroxisomes and endoplasmic reticulum (J. Yamada, 2005).

Within the ACOT enzyme family, one member in particular, ACOT7 has recently been identified as playing a role inflammation through the production of arachidonic acid (AA). It was recently proposed that ACOT7-mediated AA production may provide a complementary source of AA to the well characterised phospholipase A_2 (PLA_2) pathway (Satoru Sakuma, Usa, & Fujimoto, 2006); see Table 1 for review of Acot substrate specificity. Evidence for these observations was through experimental data showing that ACOT7 possessed high substrate specificity for AA-CoA; the gene encoding ACOT7 was highly expressed in macrophages and up-regulated when stimulated by lipopolysaccharide (LPS); and that over-expression of the enzyme lead to an increase in prostaglandin production. Together, these observations highlight a novel role of ACOT7 in inflammation through the production of arachidonic acid from the thiolytic cleavage of activated polyunsaturated omega-6 fatty acid C20:4-CoA (Forwood et al., 2007).

2. Cellular production of arachidonic acid (C20:4)

Arachidonic acid has a number of important cellular roles, namely in cell signalling, regulation of metabolic and signalling enzymes, and inflammation. Despite its importance, its methods of cellular production are not fully understood. The most well characterised cellular pathway for arachidonic acid involves its release from membrane phospholipids via the action of PLA_2, an enzyme responsible for the catalysis and hydrolysis of phospholipids at the *sn*-2 position (Sakuma et al, 2006) (see Figure 1).

Expression of PLA_2 is regulated according to the requirement for arachidonic acid and well understood. Rapid activation of PLA_2 is achieved via posttranslational modification, and enzyme activity is activated by phosphorylation (controlled by mitogen-activated protein), while prolonged expression is regulated at a transcriptional level by cytokines and growth factors such as macrophage colony stimulating factor, tumor necrosis stimulating factor-

Acot Homologue	Preferred acyl-CoA substrate
Acot1	Lauroyl and palmitoyl-CoA
Acot2	Lauroyl and palmitoyl-CoA
Acot3	Palmitoyl-CoA
Acot4	Succinyl-CoA
Acot5	Decanoyl-CoA
Acot6	Not determined
Acot7	Arachidonoyl-CoA
Acot8	Bile acids
Acot9	Myristoyl-CoA
Acot10	Myristoyl-CoA
Acot11	Not determined
Acot12	Acetyl-CoA
Acot13	Aromatic acyl-CoAs

Table 1. Substrate specificities for acyl-coA thioesterases.

alpha and glucocorticoid (Jiang et al., 2001; Satoru Sakuma, et al., 2006). While PLA_2 is well known for its role in generating AA from the cleavage of the acyl bond of membrane phospholipids in a range of cell types, several lines of evidence have recently developed to suggest that PLA_2 may not be solely responsible for controlling AA levels. For example, it was shown that AA-CoA can supply AA for prostaglandin (PG) synthesis (S. Sakuma et al., 1994), and that a novel enzymatic pathway exists whereby thioesterase cleavage of AA-CoA is responsible for supplying free AA to be utilised in the synthesis of prostaglandins (S. Sakuma, et al., 1994). A similar mechanism has also been described for controlling cellular levels of AA where it was demonstrated that AA levels were under the control of competing actions of an acyl-CoA thioesterase and synthetase, independent of the classical PLA_2 cascade (Maloberti et al., 2005). In further support of these observations, when competition on AA levels were reduced through inhibition of an AA acyl-CoA synthetase (ACS; the opposite reaction that is catalysed by Acot7), substantial increases in PG levels were observed (Castilla et al., 2004); and moreover, in an independent study, overexpression of an acyl-CoA synthetase was been shown to cause a marked increase in synthesis of AA-CoA, increased 20:4 incorporation into membrane phospholipids, reduced cellular levels of unesterified 20:4, and reduced secretion of prostaglandin E2 (PGE2) while inhibition of the ACS resulted in increased release of PGE2 (Golej et al., 2011). Thus, it is emerging that inflammation is a complex cellular process, and PLA2 is unlikely to be the sole enzymatic pathway responsible for regulating AA levels, typically kept low due to the potent biological actions of the eicosanoids (Flesch, Schonhardt, & Ferber, 1989; Irvine, 1982), and that complementary pathways exist to contribute to AA generation and synthesis of eicosanoid inflammatory mediators during an immune response. That ACOT7 is abundantly expressed in macrophages and upregulated during an immune response; has high specificity for AA-CoA; and its over-expression in LPS-simulated macrophages cause an increase in prostaglandin production, is consistent with the role of ACOT7 in inflammation through the production of AA-derived inflammatory mediators.

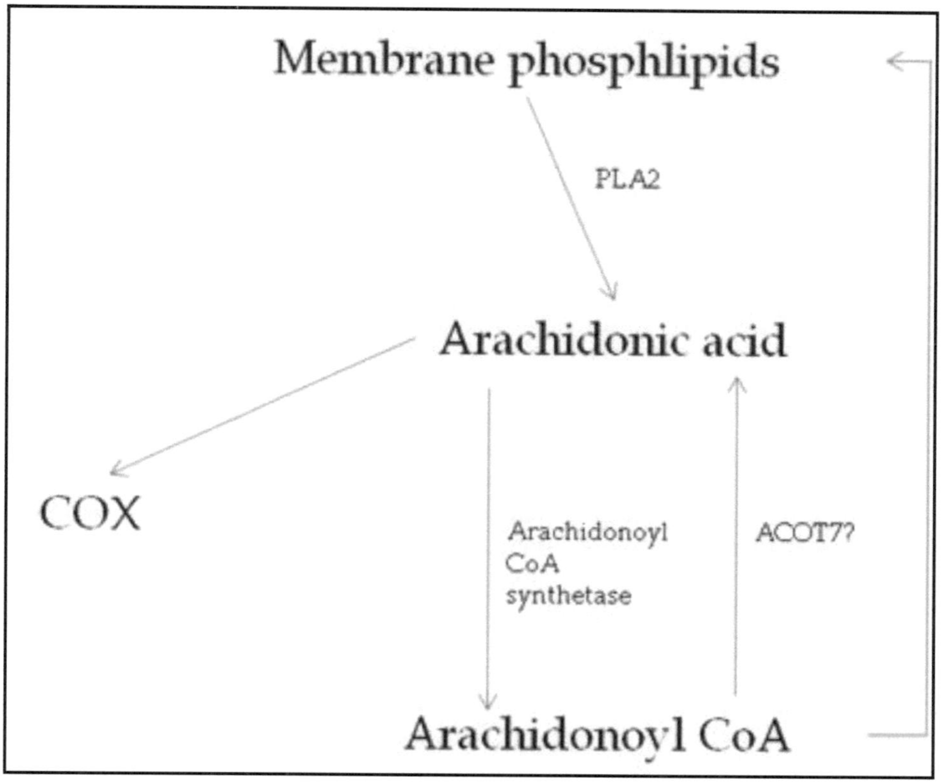

Fig. 1. The cellular pathway of arachidonic acid release involves the phospholipaseA2, and other AA-producing pathways.

2.1 Role of arachidonic acid in inflammation

Cellular production of arachidonic acid is utilized in a range of pathways, including the generation of potent mediators to initiate an inflammatory response. Two well characterised pathways important in inflammation include the cyclooxygenase (COX) and 5-Lipoxygnease pathways, and involve the conversion of arachidonic acid into prostanoids (prostaglandins, thromboxans), and leukotrienes respectively. The prostanoids include a range of arachidonic acid-derived metabolites that function to maintain body homeostasis by acting in a paracrine and autocrine fashion on cells within the vicinity of their release and are targets for the anti-inflammatory drugs including aspirin and derivatives. They typically exert their effect through activation of cell surface specific G-protein coupled receptors (GPCR), of which there are several subtypes for each prostanoid: PGD receptor (DP); PGE receptors EP1, EP2, EP3 and EP4 subtypes; PGF receptor (FP); PGI receptor (IP); and TX receptor (TP). There is also a receptor found on Th2 cells (CRTH2) that reacts to PGD_2 but belongs to the chemokine receptor family (Narumiya, 2009; Wang, Honn, & Nie, 2007).

Prostanoid production is increased during the inflammation response, particularly during acute inflammation, prior to the recruitment of leukocytes. There are a number of different prostanoids produced from the COX pathway, including prostaglandin (PG) D_2, prostaglandin E_2 (PGE_2), prostaglandin F_{2alpha} ($PGF_{2\alpha}$), prostacyclin (PGI_2) and thromboxane (TX) A_2 (Narumiya, 2009). Gilroy et al. found that PGE_2 levels are raised only during the initial phases of inflammation whilst PGD_2 becomes the predominant prostanoid during the final stages of the inflammatory response (Gilroy et al., 1999; Tilley, Coffman, & Koller, 2001).

5-lipoxygenase utilises free arachidonic acid in conjunction with 5-lipoxygenase activating-protein (FLAP), the 5-lipoxygenase activating protein, to catalyse the oxygenation of arachidonic acid into hydroperoxy-eicosatetraenoic acid (HPETE). FLAP selectively transfers arachidonic acid to 5-lipoxygenase and enhances the sequential oxygenation of this substrate to produce 5(S)-hydroperoxyeicosatetraenoic acid (5HpETE), as well as dehydration of arachidonic acid to leukotriene A_4 (LTA_4). LTA_4 can then be exported from the cell and undergo transcellular metabolism or be converted into either the pro-inflammatory LTB_4 or into a cysteinyl leukotrienes (cysLTs) LTC_4, LTD_4 or LTE_4. The cysteinyl leukotrienes are a family of bronchoconstrictive, vasoconstrictive pro-inflammatory molecules. The primary signalling method for these leukotrienes is the activation of GPCRs on cell surfaces, namely BLT_1 and BLT_2 forLTB_4, and $CysLT_1$ and $CysLT_2$ for CysLT's. Leukotrienes are thought to play a role in innate immune defence as well as a role in antimicrobial host defence. Importantly, they have been shown to play a role in respiratory diseases, such as asthma, allergies, such as anaphylaxis (Ferreira et al., 2008), as well as cardiovascular disease (Evans, Ferguson, Mosley, & Hutchinson, 2008).

Cytochrome P450 is thought to act on endogenous arachidonic acid converting it into epoxy-eicosatrienoic acids (EETs) (Piomelli, 2000). Although found primarily in the liver cytochrome P450 has also been detected in a number of different tissues such as lungs, kidney, skin, adrenal cortex and brain tissues. The implications of P450 in the brain were demonstrated by Nicholson & Renton (2005) by removing astrocytes from rat brains and demonstrating that levels of P450 are modulated by inflammation using LPS stimulation.

Peroxisome-proliferator-activated receptors (PPARs) α and γ regulate the transcription of target genes through agonist binding to the ligand-binding domain (LBD) of these genes. PPARα plays a role in fatty acid regulation, through modulating the expression of target genes, and are characterised by a high lipid catabolic activity. Jiang et al. (2001) found that clofibrate, which activates PPARα, up-regulates the expression of $cPLA_2$ and COX-2 in preadipocytes. PPARγ has been shown to play a role in the regulation of differentiation of preadipocytes into adipocytes. It was found by Murakami et al. (2001) that fatty acyl-CoA's function as antagonists for PPARα and PPARγ.

3. Acyl-CoA thioesterase activity

Acyl-CoA's perform a wide range of important cellular functions, serving as primary substrates for fatty acid degradation and lipid synthesis as well as regulators of cellular mechanisms such as ion fluxes, vesicle trafficking, protein phosphorylation and gene expression (see Figure 2 for domain organisation of Acot family members).

Most recently, the action of a specific enzyme within the ACOT enzyme family was demonstrated to act on arachidonoyl-CoA, and therefore possibly play a role in arachidonic acid production for the generation of prostanoids and leukotrienes. This is achieved by cleaving the thioester bond of activated C20:4-CoA in the general reaction described in Figure 3.

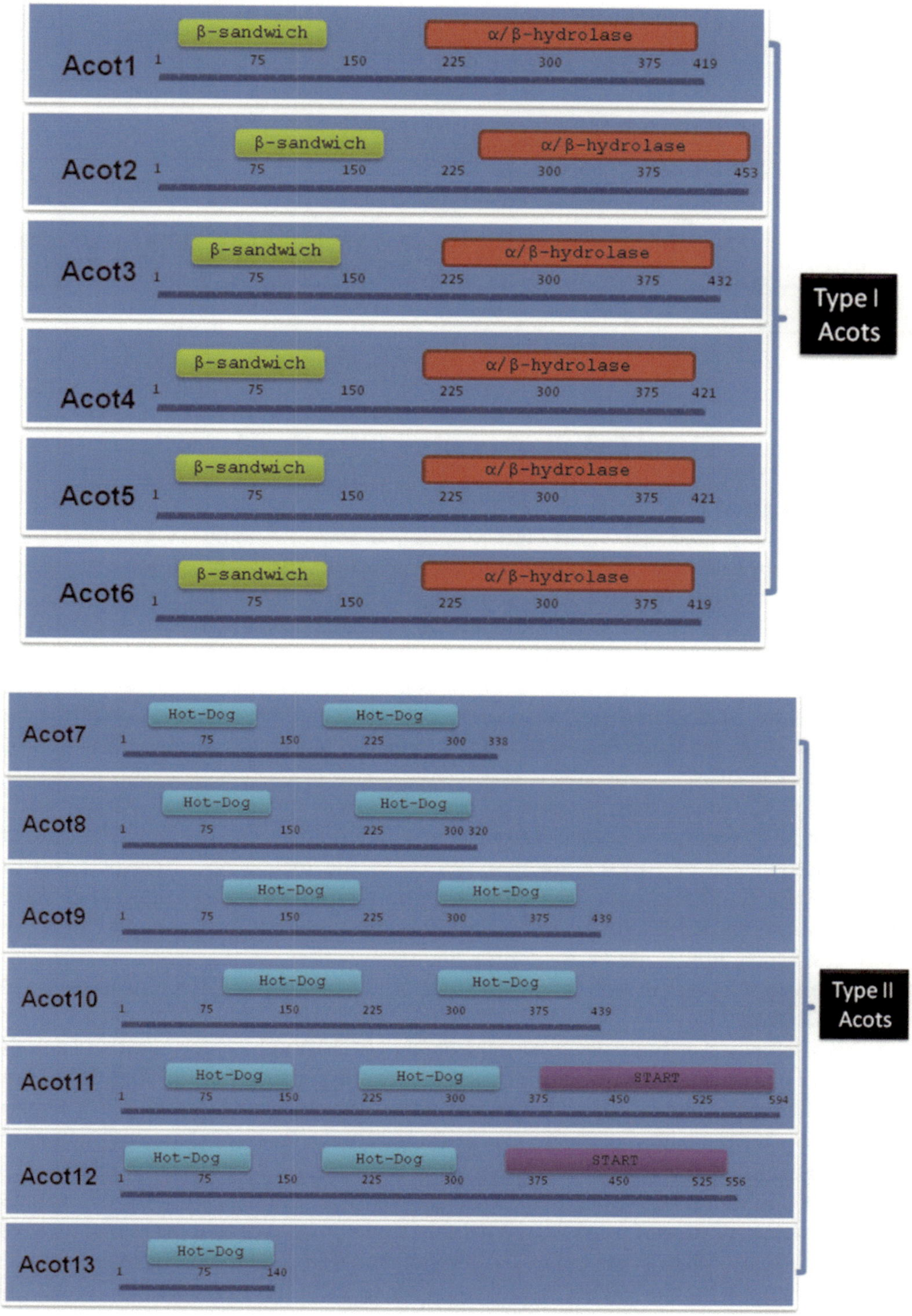

Fig. 2. Domain organisation of Acots.

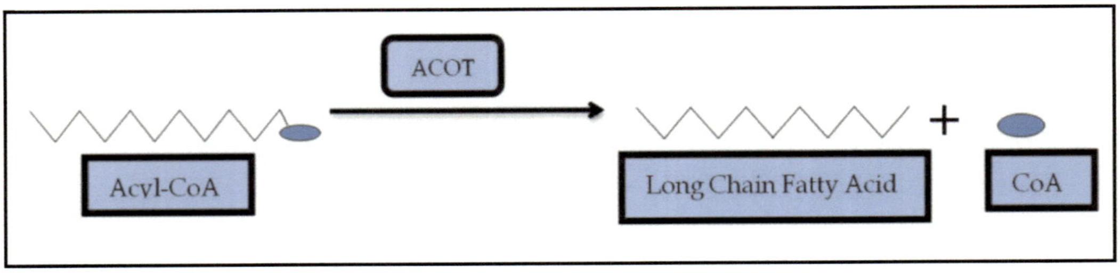

Fig. 3. ACOTs hydrolyse acyl-CoA esters to form free fatty acids and CoASH

3.1 Activity of ACOT7

It has been demonstrated that ACOT7 cleaves arachidonoyl-CoA to release CoA as CoASH and the free fatty acid arachidonic acid. Arachidonic acid is the precursor for a number of eicanosoids that enable the activation of macrophages (Kirkby, Roman, Kobe, Kellie, & Forwood, 2010), and it has been shown that ACOT7 expression is upregulated in macrophages in the presence of LPS and colony-stimulating factor 1 (CSF-1) (2007). It is from this data that the putative role of ACOT7 in inflammation was recognised. As shown in figure 4 below, ACOT7 may provide an alternative pathway for inflammation to the well characterised PLA_2-mediated pathway and a possible target for a new class of anti-inflammation therapies.

Fujita et al. (2011) found that levels of both cytosolic and mitochondrial ACOT7 within mammalian heart muscle increase in response to a high fat diet, and induce inflammation. The increased levels of ACOT7 are in response to the increasing levels of acyl-CoA imported across the mitochondrial membranes from the cytosol via the action of carnitine plamitoyltransferase (CPT). This mechanism is thought to reduce the "lipotoxic" effects of insulin resistance which leads to contractile dysfunction of the heart as the cells accumulate proinflammatory molecules such as acyl-CoA, diacylglycerol and ceramide (Fujita, et al., 2011).

ACOT7 is also known as brain acyl-CoA hydrolase (BACH) and has been purified from the brain cytosol of rats and humans and is believed to be responsible for acyl-CoA hydrolytic activity in the brain. Given the highly toxic nature of long chain acyl-CoA's, as a detergent, the activity of ACOT7 within the brain may be to reduce the levels of these within neurons (Kuramochi et al., 2002). Furthermore Takagi et al. (2006) found that ACOT7 is expressed in mouse testis and may play a role in spermatogenesis. The results of this research suggest that the regulation of ACOT7 occurs at a posttranscriptional level or that the rate of turnover in the testis is higher than in the brain. The level of ACOT7 protein was higher in the brain than the testis however the mRNA level was higher in the adult testis than the brain. The physiological significance of ACOT7 within the testis has not been determined however it is thought to scavenge cytosolic free long-chain acyl-CoA's.

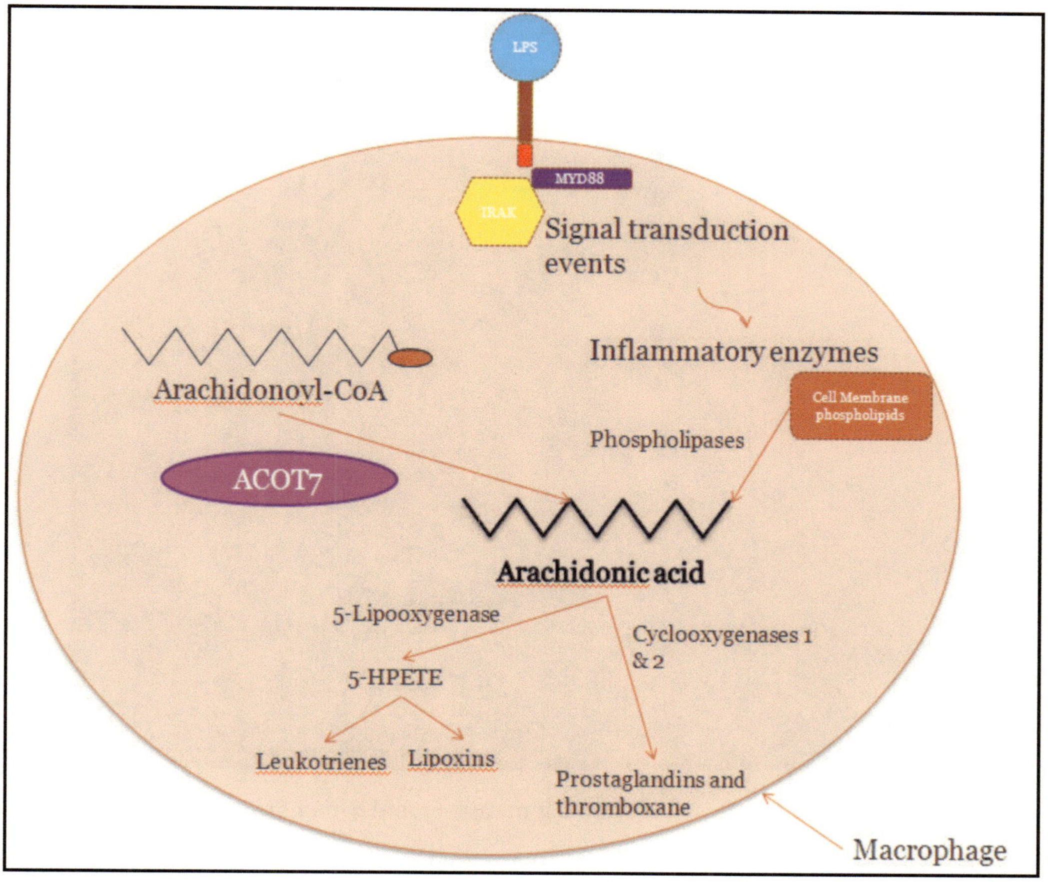

Fig. 4. Classical pathway of inflammation with role of ACOT7 in arachidonic acid production.

4. Structure of ACOT7

Structural insights into the function of ACOT7 have recently been undertaken through the cloning and high-level recombinant expression of ACOT7. Pioneering characterisation of ACOT7 was undertaken by Yamada et al. (1994) through the isolation and purification of rat liver, however high level over-expression and isolation of the enzyme required cloning of cDNA into bacterial expression vectors (Broustas, Larkins, Uhler, & Hajra, 1996; Junji Yamada et al., 1999). Serek et al. (2006) elucidated the structure of the C-terminal of the ACOT7 protein purified from *Mus musculis* by crystallising the C-terminal domain and analysing the high resolution structure using X-Ray diffraction techniques. From this data it was identified that the C-terminal domain of ACOT7 exists in a hexameric form. Forwood et al (2007) isolated and expressed both the N- and C-terminals of ACOT7. These domains were then separately crystallised and the resulting structures (in 1.8 and 2.5 Å resolution respectively) were superimposed to determine the structure of the full length ACOT7. Within the hexamer of Acot7 β-sheets from each domain form a semicontinuous antiparallel barrel with 25% of Acot7 residues involved in interdomain contacts (see Figure 5).

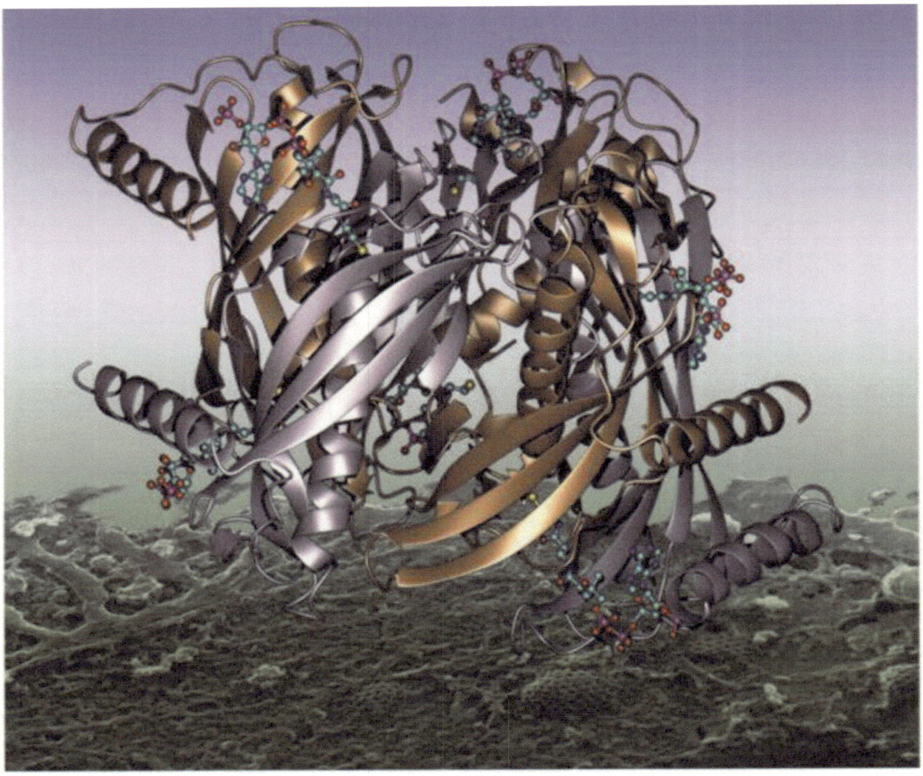

Fig. 5. Structure of full-length Acot7 showing monomer and trimer arrangement.

Wedged between the two monomers that make up the protomer are six CoA molecules, making contacts with residues from each domain. Opposite this binding site is a large hydrophobic tunnel, conserved within thioesterases that may be involved in the fatty-acid recognition and release. The individual domains are inactive when in homomeric complexes however when combined the activity can be restored to half that of the wild type enzyme. The arrangement of the N- and C-domains within ACOT7 and the positioning of the CoA molecules within the N-domain suggest that the full molecule contains three copies each of two distinct active sites in ACOT7. There are two potential active sites within ACOT7 (sites I and II, see Figure 6); these were determined via sequence analysis of mammalian ACOT7s. To assess the role that each of these active sites play in catalysis each residue was mutated to Ala and the recombinant mutant enzymes were isolated and the activity of the mutant residues determined. The mutations in site I resulted in dramatic reductions in catalytic activity, whereas the analogous mutations in site II did not affect activity. These findings demonstrated that site II were not directly involved in catalysis. Furthermore the introduction of the key catalytic residues from site I into site II resulted in a four-fold increase in catalytic activity when compared with the wild-type Acot7. Thus, Acot7 (structures of each domain presented in figure 7) is believed to contain a "half-of-sites" activity, which may regulate the enzyme by placing an upper limit on enzyme efficiency and allows the cell to regulate the cellular concentrations of AA-CoA and arachidonic acid.

5. Genetic regulation of ACOTs

The acyl-CoA thioesterase gene (*ACOT)* family encodes for two specific types of enzyme, acyl-CoA thioesterase type I and type II, which are determined by differences in structure and sequence. These two types catalyse similar reactions but share no similarity in structure or function, demonstrating that they are analogous and not homologous. They are an example of convergent evolution, whereby two molecules have evolved to fill the same need within the cell. Type I ACOT proteins are members of the α/β hydrolase fold enzyme superfamily. This superfamily also includes a number of esterase-activity-inhibiting enzymes such as carboxyl-esterase's and lipases. This group is comprised of only four genes; *ACOT1, ACOT2, ACOT4* and *ACOT6*. These proteins share a high degree of sequence homology, all forming an 80 kilobase gene cluster on chromosome 14q24.3, demonstrating that they have arisen as a result of gene duplication. Within the mouse and rat orthologues there is a similar phenomenon; *Acot1, Acot2, Acot3, Acot4, Acot5* and *Acot6* are clustered on chromosomes 12 D3 within the mouse and 6q31 within the rat. This can be seen in figure 8 below which also demonstrates the cellular compartments in which each is expressed (Brocker, Carpenter, Nebert, & Vasiliou, 2010).

Type II ACOTs are members of the 'hot dog' fold enzyme superfamily. The type II ACOTs are far less related than the type I ACOTs. There is only one type II ACOT that does not contain a double 'hot dog' domain suggesting that they may have evolved as a gene duplication event, allowing for the accommodation of bulky substrates. Type II ACOTs show highly divergent sequences making evolutionary comparisons difficult without three-dimensional structures, as structural interaction conservation does not directly correspond with residue conservation. Within the mouse genome there is an additional type II ACOT, known as *Acot10*, which shares 95% mRNA identity with ACOT9. The other seven type II ACOT genes are highly conserved among human, mouse and rat indicating that they were all present in the ancestor preceding mammalian radiation (Brocker, et al., 2010; M. C. Hunt & Alexson, 2008; Kirkby, et al., 2010).

5.1 Expression and regulation of ACOT7

The ACOT7 enzyme is highly conserved, exhibiting greater than 95% sequence homology at the amino acid level between human, mice and rats (Kuramochi et al., 2002). Transcription start sites for ACOT7 were characterised by Takagi et al. in 2004 and shown to encode a 43kDa subunit, located in the cytosol; and six isoforms comprised of 50kDa subunits, expressed at trace levels and located in the mitochondria. Independent studies have confirmed that the ACOT7 gene can generate up to seven different protein isoforms as can be seen below in figure 6 (J. Yamada, 2005). The human ACOT7 gene consists of 13 exons, with the first four of these able to be used as first exons. The most well characterised of the ACOT7 isoforms, ACOT7a, is derived from the sequence corresponding to transcription initiation at exon 2 (M. Hunt et al., 2007; Kirkby, et al., 2010).

Expression of ACOT7 has been detected in the developing mouse embryo brain as early as embryonic 11.5 days although in very low concentrations and increases until day seven following birth. Thereafter the level declined until day 28 following birth when it reached a steady state which was about 70% of its highest expression (on day 7) and identical to

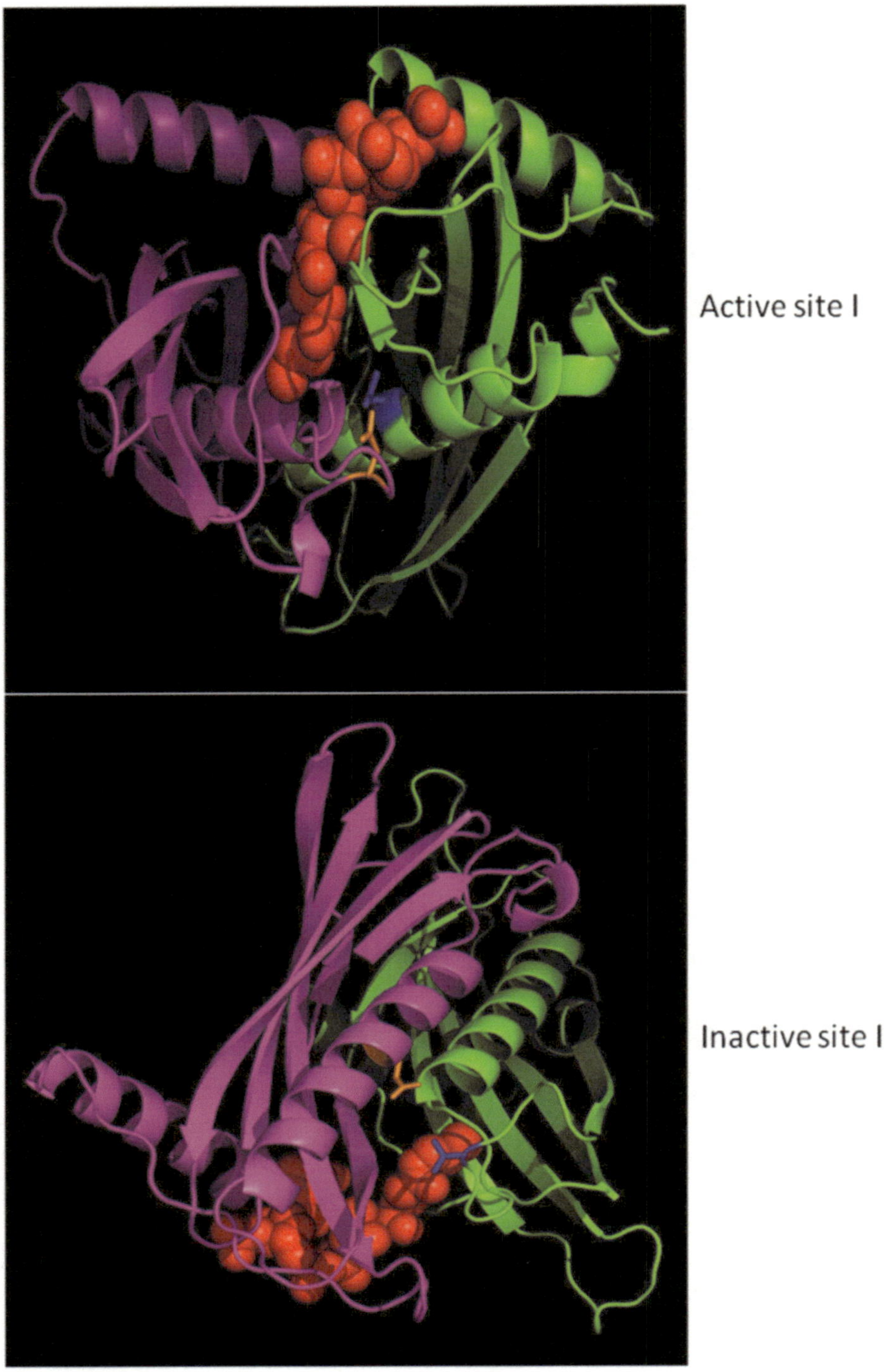

Fig. 6. Active sites of Acot7: Active site I is comprised of Asn24 from the N-domain and Asp213 from the C-domain; the analogous site (later determined to be inactive) is comprised of Glu39 from the N-domain and Thr198 from the C-domain

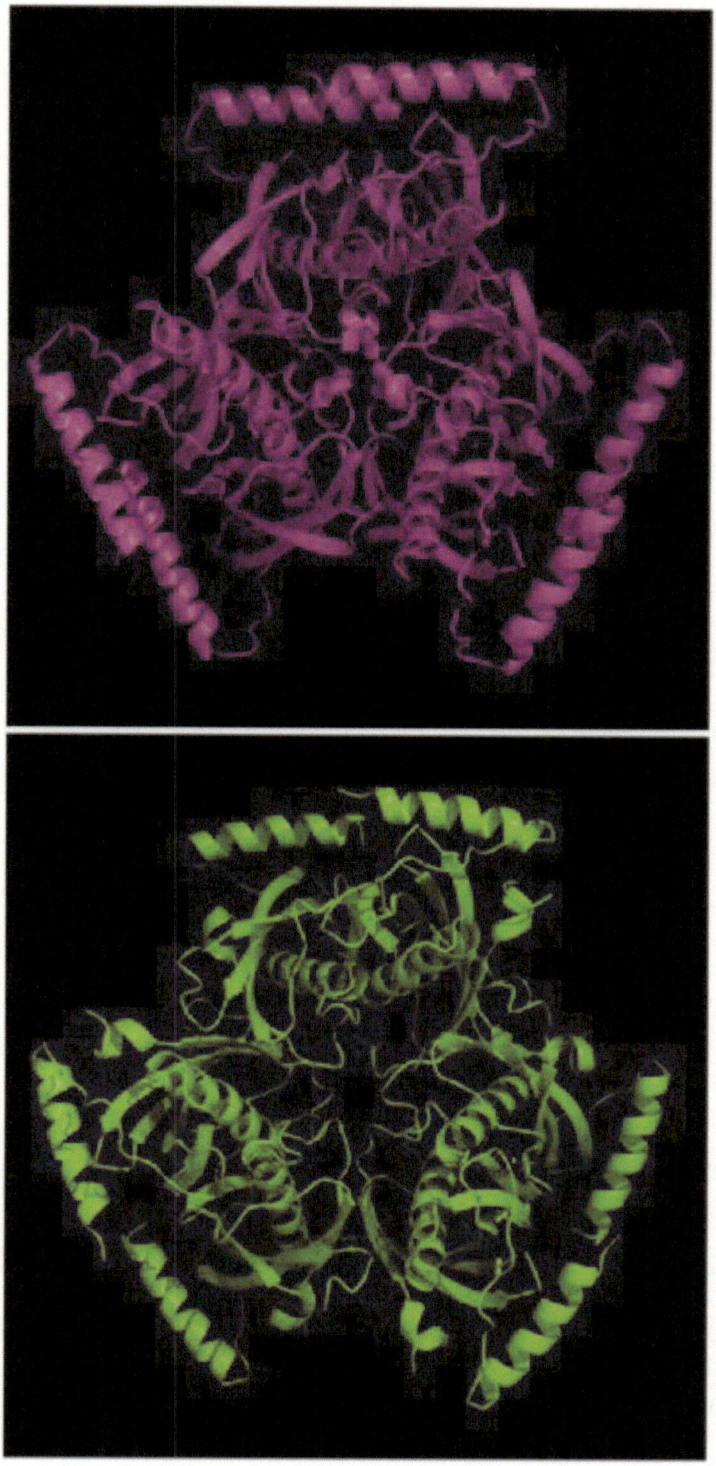

Fig. 7. (A) (B) Quaternary structure of Acot7 (N terminus) and C terminus respectively

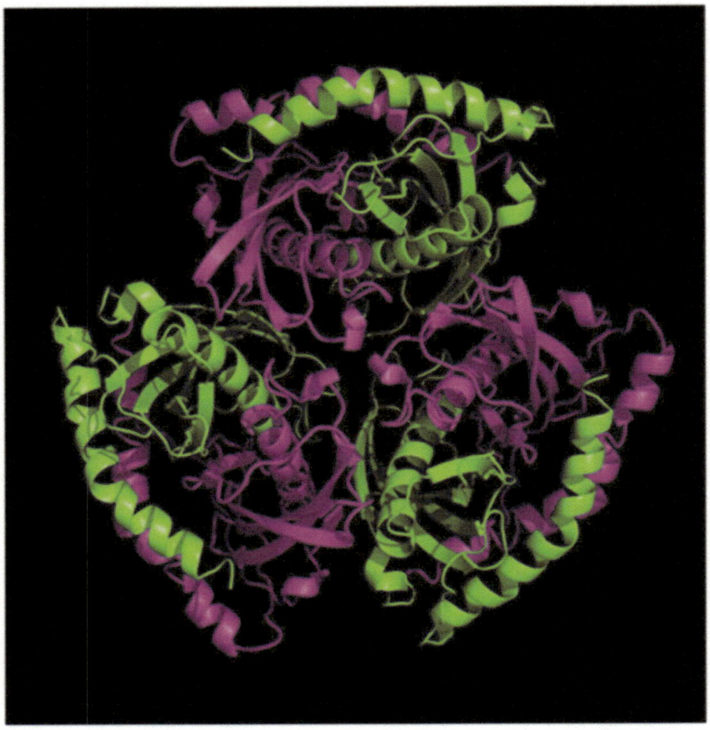

Fig. 8. Full length Acot7 demonstrating the N terminus domain (in green) and C terminus domain (in purple)

levels recorded at birth. The expression of *ACOT7* was located only in cells committed to neuronal lineage, and continues to be expressed in these cells resulting in the high expression of *ACOT7* in the adult brain (Junji Yamada, Kuramochi, Takagi, & Suga, 2004).

Research by Takagi, Suto, Suga & Yamada (2005) showed that ACOT7 gene expression is regulated by Sterol Regulatory Element-Binding Proteins (SREBPs). SREBPs form a few transcription factors which play a critical role in the regulation of cholesterol and fatty acids. Within the cell SREBPs are located in the membrane, to enter the nucleus they undergo proteolytic cleavage and their N-terminals are released as nSREBPs. Within the nucleus SREBPs bind to the sterol regulatory element (SRE) of target genes. The BACH gene promoter region contains two SRE motifs providing a binding partner for nSREBPs stimulating the production of cDNA of Acot7 (Takagi, et al., 2005).

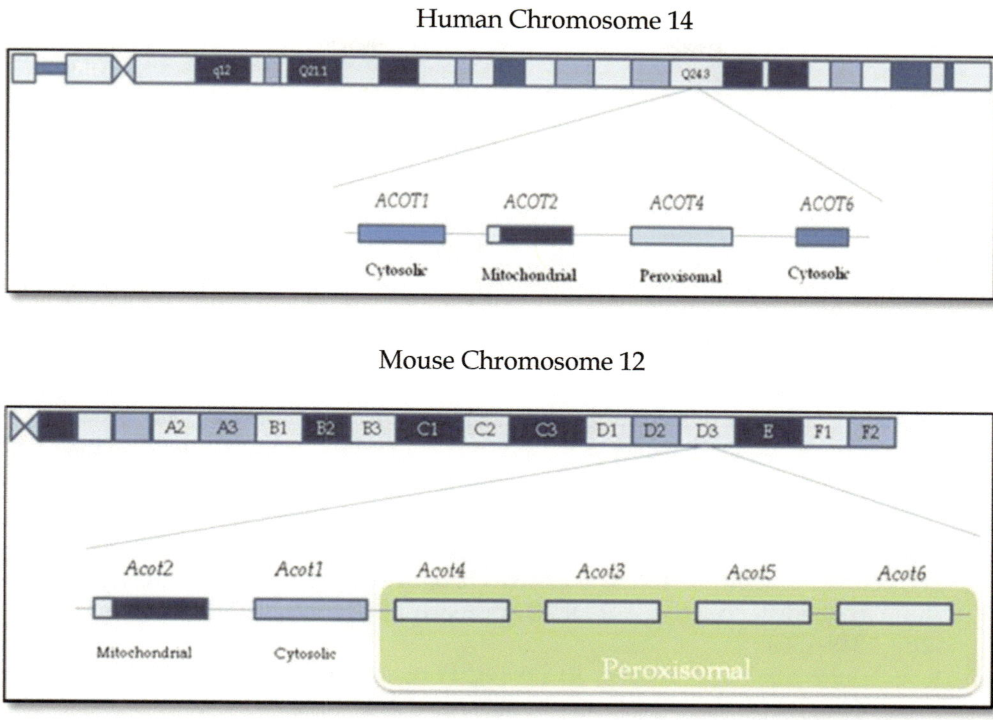

Fig. 9. The type I acyl-CoA thioesterase gene cluster is found on chromosome 14q24.3 in the human genome and chromosome 12 D3 in the mouse genome, adapted from Hunt & Alexson (2008)

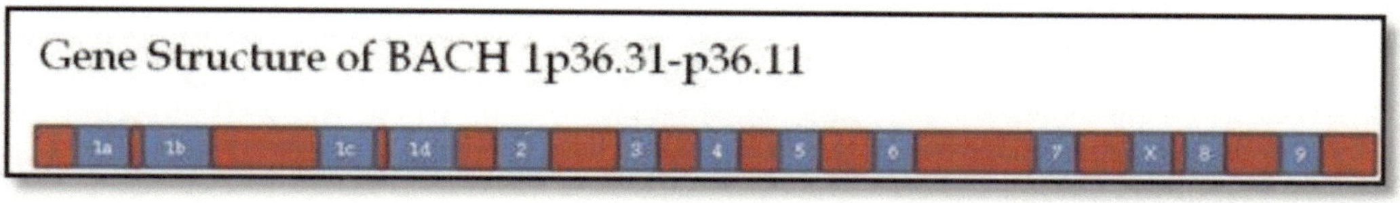

Fig. 10. Structural organisation of the human BACH gene, exons are designated by blue boxes and introns by red segments, adapted from Yamada et al. (2005)

6. Conclusion

Inflammation is a complex immune response that involves the production of eicosanoids via AA. The cellular role of ACOT7 has been extended to include the cleavage of arachidonoyl:CoA to yield arachidonic acid, and therefore may provide a mechanism for the supply of arachidonic acid from intracellular arachidonoyl-CoA. This is supported by a number of lines of evidence: ACOT7 is highly expressed in macrophages and upregulated by proinflammatory stimuli; the preferred substrate of ACOT7 is arachidonoyl-CoA and the reaction product is the central precursor for lipid inflammatory mediators; and finally, over-expression of ACOT7 in activated macrophages increases prostaglandin production. Thus, ACOT7 is able to complement the well-characterised PLA_2 AA-producing pathway, and may play a role in inflammation by producing sufficient levels of AA for eicosanoid production.

7. References

Brocker, C., Carpenter, C., Nebert, D., & Vasiliou, V. (2010). Evolutionary divergence and functions of the human acyl-CoA thioesterase gene (ACOT) family. *Human Genomics, 4*(6), 411-420.

Broustas, C., Larkins, L., Uhler, M., & Hajra, A. (1996). Molecular cloning and expression of cDNA encoding rat brain cytosolic Acyl-Coenzyme A thioester hydrolase. *The Journal of Biological Chemistry, 271*(18), 10470-10476.

Castilla, R., Maloberti, P., Castillo, F., Duarte, A., Cano, F., Cornejo Maciel, F., . . . Podesta, E. (2004). Arachidonic acid regulation of steroid synthesis: new partners in the signaling pathway of steroidogenic hormones. *Endocrine research, 30*(4), 599-606.

Evans, J. F., Ferguson, A. D., Mosley, R. T., & Hutchinson, J. H. (2008). What's all the FLAP about?: 5-lipoxygenase-activating protein inhibitors for inflammatory diseases. *Trends in Pharmacological Sciences, 29*(2), 72-78. doi: 10.1016/j.tips.2007.11.006

Ferreira, G. B., Overbergh, L., van Etten, E., Lage, K., D'Hertog, W., Hansen, D. A., . . . Waelkens, E. (2008). Protein induced changes during the maturation process of human dendritic cells: A 2 D DIGE approach. *PROTEOMICS–Clinical Applications, 2*(9), 1349-1360.

Flesch, I., Schonhardt, T., & Ferber, E. (1989). Phospholipases and acyltransferases in macrophages. *Journal of Molecular Medicine, 67*(3), 119-122.

Forwood, J. K., Thakur, A. S., Guncar, G., Marfori, M., Mouradov, D., Meng, W., . . . Martin, J. L. (2007). Structural basis for recruitment of tandem hotdog domains in acyl-CoA thioesterase 7 and its role in inflammation. *Proceedings of the National Academy of Sciences, 104*(25), 10382.

Fujita, M., Momose, A., Ohtomo, T., Nishinosono, A., Tanonaka, K., Toyoda, H., . . . Yamada, J. (2011). Upregulation of fatty acyl-CoA thioesterases in the heart and skeletal muscle of rats fed a high-fat diet. *Biological Pharmacy Bulletin, 34*(1), 87-91.

Gilroy, D. W., Colville-Nash, P., Willis, D., Chivers, J., Paul-Clark, M., & Willoughby, D. (1999). Inducible cyclooxygenase may have anti-inflammatory properties. *Nature medicine, 5*(6), 698-701.

Golej, D. L., Askari, B., Kramer, F., Barnhart, S., Vivekanandan-Giri, A., Pennathur, S., & Bornfeldt, K. E. (2011). Long-chain acyl-CoA synthetase 4 modulates prostaglandin E2 release from human arterial smooth muscle cells. *Journal of Lipid Research, 52*(4), 782.

Hunt, M., Greene, S., Hultenby, K., Svensson, L., Engberg, S., & Alexson, S. (2007). Alternative exon usage selectively determines both tissue distribution and subcellular localization of the acyl-CoA thioesterase 7 gene products. *Cellular and Molecular Life Sciences, 64*(12), 1558-1570. doi: 10.1007/s00018-007-7062-6

Hunt, M. C., & Alexson, S. E. H. (2008). Novel functions of acyl-CoA thioesterases and acyltransferases as auxiliary enzymes in peroxisomal lipid metabolism. *Progress in Lipid Research, 47*(6), 405-421. doi: 10.1016/j.plipres.2008.05.001

Irvine, R. F. (1982). How is the level of free arachidonic acid controlled in mammalian cells? *Biochemical Journal, 204*(1), 3.

Jiang, Y. J., Hatch, G. M., Mymin, D., Dembinski, T., Kroeger, E. A., & Choy, P. C. (2001). Modulation of cytosolic phospholipase A2 by PPAR activators in human preadipocytes. *Journal of Lipid Research, 42*(5), 716.

Kirkby, B., Roman, N., Kobe, B., Kellie, S., & Forwood, J. K. (2010). Functional and structural properties of mammalian acyl-coenzyme A thioesterases. *Progress in Lipid Research, 49*(4), 366-377. doi: 10.1016/j.plipres.2010.04.001

Kunishima, N., Asada, Y., Sugahara, M., Ishijima, J., Nodake, Y., Sugahara, M., . . . Sugahara, M. (2005). A Novel Induced-fit Reaction Mechanism of Asymmetric Hot Dog Thioesterase PaaI. *Journal of Molecular Biology, 352*(1), 212-228. doi: 10.1016/j.jmb.2005.07.008

Kuramochi, Y., Takagi-Sakuma, M., Kitahara, M., Emori, R., Asaba, Y., Sakaguchi, R., . . . Yamada, J. (2002). Characterization of mouse homolog of brain acyl-CoA hydrolase: molecular cloning and neuronal localization. *Molecular Brain Research, 98*(1-2), 81-92. doi: 10.1016/s0169-328x(01)00323-0

Maloberti, P., Castilla, R., Castillo, F., Maciel, F. C., Mendez, C. F., Paz, C., & Podestá, E. J. (2005). Silencing the expression of mitochondrial acyl CoA thioesterase I and acyl CoA synthetase 4 inhibits hormone induced steroidogenesis. *FEBS Journal, 272*(7), 1804-1814.

Murakami, K., Ide, T., Nakazawa, T., Mochizuki, T., & Kaowaki, T. (2001). Fatty-acyl-CoA thioesters inhibit recruitment of steroid receptor co-activator 1 to α and γ isoforms of peroxisome-proliferator-activated receptors by competing with agonists. *Biochemical Journal, 353*, 231-238.

Narumiya, S. (2009). Prostanoids and inflammation: a new concept arising from receptor knockout mice. *Journal of Molecular Medicine, 87*(10), 1015-1022. doi: 10.1007/s00109-009-0500-1

Piomelli, D. (2000). Neurophsychopharmacology: the Fifth Generation of Progress *Arachidonic Acid*

Sakuma, S., Fujimoto, Y., Doi, K., Nagamatsu, S., Nishida, H., & Fujita, T. (1994). Existence of an enzymatic pathway furnishing arachidonic acid for prostaglandin synthesis from arachidonoyl CoA in rabbit kidney medulla. *Biochemical and Biophysical Research Communications, 202*(2), 1054-1059.

Sakuma, S., Usa, K., & Fujimoto, Y. (2006). The regulation of formation of prostaglandins and arachidonoyl-CoA from arachidonic acid in rabbit kidney medulla microsomes by linoleic acid hydroperoxide. *Prostaglandins & Other Lipid Mediators, 79*(3-4), 271-277. doi: 10.1016/j.prostaglandins.2006.02.005

Serek, R., Forwood, J., Hume, D., Martin, J., & Kobe, B. (2006). Crystallisation of the C-terminal domain of the mouse brain cytosolic long-chain acyl-CoA thioesterase. *Structural Biology and Crystallisation Communications, 62*, 133-135.

Takagi, M., Ohtomo, T., Hiratsuka, K., Kuramochi, Y., Suga, T., & Yamada, J. (2006). Localization of a long-chain acyl-CoA hydrolase in spermatogenic cells in mice. *Archives of Biochemistry and Biophysics, 446*, 161-166.

Takagi, M., Suto, F., Suga, T., & Yamada, J. (2005). Sterol Regulatory Element-Binding Protein-2 modulates human brain acyl-CoA hydrolase gene transcription. *Molecular and Cellular Biochemistry, 275*(1), 199-206. doi: 10.1007/s11010-005-1990-y

Tilley, S. L., Coffman, T. M., & Koller, B. H. (2001). Mixed messages: modulation of inflammation and immune responses by prostaglandins and thromboxanes. *Journal of Clinical Investigation, 108*(1), 15-24.

Wang, M.-T., Honn, K., & Nie, D. (2007). Cyclooxygenases, prostanoids, and tumor progression. *Cancer and Metastasis Reviews, 26*(3), 525-534. doi: 10.1007/s10555-007-9096-5

Yamada, J. (2005). Long-chain acyl-CoA hydrolase in the brain. *Amino Acids, 28*(3), 273-278. doi: 10.1007/s00726-005-0181-1

Yamada, J., Kuramochi, Y., Takagi, M., & Suga, T. (2004). Expression of acyl-CoA hydrolase in the developing mouse brain. *Neuroscience Letters, 355*(1-2), 89-92. doi: 10.1016/j.neulet.2003.10.049

Yamada, J., Kurata, A., Hirata, M., Taniguchi, T., Takama, H., Furihata, T., . . . Suga, T. (1999). Purification, molecular cloning, and genomic organisation of human brain long-chain acyl-CoA hydrolase. *Journal of Biochemistry, 126*, 1013-1019.

Yamada, J., Matsumoto, I., Furihata, T., Sakuma, M., & Suga, T. (1994). Purification and properties of long-chain Acyl-CoA hydrolases from the liver cytosol of rats treated with peroxisome proliferator. *Archives of Biochemistry and Biophysics, 308*(1), 118-125.

Part 11

Inflammatory Bowel Disease

11

The Effects of n-3 Polyunsaturated Fatty Acid-Rich Salmon on Inflammatory Bowel Diseases

Nicole C. Roy[1,2,3], Nadja Berger[1,2,3], Emma N. Bermingham[1,3], Warren C. McNabb[2,3,4] and Janine M. Cooney[3,5]

[1]*Food Nutrition & Health Team, AgResearch Grasslands, Palmerston North*
[2]*The Riddet Institute, Massey University, Palmerston North*
[3]*Nutrigenomics New Zealand*
[4]*AgResearch Grasslands, Palmerston North*
[5]*Biological Chemistry & Bioactives, Food Innovation, Plant & Food Research Ruakura, Hamilton*
New Zealand

1. Introduction

Inflammatory Bowel Disease (IBD) is a disorder of the gastrointestinal tract that is characterised by chronic inflammation, with high incidence in Westernised countries (Yamamoto et al., 2009). Long-chain n-3 polyunsaturated fatty acids (PUFA), in particular docosahexaenoic acid (DHA) and eicosapentaenoic acid (EPA), are purported to be important for maintaining health and protection against disease (Connor, 2000). They exhibit beneficial effects with respect to cardiovascular diseases, rheumatoid arthritis, inflammatory diseases and neurodegenerative illnesses (Wahrburg, 2004). PUFA can modulate the inflammatory response (Calder, 2008) and could therefore be an important factor in the course of IBD. Several studies have tested the anti-inflammatory potential of pure n-3 PUFA extracts, fish oil and whole fish, however, the results of these studies are inconsistent (effects of dietary n-3 PUFA on animal models of colitis reviewed in Calder, 2008; effects of dietary n-3 PUFA in intervention studies with IBD patients reviewed in Ferguson et al., 2010). Nevertheless, experimental evidence (Knoch et al., 2009) has shown potential anti-inflammatory effects of dietary EPA supplementation, a nutrient which is found in high levels in salmon. Furthermore, New Zealand IBD patients recorded a higher tolerance to salmon compared with other foods on the basis of a food frequency questionnaire (Triggs et al., 2010) and salmon has shown beneficial effects for patients with mild IBD (Grimstad et al., 2011). Various factors play a role in the development of IBD, however, the focus of this review is the effect of dietary n-3 PUFA and n-3 PUFA-rich food such as salmon.

2. Background

2.1 Inflammation in inflammatory bowel disease

The inflammatory response is the beginning of an immunological process and is necessary to protect the body against invading pathogens and toxins. The response is typified by activation/production of at least the following four classes of active molecules (Chapkin et al., 2009): (i) adhesions molecules (*e.g.* vascular cell adhesion molecule-1 (VCAM-1), intercellular adhesion molecule-1 (ICAM-1) and E-selectin) on the surface of endothelial cells, allowing leukocyte binding and subsequent diapedesis; (ii) inflammatory cytokines (*e.g.* tumor necrosis factor alpha (TNFα), interleukin (IL) 1, IL6 and IL8); (iii) arachidonic acid (AA)-derived eicosanoids; and (iv) inflammatory mediators (*e.g.* platelet activating factor). The activation/production of these molecules must be ordered and controlled to avoid excessive damage to host tissue and chronic inflammatory disorders (Calder, 2006). This defect in resolving inflammation and returning the target tissue back to homeostasis is a hallmark of IBD (Chapkin et al., 2009). While the rate of new cases of IBD is beginning to stabilise in high-incidence areas, including northern Europe and North America, countries with traditionally low occurrence rates (*e.g.* southern Europe, Asia and developing countries) are reporting an increased rate of new patients (Loftus, 2004). Ulcerative colitis (UC) and Crohn's disease (CD) are the two most common forms of IBD and although the two forms have distinctive characteristics, they share many common symptoms and can be difficult to distinguish clinically (Lee & Buchman, 2009; Teitelbaum & Allan Walker, 2001). The aetiology of IBD is largely unknown, but it is generally accepted that genetic factors and the environment play a role (Ferguson, 2010; Hanauer, 2006; Lee & Buchman, 2009). Furthermore, the tolerance of the mucosal immune system to the commensal intestinal microbiota is disrupted and dysregulation of the immune system occurs (Duchmann et al., 1995).

Observations in twin studies have highlighted that susceptibility to IBD, in particular CD, is inherited (Bouma & Strober, 2003). The genetics of IBD is complex and it is suggested that variations in key genes, for example single-nucleotide polymorphisms (SNPs), play a role. SNPs are genetic variations in the DNA sequence, whereby only a single nucleotide is changed. Approximately seven million common SNPs have been found across the human population (Hinds et al., 2005). While only a few of these may have a functional effect (Stover, 2006), some variations can affect health or even cause disease (Lee & Buchman, 2009). Currently, 99 susceptibility loci/genes are known to contribute susceptibly to IBD (Lees et al., 2011). One of the first susceptibility loci was found to be a polymorphism of the caspase recruitment domain family member 15 (CARD15) gene, which encodes the protein nucleotide-binding oligomerization domain 2 (NOD2) (Hugot et al., 1996; Hugot et al., 2001).

Environmental factors such as dietary changes, smoking, oral contraceptives, appendectomy and stress can affect the development of IBD (Krishnan & Korzenik, 2002; Loftus, 2004). In the last three decades, the incidence of IBD in Japan has increased sharply, correlating with changes in dietary preferences towards a Western-type diet (Yamamoto et al., 2009). This implies that dietary choice is an important factor in the development of IBD. The lipid profile of Western-type diets features excessive amounts of saturated fats and n-6 PUFA, but a deficiency of n-3 PUFA. This imbalance leads to an altered n-6/n-3 ratio, which may promote the pathogenesis of many diseases including IBD (Simopoulos, 2008). Thus increasing the n-3 PUFA intake and lowering the ratio of n-6/n-3 PUFA in the diet may reduce the risk of developing chronic diseases.

The molecular mechanisms underlying the interaction of nutrients including n-3 PUFA with an individual's genome are very complex, and also poorly understood (Stover, 2006; Weaver et al., 2009). To improve the understanding of these gene-diet interactions, the field of nutrigenomics has evolved with the aim of developing a personalised strategy for health maintenance or disease treatment (Ferguson, 2010). In nutrigenomics research, nutrients are considered signalling molecules that can target the cellular sensor system and therefore subsequently influence gene expression, protein expression and metabolite production (Subbiah, 2008). These dietary signals can cause changes in the organism, tissue or single cells and subsequently influence homeostasis (Müller & Kersten, 2003).

2.2 Dietary intake of lipids

2.2.1 Fatty acids

Fatty acids form the major component of dietary fats, and dietary sources range from free fatty acids to phospholipids, sterols and triacylglycerol (TG) (Ratnayake & Galli, 2009). The term fatty acid describes a carboxylic acid with an aliphatic chain that can be saturated or unsaturated. The degree of un-saturation is addressed by the number of double bonds between the carbon atoms of a fatty acid. A fatty acid that contains two or more double bonds between the carbon atoms is classified as polyunsaturated, while monounsaturated fatty acids (MUFA) contain only one double bond. The classification into n-3 and n-6 PUFA is based on the position of the first double bond, starting from the terminal methyl end. In general, short-chain unsaturated fatty acids refer to 19 or fewer carbon atoms, long-chain to 20-24 carbon atoms and very-long-chain to 25 or more. The reactivity of fatty acids increases with double bonds; therefore, saturated fatty acids are more stable and have a longer shelf life than unsaturated ones (Ratnayake & Galli, 2009).

The dietary intake of lipids is predominately through TG, which is the vast majority of lipid found in vegetable oils and animal fats (Ratnayake & Galli, 2009). TG are characterised by a glycerol backbone connected to three molecules of fatty acids (sn-1, sn-2 and sn-3, starting from the top of the glycerol), whereby the three hydroxyl groups from the glycerol backbone form an ester bond with the carboxyl groups from fatty acids (Fahy et al., 2005). Nutritionally, the distribution of fatty acids over the three sn-positions changes biological activity and absorption pattern, whereas the composition of sn-2 is of importance due to facilitated absorption (Ratnayake & Galli, 2009). In Atlantic salmon, the TG in the depot fat comprise ~70% DHA on sn-2 position, whereas EPA is nearly randomly distributed (40% on sn-2) (Aursand et al., 1995). In order to be absorbed by the gastrointestinal tract lining, TG need to be digested, *i.e.* broken down into smaller components (Ratnayake & Galli, 2009). The small intestine is the main site for fat digestion, where the pancreatic lipase hydrolyses TG at sn-1 and sn-3 position, yielding final products of 2-monoacylglycerols and free fatty acids (Mu & Porsgaard, 2005). Free fatty acids are directly absorbed through the intestinal wall and 2-monoacylglycerols form micelles that further diffuse to the epithelial cells, where they leave the micelles and enter epithelial cells by diffusion. In the enterocytes, they are transported to the endoplasmic reticulum in association with a fatty acid binding protein (FABP) and are re-synthesised to TG. Newly synthesized TG are transported out of the enterocyte and enter the bloodstream *via* the lymph vessels in the form of chylomicrons. In the bloodstream, the TG of the chylomicrons are hydrolysed to free fatty acids and glycerol that then pass through the capillary walls to be used by cells as the major substrates for energy production and storage (Ratnayake & Galli, 2009). Some fatty acids (*e.g.* DHA, EPA and AA) have additional roles in modulating the structural and functional properties of cells (Galli & Calder, 2009).

2.2.2 Fatty acid metabolism

Due to its abundance in food, many human populations over-consume n-6, but consequently lack long-chain n-3 PUFA (Calder, 2006; Ratnayake & Galli, 2009), resulting in an n-6/n-3 ratio of ~10:1 to 20-25:1, which may promote the pathogenesis of many diseases including inflammatory disorders (Simopoulos, 1991). Whereas humans evolved on a diet with a ratio of ~1:1 (Simopoulos, 2008), a ratio of 4:1 is recommended as optimal (Wall et al., 2010), but this may vary with disease state (Simopoulos, 2008). It has been suggested that lowering the n-6/n-3 ratio in the diet should be achieved by increasing the amount of n-3 PUFA rather than by simply reducing n-6 PUFA, which may reduce the risk of developing chronic diseases (Camuesco et al., 2005; Simopoulos, 2008). The long-chain PUFA AA, EPA and DHA are supplied to tissues from dietary sources, either *via* direct supplementation or *via* the consumption of the precursor PUFA linoleic acid (LA; n-6 pathway) and α-linolenic acid (ALA; n-3 pathway). LA and ALA cannot be synthesised in the human body, but can be metabolised to longer-chain fatty acids. This conversion of LA and ALA occurs *via* several elongation and desaturation steps (Fig. 1), with competition for the same enzymes on both pathways (Calder & Yaqoob, 2009). LA, the parent fatty acid on the n-6 PUFA pathway, is metabolised to AA, whereas ALA on the n-3 PUFA pathway is metabolised to EPA and further to DHA. However, as the conversion of ALA to EPA is limited and further conversion to DHA is even lower (Burdge & Calder, 2005; Garg et al., 2006), direct DHA and EPA supplementation is more effective than *de-novo* synthesis in increasing long-chain n-3 PUFA concentrations in the cell membrane (Hamilton et al., 2005).

3. Putative mechanisms of action

Long-chain PUFA are taken up by inflammatory cells and incorporated into membrane phospholipids (Leslie, 2004). Membrane phospholipids of inflammatory cells from humans consuming Western-type diets possess a relatively high amount (>20%) of n-6 PUFA, whereas long-chain n-3 PUFA represent less than 1% of fatty acids (Calder, 2006). The result

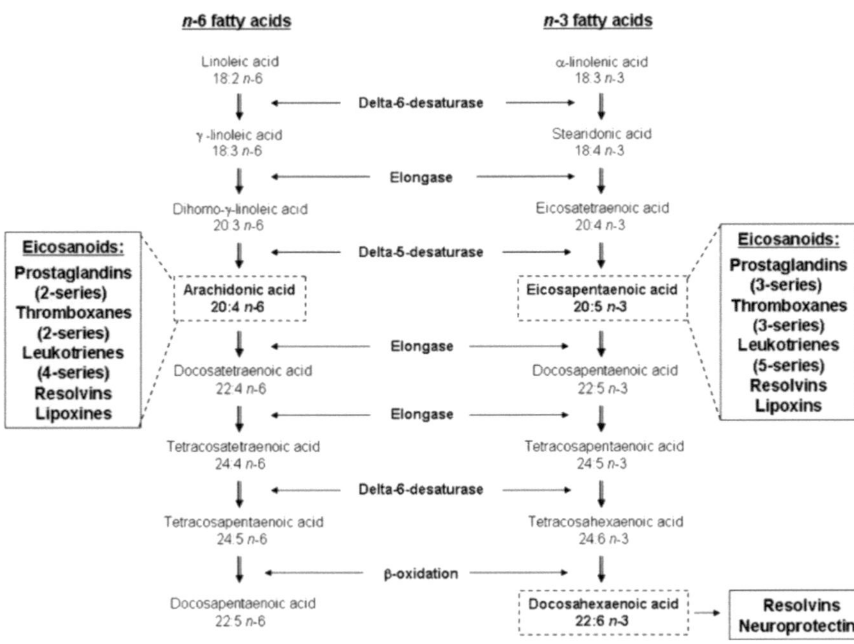

Fig. 1. Metabolism of n-6 and n-3 PUFA from precursor fatty acids (Wall et al., 2010)

is an unbalanced n-6/n-3 ratio which can promote a pro-inflammatory phenotype. The dietary intake of foods rich in EPA and DHA results in membrane replacement of n-6 PUFA in a time and dose-dependent manner, which may contribute to anti-inflammatory effects (Calder, 2009). How an elevated dietary intake of n-3 PUFA exerts its beneficial effects is not fully understood, but the putative mechanisms of action of n-3 PUFA are illustrated in Fig. 2. These include alterations in (i) cell membrane lipid bi-layer composition; (ii) gene expression; and (iii) lipid mediator metabolism (Chapkin et al., 2009). The overall physiological outcome depends on several factors, for example, the quantity and chemistry of the fat ingested, the cells present, cell-specific fatty acid metabolism (oxidative pathways, kinetics, and competing reactions) or the nature of the stimulus (Calder et al., 2009; Jump & Clarke, 1999). However, the different effects of DHA versus EPA are not well studied (Chapkin et al., 2009).

Lipid rafts are complex micro-domains in the cell membrane that appear to serve as platforms for receptor-mediated signal transduction (Calder & Yaqoob, 2007; Chapkin et al., 2009). When incorporated into cell membrane phospholipids, n-3 PUFA can increase membrane fluidity (Li et al., 2005), however, lipid rafts are far more sensitive to the incorporation of n-3 PUFA than non-raft domains (Rockett et al., 2011). A modulation of the lipid composition in rafts is associated with altered signalling pathways (Li et al., 2005; Schley et al., 2007; Stulnig et al., 2001).

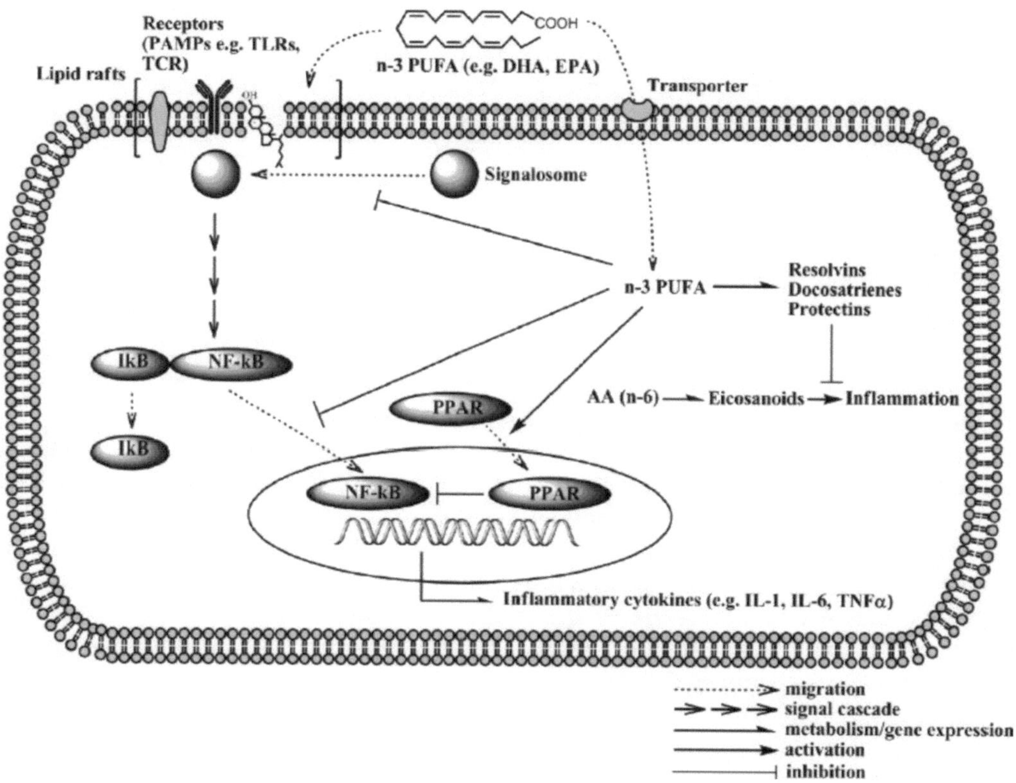

Fig. 2. Putative mechanism of action of PUFA. These include alterations in lipid mediator synthesis, gene expression, lipid composition in cell membrane and signal transduction (Chapkin et al., 2009)

Dietary n-3 PUFA can be transported into the cell *via* passive diffusion or active protein-mediated transport (Bordoni et al., 2006), depending on the chain size. Longer-chain fatty acids are actively transported *via* fatty acid transport proteins (FATP) 1-6 and/or CD36 (Bordoni et al., 2006; Heimerl et al., 2006). Inside the cell, n-3 PUFA can give rise to the anti-inflammatory lipid mediators resolvins and protectins (Serhan et al., 2008) and in turn competitively inhibit the production of mainly pro-inflammatory eicosanoids from AA. Furthermore, alterations in gene expression by n-3 PUFA can be mediated by interaction with transcription factors. For example, the activation of peroxisome proliferator-acitvated receptors (PPARs) can suppress nuclear factor-kappaB (NFκB) translocation and thereby inhibit the expression levels of pro-inflammatory cytokine genes (*e.g.* IL1 or TNFα) (Chapkin et al., 2009).

3.1 The formation of lipid mediators from fatty acids

Lipid mediators including eicosanoids, resolvins and protectins are regulators of inflammation and are generated from long-chain PUFA (Fig. 1) (Calder, 2009). The biological activity and potency of lipid mediators is dependent on the PUFA substrate. The n-6 PUFA AA gives rise to several eicosanoids (*e.g.* series-2 prostaglandins and thromboxanes, series-4 leukotrienes), hydroperoxy- and hydroxy-eicosatetraenoic derivatives and lipoxins. The majority of eicosanoids derived from AA are pro-inflammatory; however, prostaglandin E_2 and lipoxin have been shown to exert anti-inflammatory effects (Calder, 2008). EPA is the substrate for the anti-inflammatory eicosanoids and resolvins (*e.g.* series-3 prostaglandins and thromboxanes and series-5 leukotrienes) and hydroperoxy- and hydroxy-eicosapentaenoic derivatives. DHA gives rise to anti-inflammatory and pro-resolution mediators (*e.g.* resolvins and neuroprotectin) (Wall et al., 2010). The enzymes which catalyse these conversions are at least two cyclooxygenase (COX) and several lipoxygenase (LOX) enzymes (Calder et al., 2009), thus an elevated n-3 PUFA intake can lead to competitive inhibition of eicosanoid production from AA. Consequently, the pattern of lipid mediator production can be modulated towards a decrease in mainly pro-inflammatory eicosanoids from n-6 PUFA and an increase in anti-inflammatory resolvins from EPA and DHA (Calder, 2008; Calder, 2009).

3.2 Modulation of gene expression by polyunsaturated fatty acids

As well as altering lipid mediator synthesis, dietary fatty acids can affect gene expression and subsequently influence metabolism, growth and cell differentiation (Jump & Clarke, 1999). The mechanisms for these influences may be *via* intermediate molecules (*e.g.* transcription factors, nuclear hormone receptors and lipid secondary messengers) that subsequently alter gene expression, or a direct interaction with target genes (Deckelbaum et al., 2006). The expression levels of genes encoding several key proteins involved in inflammation, lipid metabolism and energy utilisation have been identified to be modulated by n-3 PUFA (Deckelbaum et al., 2006).

3.2.1 Gene expression changes underlying intestinal inflammation

Differences in gene expression and metabolic pathways underlying intestinal inflammation can be characterised when inflamed colon tissue from interleukin-10 gene-deficient (*Il10*$^{-/-}$) mice is compared to colon tissue from healthy control mice. The gene expression levels in *Il10*$^{-/-}$ mice on a control diet were mainly increased in the inflammatory and immune response pathway, with pro-inflammatory genes encoding cytokines (*e.g.* Il1β and TNFα) or chemokine receptors (*e.g.* Ccr5) as examples (Table 2) (Knoch et al., 2009). Decreased expression levels were observed for genes involved in fatty acid metabolism and xenobiotic metabolism (Table 1) (Knoch et al., 2009). The decreased expression levels of genes associated with fatty acid oxidation may have a role in disease progression (Knoch et al., 2009) and have also been observed in colon tissue of IBD patients (Heimerl et al., 2006). Decreased mRNA levels of genes involved in xenobiotic metabolism were observed in *Il10*$^{-/-}$ mice. Detoxification and biotransformation alter xenobiotics, *i.e.* foreign compounds (Jakoby & Ziegler, 1990), and a dysfunction of these mechanisms exposes enterocytes to toxic luminal antigens (Langmann & Schmitz, 2006), promoting local injury (Sartor, 1995) and contributing to the pathophysiology of IBD (Crotty, 1994; Langmann & Schmitz, 2006). Expression levels of genes encoding tight junction proteins were decreased in colon tissue of *Il10*$^{-/-}$ mice (Knoch et al., 2009). Tight junctions are intercellular barriers that regulate the transport of large molecules between the intestinal epithelial cells (Balda et al., 1992) and a dysfunction leads to impaired intestinal integrity and increased permeability ('leaky gut') (Forster, 2008). A non-invasive method to assess intestinal permeability is the urinary measurement after an oral dose of sugar probes, for example sucralose, mannitol and lactulose (Arrieta et al., 2006; Farhadi et al., 2003). In *Il10*$^{-/-}$ mice, it was found that the ratio of lactulose/mannitol, a marker of small intestinal barrier permeability, was increased compared to control mice (Arrieta et al., 2009). The urinary excretion of sucralose, which indicates colonic damage, was also increased in *Il10*$^{-/-}$ mice.

Gene family (genes) down-regulated in the *Il10*$^{-/-}$ mouse compared to WT	Pathways influenced in the *Il10*$^{-/-}$ mouse compared to WT	The effect of PUFA on gene expression during intestinal inflammation		Reference
		EPA (*Il10*$^{-/-}$)	AA (*Il10*$^{-/-}$)	
ATP-binding cassette (Abca1, Abcb1α (mdr1a), Abcc3)	Xenobiotic metabolism	Up	Up	A, C
Cytochrome P450 (Cyp2c40, Cyp2e1)	Xenobiotic metabolism	Up	Up	A, B, C
Glutathione S-transferase (Gsta4, Gstt1, Gstm1)	Xenobiotic metabolism	Up	Up	A, B, C
Interleukin (Il6)	Immune and inflammatory response	Down*	Down	B
Peroxisome proliferator-activated receptor (PPARα)	Immune and inflammatory response	Up		A, C

Table 1. Selected genes and their associated pathways that are down-regulated in the *Il10*$^{-/-}$ mouse model, compared to wild-type (WT) mice, and the effects of polyunsaturated fatty acids in mouse models of intestinal inflammation (Table constructed with information from (A) Knoch et al., 2009; (B) Knoch et al., 2010a; (C) Reiff et al., 2009). (*) indicates a non-significant change.

Gene family (genes) up-regulated in the *Il10*$^{-/-}$ mouse compared to WT	Pathways influenced in the *Il10*$^{-/-}$ mouse compared to WT	The effect of PUFA on gene expression during intestinal inflammation			Reference
		EPA (*Il10*$^{-/-}$)	AA (*Il10*$^{-/-}$)	DHA (BALB/c + DSS)	
S100 calcium binding protein (S100a8, S100a9)	Oxidative stress response	Up*	Down	Down	A, B
Tumor necrosis factor alpha (TNFα)	Immune and inflammatory response	Down*	Down		B, C, D, E
Tumor necrosis factor receptor superfamily, member 1b (Tnfrsf1β)	Immune and inflammatory response	Down	Down*	Down	A, B, D, E
Prostaglandin-endoperoxide synthase 2 (COX-2) (PTGS2)	Immune and inflammatory response	Down*	Down		C
Chemokine (C-C motif) receptor (Ccr5, Ccr7)	Immune and inflammatory response	Down			B
Interleukin (Il1β)	Immune and inflammatory response		Down	Down	A, B, C
Matrix metallopeptidase (Mmp3, Mmp9, Mmp13)	Leukocyte extravasation signalling		Down	Down	A, B, C

Table 2. Selected genes and their associated pathways that are up-regulated in the *Il10*$^{-/-}$ mouse model, compared to wild-type (WT) mice, and the effects of polyunsaturated fatty acids in mouse models of intestinal inflammation (Table constructed with information from (A) Cho et al., 2011; (B) Knoch et al., 2009; (C) Knoch et al., 2010a; (D) Knoch et al., 2010b; (E) Reiff et al., 2009). (*) indicates a non-significant change.

3.2.2 Modulation of gene expression by polyunsaturated fatty acids

PUFA-enriched diets were partly able to reduce expression levels of genes associated with inflammation (Table 1 and Table 2) (Cho et al., 2011; Deckelbaum et al., 2006; Knoch et al., 2009; Knoch et al., 2010a; Knoch et al., 2010b; Reiff et al., 2009). As illustrated in Table 1, expression levels of the PPARα gene were increased by EPA-enriched diets. This is supported by a study in a pig model of IBD, where dietary LA increased colonic PPARγ gene expression levels and dietary n-3 PUFA activated PPARδ (Bassaganya-Riera & Hontecillas, 2006). In this study (Bassaganya-Riera & Hontecillas, 2006), the onset of

experimental IBD was either delayed (PPARγ activation) or colonic regeneration and clinical remission accelerated (PPARδ activation). The expression levels of the gene encoding for the S100a8 protein, associated with neutrophil activation (Ryckman et al., 2003), was increased in UC patients compared to healthy subjects (Dieckgraefe et al., 2000). Its expression level was also increased in mice with experimental colitis compared to healthy mice; DHA- and AA-enriched diets were able to reduce increased S100a8 gene expression levels in *Il10*$^{-/-}$ mice, however, EPA-enriched diets were not (Cho et al., 2011; Knoch et al., 2009).
The transcription factors NFκB and PPARs are reported to be modulated in inflammatory states and by dietary PUFA (Calder, 2008; Chapkin et al., 2009; Wall et al., 2010). NFκB is a regulator of the inflammatory response and oxidative stress (Hassan et al., 2010) and its activation is triggered by extracellular inflammatory stimuli, followed by translocation of NFκB to the nucleus and an increase in expression levels of genes associated with inflammation (*e.g.* the cytokines IL1, IL6 or TNFα) (Calder, 2008). Fatty acids and eicosanoids are natural ligands of PPARs. When activated by ligand binding, PPARs dimerise with the retinoid X receptor (RXR) and the dimer subsequently binds to specific response elements (PPREs) within promoter regions of target genes, thus modulating transcription of the genes (Berger & Moller, 2002). The three isotypes PPARα, PPARβ/γ and PPARδ are encoded by different genes and exhibit broad, isotype-specific tissue expression patterns (Michalik et al., 2006). PPARγ activity can be inhibited by TNFα which consequently is associated with the pathogenesis of inflammation (Ye, 2008). PPARα was shown to be an important transcriptional regulator in the small intestine (Buenger et al., 2007) and reduced NFκB gene expression levels (Knoch et al., 2009). DHA and EPA are natural ligands of PPARα and its activation can trigger fatty acid oxidation, thus a deficiency in PPARα resulted in a dysfunction of hepatic fatty acid uptake and oxidation in an animal model (Lee & Kim, 2010).

3.3 Modulation of protein expression by polyunsaturated fatty acids

The analysis of gene expression explains only a part of the observed phenotype, as the increase or decrease of expression levels of a gene that code for a certain protein does not necessarily result in changed protein abundance (Ideker et al., 2001). Several influences, including the degradation of mRNA, post-translational modifications and the rate of degradation of the protein, can affect protein abundance. While there is published research on the effects of fatty acids on gene expression, there is less data available on its effects on protein expression. Proteomic analysis for IBD patients exists (Shkoda et al., 2007; Zhao et al., 2011) and has identified distinctive patterns in protein expression compared to healthy subjects. The studies showed that the biological processes inflammatory response and oxidative stress, signal transduction, energy generation including lipid metabolism and cell apoptosis were influenced (Shkoda et al., 2007; Zhao et al., 2011). How n-3 PUFA can influence protein expression in *Il10*$^{-/-}$ mice should therefore provide further insights into the putative molecular mechanisms behind the observed phenotypical changes between *Il10*$^{-/-}$ and control mice.

4. The role of foods in IBD

Minor components in foods such as antioxidants or PUFA are necessary for several processes in the human body (Visioli et al., 2003). The use of pure extracts of these components has occasionally been promoted and the effects of these single nutrients have been reviewed. For example, curcumin (a polyphenolic compound found in some foods such as the spice turmeric), reduced histological signs of colonic inflammation and the expression levels of genes in pro-inflammatory pathways in a mouse model of IBD (Nones et al., 2009). The influences of dietary PUFA supplementation on mice with chronic colitis were studied by Knoch et al. (2009; 2010a) and Roy et al. (2007). The results of these experiments showed mild anti-inflammatory effects for both n-3 and n-6 PUFA, the former *via* the activation of a PPARα transcription factor. However, single nutrients may exert different protective effects than whole foods which provide these components. Possible anti-inflammatory features of extracted long-chain n-3 PUFA (Calder, 2009; Knoch et al., 2009; Knoch et al., 2010a; Roy et al., 2007) may function differently when in a food matrix (Kris-Etherton & Hill, 2008). Dietary n-3 PUFA can be ingested as highly purified extracts of single n-3 PUFA, fish oil (mixture of PUFA) or marine fish (nutrient package and rich in n-3 PUFA). One of the advantages in the consumption of whole fish is nutritional diversity, which favours possible synergistic effects (He, 2009; Rudkowska et al., 2010).

4.1 The benefits of dietary fish intake

Compared to other foods, marine fish (especially salmon and tuna) are naturally rich in long-chain n-3 PUFA (Mozaffarian, 2006). Early evidence of potential health benefits of fish was found in the dietary habits of Greenland Eskimos (Bang et al., 1976). The food consumed by Eskimos is mostly of marine origin and provides high amounts of long-chain n-3 PUFA including EPA and DHA. An important correlation between dietary fish intake and a lower risk of coronary atherosclerotic diseases was found (Bang et al., 1976).

Long-chain n-3 PUFA accumulates in fish through the food chain (Sargent, 1997). The basis of the food chain is marine phytoplankton, which synthesises long-chain n-3 PUFA by conversion of LA to ALA (Hamilton et al., 2005). The uptake of phytoplankton by marine zooplankton leads to the accumulation of n-3 PUFA in the phospholipids of cellular membranes and through the ingestion of zooplankton, n-3 PUFA accumulates in fish. In general, deep water fish including salmon, herring, mackerel or tuna are classified as oily fish, with the main fat storage being the flesh. The lipid reserves of lean fish, for example cod, haddock or whiting, are in the liver. Cod liver is therefore a rich source of n-3 PUFA, as well as the fillets of salmon, herring etc. (Sargent, 1997). The n-3 PUFA content in fish varies with species, age, size, reproduction stage, season, geographical location and diet (Larsen et al., 2010).

The advantage of whole fish consumption compared to supplements is nutritional diversity. A common problem in IBD is malnutrition, caused by for example poor dietary intake or impaired nutrient absorption (O'Sullivan & O'Morain, 2006). Fish could compensate for the micronutrient deficiencies and provide a mechanism to elevate the levels of several minerals and vitamins. Of particular clinical relevance are deficiencies in calcium, vitamin D and B12, folate (Goh & O'Morain, 2003), zinc (Hendricks & Walker, 1988) and vitamin B6 (Saibeni et al., 2003), which are all contained in fish (Sidhu, 2003). Several of these micronutrients were able to suppress inflammation in rodents with experimental colitis. For example, vitamin E protected the rat colon from oxidative stress, which is associated with inflammation (González et al., 2001). Oxidised PUFA can activate transcription factors such as NFκB and subsequently trigger pro-inflammatory gene expression, whereby vitamin E as an antioxidant compound in salmon might prevent oxidation and in turn NFκB activation

(Calder et al., 2009). The supplementation of vitamin D and calcium showed protective effects in *Il10*$^{-/-}$ mice (associated with TNFα pathway) (Zhu et al., 2005) and selenium protected rats with experimental colitis (Tirosh et al., 2007). Furthermore, fish is also an excellent source of amino acids, such as taurine, arginine and glutamine, which may contribute to anti-inflammatory effects (He, 2009; Rudkowska et al., 2010).

A positive association of salmon with IBD has been identified among New Zealand CD patients (Triggs et al., 2010). 446 patients rated food items and their effects on disease symptoms. No single food item was considered beneficial in all cases, however a small number of foods were frequently perceived to be beneficial, including white fish, salmon and tuna. These results indicated that salmon was perceived to be one of the most beneficial foods for those patients. Furthermore, intervention studies involving patients with active CD showed a favourable influence of salmon on IBD. After 8 weeks of a dietary intake of 600 g Atlantic salmon per week, the clinical colitis activity index was improved and the n-3/n-6 ratio increased (Grimstad et al., 2011). Another study (Pot et al., 2010) revealed that after 6 months, patients with previous colorectal adenomas or non-active UC showed partially decreased inflammation markers. The patients consumed either fatty (farmed salmon) or lean fish (Icelandic cod) in 2 x 150 g portions per week. Interestingly, the consumption of cod (lean fish) showed the same results as the salmon group, suggesting that not only oily fish, but also lean fish can exert anti-inflammatory effects (Pot et al., 2010).

4.2 Whole foods vs. supplements

Bioavailability is defined as "the proportion of a drug or other substance which enters the circulation when introduced into the body and so is able to have an active effect"(Oxford Dictionaries, 2010). Dietary n-3 PUFA can be provided by fatty fish, fish oil capsules or *via* foods enriched with n-3 PUFA (*e.g.* milk and meat) (Kitessa et al., 2001; Knowles et al., 2004; Ponnampalam et al., 2002), however its bioavailability may differ between these formats. Fish intake may increase the bioavailability of n-3 PUFA because: (i) the ingestion of whole foods is followed by a more effective activation of digestion/absorption in the intestine compared to capsules (Elvevoll et al., 2006; Galli & Calder, 2009; Visioli et al., 2003); (ii) lipids in fish are mostly in form of TG, with n-3 PUFA mostly in position sn-2, which facilitates absorption (Aursand et al., 1995; Ratnayake & Galli, 2009); and (iii) the bioavailability of EPA is improved when co-ingested with a high-fat meal (Lawson & Hughes, 1988a). Human studies have found that the n-3 PUFA within salmon are more efficient at increasing n-3 PUFA levels in serum and plasma compared to fish oil capsules (Elvevoll et al., 2006; Visioli et al., 2003). However, this contrasts to results from Arterburn et al. (2008), who found that algal-oil capsules and cooked salmon are nutritionally equivalent sources of DHA, thus representing an alternative to fish. The results of these studies (Arterburn et al., 2008; Elvevoll et al., 2006; Visioli et al., 2003) may depend on several factors, for example genetic differences in the individual subjects, but also on the oxidation rate of n-3 PUFA in capsules or differences in encapsulation (*e.g.* hard vs. soft gelatine capsules) (Ferguson et al., 2010).

5. Limitations

Dietary recommendations of two servings of fish per week require unlimited sources of fish. However, wild-caught fish are finite and some species are already classified as over-fished

(Naylor et al., 2000). Producing farmed fish in aquacultures may not be sustainable long-term. Apart from water pollution or habitat destruction, aquacultures require large inputs of wild fish for feed (Jenkins et al., 2009; Naylor et al., 2000). For example, the production of one kilogram of farmed fish, raised on feeds fortified with fish meal and oil, requires approximately three kilograms of wild fish (Naylor et al., 2000). To lower fish input in feed, n-3 PUFA-rich fish oil was replaced by n-3 PUFA-deficient vegetable oil. However, this resulted in lower levels of n-3 PUFA in salmon flesh, which would therefore not serve the purpose of increasing DHA and EPA in the human diet.

For those who do not wish to consume fish, enrichment of foods which are not naturally rich in long-chain n-3 PUFA is an option (Bermingham et al., 2008; Calder & Yaqoob, 2009; Whelan et al., 2009). These include n-3 PUFA-enriched eggs, meat (Knowles et al., 2004; Ponnampalam et al., 2002) or milk (Kitessa et al., 2001) that can be produced by bio-fortification (feeding the animal n-3 PUFA-rich feeds) or post-harvest modification of foods (n-3 PUFA-rich oils into foods) (Bermingham et al., 2008; Whelan et al., 2009). However in most cases, fish oils are used for elevating the n-3 PUFA levels. In order to reduce pressure on wild fish stocks, it is important to find an alternative source of n-3 PUFA. A possible solution could be DHA-rich algal oil, which is considered as plant-derived, thus also appropriate for vegetarians for direct supplementation (Whelan & Rust, 2006).

Evidence for the protective effects of n-3 PUFA is inconsistent, possibly due to various factors (Ferguson et al., 2010). *In vitro* models can not mimic the complexity of an entire organism, which makes the use of animal models necessary. However, disease pathogenesis differs across animal models, thus making it difficult to compare results (Hegazi et al., 2003; Hegazi et al., 2006). Diets enriched with n-3 PUFA which are fed to animals differ in their sources and range from highly purified extracts of single PUFA (*i.e.* DHA or EPA) to fish oil and marine fish. Although these sources generally represent an excess of n-3 PUFA, bioavailability might change with the form provided (*e.g.* free fatty acids, ethyl esters, TG or embedded in a food matrix) (Lawson & Hughes, 1988b). Additionally, the time point of supplying the PUFA diets may be an important factor for the outcome of the study (Ramakers et al., 2008). As a preventive approach, the feeding of diets prior to colitis induction could exert different effects when compared with a therapeutic approach, in which the diets are fed when colitis is already present (Ramakers et al., 2008). An important factor is the dose of the supplemented n-3 PUFA. Trebble et al. (2003) demonstrated that the production of the pro-inflammatory cytokines TNFα and IL6 by cells appear to follow a 'U-shaped' dose response when n-3 PUFA supplementation was present. In this study, the supplementation of dietary fish oil in healthy humans resulted in a significantly decreased TNFα and IL6 production of the peripheral blood mononuclear cells at the lowest level (0.3 g n-3 PUFA per day). A maximum inhibition was observed at intermediate levels (1.0 g n-3 PUFA per day), but the least inhibition at highest supplementation levels (2.0 g n-3 PUFA per day). Thus, the dose of the dietary n-3 PUFA may considerably influence the outcome of n-3 PUFA supplementation studies (Trebble et al., 2003). A possible explanation for the observations might be found in the molecular mechanisms by which n-3 PUFA influences cell function, *i.e.* altered eicosanoid synthesis, signal transduction or gene expression. It is hypothesised that those mechanisms have maximum effects at different intake levels of n-3 PUFA and thus a 'U-shaped' dose-response curve results (Trebble et al., 2003).

6. Conclusion

Fish is high in protein, low in saturated fat and it provides high amounts of n-3 PUFA (He, 2009). Therefore, as part of a healthy lifestyle, fish should be consumed at least twice per week, and one of these servings should be oily fish (Kris-Etherton & Hill, 2008; Scientific Advisory Committee on Nutrition/Committee on Toxicity, 2004). The underlying molecular mechanisms by which salmon-containing diets influence intestinal inflammation are not well known. In *Il10*$^{-/-}$ mice, pure EPA can reduce colon inflammation and regulate gene and protein expression involved in various pathways (Knoch et al., 2009), leaving a unique dietary signature. A genome-wide approach can be applied with the use of 'omics'-technologies - transcriptomics (gene expression analysis) and proteomics (protein expression analysis) - to identify metabolic pathways and key gene/protein regulatory 'hubs' which are responsive to n-3 PUFA-enriched diets, and through which anti-inflammatory effects are exerted. A metabolomic approach can be used to identify metabolites in mouse urine and plasma samples that are influenced by the n-3 PUFA-enriched diets. These metabolites could serve as biomarkers for future human clinical intervention studies to assess the effect of these diets non-invasively. Future studies need to determine if the dietary intake of salmon is more beneficial than fish oil (mixture of n-3 PUFA) or single n-3 PUFA (*i.e.* DHA or EPA). Further, if the intake of fish has anti-inflammatory effects, can these be attributed to DHA or EPA, a combination, or synergistic effects with other nutrients?

7. Acknowledgement

This study is part of Nutrigenomics New Zealand, a collaboration between AgResearch, Plant and Food Research, and The University of Auckland, and is primarily funded by the New Zealand Ministry of Science and Innovation (MSI). Nadja Berger's PhD Fellowship is funded by AgResearch within the Nutrigenomics New Zealand partnership. The authors would like to thank Denise Martin and Dr Matthew Barnett (AgResearch) for manuscript reviewing.

8. References

Arrieta, M.C., Bistritz, L. & Meddings, J.B. (2006). Alterations in intestinal permeability. *Gut*, Vol. 55, No. 10, pp. 1512-1520, ISSN: 0017-5749

Arrieta, M.C., Madsen, K., Doyle, J. & Meddings, J. (2009). Reducing small intestinal permeability attenuates colitis in the IL10 gene-deficient mouse. *Gut*, Vol. 58, No. 1, pp. 41-48, ISSN: 1468-3288

Arterburn, L.M., Oken, H.A., Hall, E.B., Hamersley, J., Kuratko, C.N. & Hoffman, J.P. (2008). Algal-oil capsules and cooked salmon: Nutritionally equivalent sources of docosahexaenoic acid. *Journal of the American Dietetic Association*, Vol. 108, No. 7, pp. 1204-1209, ISSN: 0002-8223

Aursand, M., Jorgensen, L. & Grasdalen, H. (1995). Positional distribution of omega-3-fatty-acids in marine lipid triacylglycerols by high-resolution C-13 nuclear-magnetic-resonance spectroscopy. *Journal of the American Oil Chemists Society*, Vol. 72, No. 3, pp. 293-297, ISSN: 0003-021X

Balda, M.S., Fallon, M.B., Van Itallie, C.M. & Anderson, J.M. (1992). Structure, regulation, and pathophysiology of tight junctions in the gastrointestinal tract. *Yale J Biol Med*, Vol. 65, No. 6, pp. 725-735, ISSN: 0044-0086

Bang, H.O., Dyerberg, J. & Hjoorne, N. (1976). The composition of food consumed by Greenland Eskimos. *Acta Med Scand*, Vol. 200, No. 1-2, pp. 69-73, ISSN: 0001-6101

Bassaganya-Riera, J. & Hontecillas, R. (2006). CLA and n-3 PUFA differentially modulate clinical activity and colonic PPAR-responsive gene expression in a pig model of experimental IBD. *Clinical Nutrition*, Vol. 25, No. 3, pp. 454-465, ISSN: 0261-5614

Berger, J. & Moller, D.E. (2002). The mechanisms of action of PPARs. *Annu Rev Med*, Vol. 53, pp. 409-435, ISSN: 0066-4219

Bermingham, E., Roy, N., Anderson, R., Barnett, M., Knowles, S.O. & McNabb, W. (2008). Smart Foods from the pastoral sector - implications for meat and milk producers. *Austral J Experimental Agriculture*, Vol. 48, pp. 726-734

Bordoni, A., Di Nunzio, M., Danesi, F. & Biagi, P.L. (2006). Polyunsaturated fatty acids: From diet to binding to PPARs and other nuclear receptors. *Genes Nutr*, Vol. 1, No. 2, pp. 95-106, ISSN: 1555-8932

Bouma, G. & Strober, W. (2003). The immunological and genetic basis of inflammatory bowel disease. *Nat Rev Immunol*, Vol. 3, No. 7, pp. 521-533, ISSN: 1474-1733

Buenger, M., van den Bosch, H.M., van der Meijde, J., Kersten, S., Hooiveld, G.J.E.J. & Mueller, M. (2007). Genome-wide analysis of PPAR(alpha) activation in murine small intestine. *Physiol Genomics*, Vol. 30, pp. 192-204

Burdge, G.C. & Calder, P.C. (2005). Conversion of alpha-linolenic acid to longer-chain polyunsaturated fatty acids in human adults. *Reprod Nutr Dev*, Vol. 45, No. 5, pp. 581-597, ISSN: 0926-5287

Calder, P.C. (2006). Polyunsaturated fatty acids and inflammation. *Prostaglandins Leukot Essent Fatty Acids*, Vol. 75, pp. 197-202

Calder, P.C. & Yaqoob, P. (2007). Lipid rafts - composition, characterization, and controversies. *J Nutr*, Vol. 137, No. 3, pp. 545-547, ISSN: 0022-3166

Calder, P.C. (2008). Polyunsaturated fatty acids, inflammatory processes and inflammatory bowel disease. *Mol Nutr Food Res*, Vol. 52, pp. 885-897

Calder, P.C., Albers, R., Antoine, J.M., Blum, S., Bourdet-Sicard, R., Ferns, G.A., Folkerts, G., Friedmann, P.S., Frost, G.S., Guarner, F., Lovik, M., Macfarlane, S., Meyer, P.D., M'Rabet, L., Serafini, M., van Eden, W., van Loo, J., Vas Dias, W., Vidry, S., Winklhofer-Roob, B.M. & Zhao, J. (2009). Inflammatory disease processes and interactions with nutrition. *Br J Nutr*, Vol. 101, No. Suppl S1, pp. S1-45, ISSN: 1475-2662

Calder, P.C. & Yaqoob, P. (2009). Omega-3 polyunsaturated fatty acids and human health outcomes. *Biofactors*, Vol. 35, No. 3, pp. 266-272, ISSN: 0951-6433

Calder, P.C. (2009). Polyunsaturated fatty acids and inflammatory processes: New twists in an old tale. *Biochimie*, Vol. 91, pp. 791-795

Camuesco, D., Galvez, J., Nieto, A., Comalada, M., Rodriguez-Cabezas, M.E., Concha, A., Xaus, J. & Zarzuelo, A. (2005). Dietary olive oil supplemented with fish oil, rich in EPA and DHA (n-3) polyunsaturated fatty acids, attenuates colonic inflammation in rats with DSS-induced colitis. *Journal of Nutrition*, Vol. 135, No. 4, pp. 687-694, ISSN: 0022-3166

Chapkin, R.S., Kim, W., Lupton, J.R. & McMurray, D.N. (2009). Dietary docosahexaenoic and eicosapentaenoic acid: Emerging mediators of inflammation. *Prostaglandins, Leukotrienes and Essential Fatty Acids*, Vol. 81, pp. 187-191

Cho, J.Y., Chi, S.G. & Chun, H.S. (2011). Oral administration of docosahexaenoic acid attenuates colitis induced by dextran sulfate sodium in mice. *Molecular Nutrition & Food Research*, Vol. 55, No. 2, pp. 239-246, ISSN: 1613-4125

Connor, W.E. (2000). Importance of n-3 fatty acids in health and disease. *American Journal of Clinical Nutrition*, Vol. 71, No. 1, pp. 171S-175S, ISSN: 0002-9165

Crotty, B. (1994). Ulcerative colitis and xenobiotic metabolism. *The Lancet*, Vol. 343, No. 8888, pp. 35-38, ISSN: 0140-6736

Deckelbaum, R.J., Worgall, T.S. & Seo, T. (2006). N-3 fatty acids and gene expression. *Am J Clin Nutr*, Vol. 83, No. 6 Suppl, pp. 1520S-1525S, ISSN: 0002-9165

Dieckgraefe, B., Stenson, W., Korzenik, J., Swanson, P. & Harrington, C. (2000). Analysis of mucosal gene expression in inflammatory bowel disease by parallel oligonucleotide arrays. *Physiological Genomics*, Vol. 4, pp. 1-11, ISSN: 1094-8341

Duchmann, R., Kaiser, I., Hermann, E., Mayet, W., Ewe, K. & Meyer zum Buschenfelde, K.H. (1995). Tolerance exists towards resident intestinal flora but is broken in active inflammatory bowel disease (IBD). *Clin Exp Immunol*, Vol. 102, No. 3, pp. 448-455, ISSN: 0009-9104

Elvevoll, E.O., Barstad, H., Breimo, E.S., Brox, J., Eilertsen, K.E., Lund, T., Olsen, J.O. & Osterud, B. (2006). Enhanced incorporation of n-3 fatty acids from fish compared with fish oils. *Lipids*, Vol. 41, No. 12, pp. 1109-1114, ISSN: 0024-4201

Fahy, E., Subramaniam, S., Brown, H.A., Glass, C.K., Merrill, A.H., Jr., Murphy, R.C., Raetz, C.R., Russell, D.W., Seyama, Y., Shaw, W., Shimizu, T., Spener, F., van Meer, G., VanNieuwenhze, M.S., White, S.H., Witztum, J.L. & Dennis, E.A. (2005). A comprehensive classification system for lipids. *J Lipid Res*, Vol. 46, No. 5, pp. 839-861, ISSN: 0022-2275

Farhadi, A., Banan, A., Fields, J. & Keshavarzian, A. (2003). Intestinal barrier: an interface between health and disease. *J Gastroenterol Hepatol*, Vol. 18, No. 5, pp. 479-497, ISSN: 0815-9319

Ferguson, L.R., Smith, B.G. & James, B.J. (2010). Combining nutrition, food science and engineering in developing solutions to Inflammatory bowel diseases - omega-3 polyunsaturated fatty acids as an example. *Food & Function*, Vol. 1, No. 1, pp. 60-72, ISSN: 2042-6496

Ferguson, L.R. (2010). Nutrigenomics and inflammatory bowel diseases. *Expert Review of Clinical Immunology*, Vol. 6, No. 4, pp. 573-583, ISSN: 1744-666X

Forster, C. (2008). Tight junctions and the modulation of barrier function in disease. *Histochem Cell Biol*, Vol. 130, No. 1, pp. 55-70, ISSN: 0948-6143

Galli, C. & Calder, P.C. (2009). Effects of fat and fatty acid intake on inflammatory and immune responses: A critical review. *Ann Nutr Metab*, Vol. 55, pp. 123-139

Garg, M.L., Wood, L.G., Singh, H. & Moughan, P.J. (2006). Means of delivering recommended levels of long chain n-3 polyunsaturated fatty acids in human diets. *Journal of Food Science*, Vol. 71, No. 5, pp. R66-R71, ISSN: 0022-1147

Goh, J. & O'Morain, C.A. (2003). Nutrition and adult inflammatory bowel disease. *Alimentary Pharmacology & Therapeutics*, Vol. 17, No. 3, pp. 307-320, ISSN: 1365-2036

González, R., Sanchez de Medina, F., Gálvez, J., Rodriguez-Cabezas, J., Duarte, J. & Zarzuelo, A. (2001). Dietary vitamin E supplementation protects the rat large intestine from experimental inflammation. *International journal for vitamin and nutrition research*, Vol. 71, No. 4, pp. 243-250, ISSN: 0300-9831

Grimstad, T., Berge, R.K., Bohov, P., Skorve, J., Goransson, L., Omdal, R., Aasprong, O.G., Haugen, M., Meltzer, H.M. & Hausken, T. (2011). Salmon diet in patients with active ulcerative colitis reduced the simple clinical colitis activity index and increased the anti-inflammatory fatty acid index - a pilot study. *Scand J Clin Lab Invest*, Vol. 71, No. 1, pp. 68-73, ISSN: 1502-7686

Hamilton, M.C., Hites, R.A., Schwager, S.J., Foran, J.A., Knuth, B.A. & Carpenter, D.O. (2005). Lipid composition and contaminants in farmed and wild salmon. *Environ Sci Technol*, Vol. 39, No. 22, pp. 8622-8629, ISSN: 0013-936X

Hanauer, S.B. (2006). Inflammatory bowel disease: Epidemiology, pathogenesis, and therapeutic opportunities. *Inflammatory Bowel Diseases*, Vol. 12, pp. S3-S9, ISSN: 1078-0998

Hassan, A., Ibrahim, A., Mbodji, K., Coeffier, M., Ziegler, F., Bounoure, F., Chardigny, J.M., Skiba, M., Savoye, G., Dechelotte, P. & Marion-Letellier, R. (2010). An {alpha}-linolenic acid-rich formula reduces oxidative stress and inflammation by regulating NF-{kappa}B in rats with TNBS-induced colitis. *J Nutr*, Vol. 140, pp. 1714-1721, ISSN: 1541-6100

He, K. (2009). Fish, long-chain omega-3 polyunsaturated fatty acids and prevention of cardiovascular disease-eat fish or take fish oil supplement? *Progress in Cardiovascular Diseases*, Vol. 52, No. 2, pp. 95-114, ISSN: 0033-0620

Hegazi, R.A.F., Mady, H.H., Melhem, M.F., Sepulveda, A.R., Mohi, M. & Kandil, H.M. (2003). Celecoxib and rofecoxib potentiate chronic colitis and premalignant changes in interleukin 10 knockout mice. *Inflammatory Bowel Diseases*, Vol. 9, No. 4, pp. 230-236, ISSN: 1078-0998

Hegazi, R.A.F., Saad, R.S., Mady, H., Matarese, L.E., O'Keefe, S. & Kandil, H.M. (2006). Dietary fatty acids modulate chronic colitis, colitis-associated colon neoplasia and COX-2 expression in IL-10 knockout mice. *Nutrition*, Vol. 22, No. 3, pp. 275-282, ISSN: 0899-9007

Heimerl, S., Moehle, C., Zahn, A., Boettcher, A., Stremmel, W., Langmann, T. & Schmitz, G. (2006). Alterations in intestinal fatty acid metabolism in inflammatory bowel disease. *Biochimica Et Biophysica Acta-Molecular Basis of Disease*, Vol. 1762, No. 3, pp. 341-350, ISSN: 0925-4439

Hendricks, K.M. & Walker, W.A. (1988). Zinc Deficiency in Inflammatory Bowel Disease. *Nutrition Reviews*, Vol. 46, No. 12, pp. 401-408, ISSN: 1753-4887

Hinds, D.A., Stuve, L.L., Nilsen, G.B., Halperin, E., Eskin, E., Ballinger, D.G., Frazer, K.A. & Cox, D.R. (2005). Whole-genome patterns of common DNA variation in three human populations. *Science*, Vol. 307, No. 5712, pp. 1072-1079, ISSN: 0036-8075

Hugot, J.P., Laurent-Puig, P., Gower-Rousseau, C., Olson, J.M., Lee, J.C., Beaugerie, L., Naom, I., Dupas, J.L., Van Gossum, A., Orholm, M., Bonaiti-Pellie, C., Weissenbach, J., Mathew, C.G., Lennard-Jones, J.E., Cortot, A., Colombel, J.F. & Thomas, G. (1996). Mapping of a susceptibility locus for Crohn's disease on chromosome 16. *Nature*, Vol. 379, No. 6568, pp. 821-823, ISSN: 0028-0836

Hugot, J.P., Chamaillard, M., Zouali, H., Lesage, S., Cezard, J.P., Belaiche, J., Almer, S., Tysk, C., O'Morain, C.A., Gassull, M., Binder, V., Finkel, Y., Cortot, A., Modigliani, R., Laurent-Puig, P., Gower-Rousseau, C., Macry, J., Colombel, J.F., Sahbatou, M. & Thomas, G. (2001). Association of NOD2 leucine-rich repeat variants with susceptibility to Crohn's disease. *Nature*, Vol. 411, No. 6837, pp. 599-603, ISSN: 0028-0836

Ideker, T., Galitski, T. & Hood, L. (2001). A new approach to decoding life: Systems biology. *Annual Review of Genomics and Human Genetics*, Vol. 2, pp. 343-372, ISSN: 1527-8204

Jakoby, W.B. & Ziegler, D.M. (1990). The enzymes of detoxication. *Journal of Biological Chemistry*, Vol. 265, No. 34, pp. 20715-20718

Jenkins, D.J.A., Sievenpiper, J.L., Pauly, D., Sumaila, U.R., Kendall, C.W.C. & Mowat, F.M. (2009). Are dietary recommendations for the use of fish oils sustainable? *Canadian Medical Association Journal*, Vol. 180, No. 6, pp. 633-637, ISSN: 0820-3946

Jump, D.B. & Clarke, S.D. (1999). Regulation of gene expression by dietary fat. *Annual Review of Nutrition*, Vol. 19, pp. 63-90, ISSN: 0199-9885

Kitessa, S.M., Gulati, S.K., Ashes, J.R., Fleck, E., Scott, T.W. & Nichols, P.D. (2001). Utilisation of fish oil in ruminants - II. Transfer of fish oil fatty acids into goats' milk. *Animal Feed Science and Technology*, Vol. 89, No. 3-4, pp. 201-208, ISSN: 0377-8401

Knoch, B., Barnett, M.P.G., Zhu, S., Park, Z.A., Nones, K., Dommels, Y.E.M., Knowles, S.O., McNabb, W. & Roy, N.C. (2009). Genome-wide analysis of dietary eiosapentaenoic acid- and oleic acid-induced modulation of colon inflammation in interleukin-10-deficient mice. *J Nutrigenet Nutrigenomics*, Vol. 2, pp. 9-28

Knoch, B., Barnett, M.P., McNabb, W.C., Zhu, S., Park, Z.A., Khan, A. & Roy, N.C. (2010a). Dietary arachidonic acid-mediated effects on colon inflammation using transcriptome analysis. *Mol Nutr Food Res*, Vol. 54, No. 1 Suppl, pp. S62-74, ISSN: 1613-4133

Knoch, B., Barnett, M.P.G., Cooney, J., McNabb, W.C., Barraclough, D., Laing, W., Zhu, S.T., Park, Z.A., MacLean, P., Knowles, S.O. & Roy, N.C. (2010b). Molecular characterization of the onset and progression of colitis in inoculated interleukin-10 gene-deficient mice: A role for PPAR alpha. *Ppar Research*, ISSN: 1687-4757

Knowles, S.O., Grace, N.D., Knight, T.W., McNabb, W.C. & Lee, J. (2004). Adding nutritional value to meat and milk from pasture-fed livestock. *New Zealand Veterinary Journal*, Vol. 52, No. 6, pp. 342-351, ISSN: 0048-0169

Kris-Etherton, P.M. & Hill, A.M. (2008). N-3 fatty acids: food or supplements? *J Am Diet Assoc*, Vol. 108, No. 7, pp. 1125-1130, ISSN: 0002-8223

Krishnan, A. & Korzenik, J.R. (2002). Inflammatory bowel disease and environmental influences. *Gastroenterology Clinics of North America*, Vol. 31, No. 1, pp. 21-39, ISSN: 0889-8553

Langmann, T. & Schmitz, G. (2006). Loss of detoxification in inflammatory bowel disease. *Nature Clinical Practice Gastroenterology & Hepatology*, Vol. 3, No. 7, pp. 358-359, ISSN: 1743-4378

Larsen, D., Quek, S.Y. & Eyres, L. (2010). Effect of cooking method on the fatty acid profile of New Zealand king salmon (*Oncorhynchus tshawytscha*). *Food Chem*, Vol. 119, pp. 785-790

Lawson, L.D. & Hughes, B.G. (1988a). Absorption of eicosapentaenoic acid and docosahexaenoic acid from fish oil triacylglycerols or fish oil ethyl-esters co-ingested with a high-fat meal. *Biochemical and Biophysical Research Communications*, Vol. 156, No. 2, pp. 960-963, ISSN: 0006-291X

Lawson, L.D. & Hughes, B.G. (1988b). Human absorption of fish oil as triacylglycerols, free acids, or ethyl-esters. *Biochemical and Biophysical Research Communications*, Vol. 152, No. 1, pp. 328-335, ISSN: 0006-291X

Lee, G. & Buchman, A.L. (2009). DNA-driven nutritional therapy of inflammatory bowel disease. *Nutrition*, Vol. 25, pp. 885-891

Lee, W.H. & Kim, S.G. (2010). AMPK-dependent metabolic regulation by PPAR agonists. *Ppar Research*, Vol. 2010

Lees, C.W., Barrett, J.C., Parkes, M. & Satsangi, J. (2011). New IBD genetics: common pathways with other diseases. *Gut*

Leslie, C.C. (2004). Regulation of arachidonic acid availability for eicosanoid production. *Biochem Cell Biol*, Vol. 82, No. 1, pp. 1-17, ISSN: 0829-8211

Li, Q., Wang, M., Tan, L., Wang, C., Ma, J., Li, N., Li, Y., Xu, G. & Li, J. (2005). Docosahexaenoic acid changes lipid composition and interleukin-2 receptor signaling in membrane rafts. *J Lipid Res*, Vol. 46, No. 9, pp. 1904-1913

Loftus, E.V. (2004). Clinical epidemiology of inflammatory bowel disease: Incidence, prevalence, and environmental influences. *Gastroenterology*, Vol. 126, No. 6, pp. 1504-1517, ISSN: 0016-5085

Michalik, L., Auwerx, J., Berger, J., Chatterjee, V., Glass, C., Gonzalez, F., Grimaldi, P., Kadowaki, T., Lazar, M. & O'Rahilly, S. (2006). International Union of Pharmacology. LXI. Peroxisome proliferator-activated receptors. *Pharmacol Rev*, Vol. 58, No. 4, pp. 726-741, ISSN: 0031-6997

Mozaffarian, D. (2006). Fish intake, contaminants, and human health: Evaluating the risks and the benefits. Part 2 - Health risks and optimal intakes. *CardiologyRounds*, Vol. 10, No. 9

Mu, H. & Porsgaard, T. (2005). The metabolism of structured triacylglycerols. *Prog Lipid Res*, Vol. 44, No. 6, pp. 430-448, ISSN: 0163-7827

Müller, M. & Kersten, S. (2003). Nutrigenomics: Goals and strategies. *Genetics*, Vol. 4, pp. 315-322

Naylor, R.L., Goldburg, R.J., Primavera, J.H., Kautsky, N., Beveridge, M.C.M., Clay, J., Folke, C., Lubchenco, J., Mooney, H. & Troell, M. (2000). Effect of aquaculture on world fish supplies. *Nature*, Vol. 405, No. 6790, pp. 1017-1024, ISSN: 0028-0836

Nones, K., Dommels, Y.E., Martell, S., Butts, C., McNabb, W.C., Park, Z.A., Zhu, S., Hedderley, D., Barnett, M.P. & Roy, N.C. (2009). The effects of dietary curcumin and rutin on colonic inflammation and gene expression in multidrug resistance gene-deficient (mdr1a-/-) mice, a model of inflammatory bowel diseases. *Br J Nutr*, Vol. 101, No. 2, pp. 169-181, ISSN: 1475-2662

O'Sullivan, M. & O'Morain, C. (2006). Nutrition in inflammatory bowel disease. *Best Practice & Research in Clinical Gastroenterology*, Vol. 20, No. 3, pp. 561-573, ISSN: 1521-6918

Oxford Dictionaries. (2010). Bioavailability, In: *Oxford Dictionaries*, 22 February 2011, Available from: http://oxforddictionaries.com/view/entry/m_en_gb0078450

Ponnampalam, E.N., Sinclair, A.J., Egan, A.R., Ferrier, G.R. & Leury, B.J. (2002). Dietary manipulation of muscle long-chain omega-3 and omega-6 fatty acids and sensory properties of lamb meat. *Meat Science*, Vol. 60, No. 2, pp. 125-132, ISSN: 0309-1740

Pot, G.K., Geelen, A., Majsak-Newman, G., Harvey, L.J., Nagengast, F.M., Witteman, B.J.M., van de Meeberg, P.C., Hart, A.R., Schaafsma, G., Lund, E.K., Rijkers, G.I. & Kampman, E. (2010). Increased consumption of fatty and lean fish reduces serum c-reactive protein concentrations but not inflammation markers in feces and in colonic biopsies. *Journal of Nutrition*, Vol. 140, No. 2, pp. 371-376, ISSN: 0022-3166

Ramakers, J.D., Mensink, R.P., Verstege, M.I., Velde, A.A.T. & Plat, J. (2008). An arachidonic acid-enriched diet does not result in more colonic inflammation as compared with fish oil- or oleic acid-enriched diets in mice with experimental colitis. *British Journal of Nutrition*, Vol. 100, No. 2, pp. 347-354, ISSN: 0007-1145

Ratnayake, W.M. & Galli, C. (2009). Fat and fatty acid terminology, methods of analysis and fat digestion and metabolism: a background review paper. *Ann Nutr Metab*, Vol. 55, No. 1-3, pp. 8-43, ISSN: 1421-9697

Reiff, C., Delday, M., Rucklidge, G., Reid, M., Duncan, G., Wohlgemuth, S., Hormannsperger, G., Loh, G., Blaut, M., Collie-Duguid, E., Haller, D. & Kelly, D. (2009). Balancing inflammatory, lipid, and xenobiotic signaling pathways by VSL#3, a biotherapeutic agent, in the treatment of Inflammatory Bowel Disease. *Inflammatory Bowel Diseases*, Vol. 15, No. 11, pp. 1721-1736, ISSN: 1078-0998

Rockett, B.D., Franklin, A., Harris, M., Teague, H., Rockett, A. & Shaikh, S.R. (2011). Membrane raft organization is more sensitive to disruption by (n-3) PUFA than nonraft organization in EL4 and B cells. *The Journal of Nutrition*, Vol. 141, No. 6, pp. 1041-1048

Roy, N.C., Barnett, M.P.G., Knoch, B., Dommels, Y. & McNabb, W. (2007). Nutrigenomics applied to an animal model of inflammatory bowel disease: Transciptomic analysis of the effects of eicosapentaenoic acid- and arachidonic acid-enriched diets. *Mutat Res*, Vol. 622, pp. 103-116

Rudkowska, I., Marcotte, B., Pilon, G., Lavigne, C., Marette, A. & Vohl, M.C. (2010). Fish nutrients decrease expression levels of tumor necrosis factor-alpha in cultured human macrophages. *Physiological Genomics*, Vol. 40, No. 3, pp. 189-194, ISSN: 1094-8341

Ryckman, C., Vandal, K., Rouleau, P., Talbot, M. & Tessier, P.A. (2003). Proinflammatory activities of S100: Proteins S100A8, S100A9, and S100A8/A9 induce neutrophil chemotaxis and adhesion. *Journal of Immunology*, Vol. 170, No. 6, pp. 3233-3242, ISSN: 00221767

Saibeni, S., Cattaneo, M., Vecchi, M., Zighetti, M.L., Lecchi, A., Lombardi, R., Meucci, G., Spina, L. & Franchis, R. (2003). Low vitamin B6 plasma levels, a risk factor for thrombosis, in Inflammatory Bowel Disease: Role of inflammation and correlation with acute phase reactants. *Am J Gastroenterol*, Vol. 98, No. 1, pp. 112-117, ISSN: 0002-9270

Sargent, J.R. (1997). Fish oils and human diet. *British Journal of Nutrition*, Vol. 78, No. 1, pp. S5-S13, ISSN: 0007-1145

Sartor, R.B. (1995). Current concepts of the etiology and pathogenesis of ulcerative colitis and Crohn's disease. *Gastroenterol Clin North Am*, Vol. 24, No. 3, pp. 475-507, ISSN: 0889-8553

Schley, P.D., Brindley, D.N. & Field, C.J. (2007). (n-3) PUFA alter raft lipid composition and decrease epidermal growth factor receptor levels in lipid rafts of human breast cancer cells. *The Journal of Nutrition*, Vol. 137, No. 3, pp. 548-553

Scientific Advisory Committee on Nutrition/Committee on Toxicity (2004). Advice on fish consumption: Benefits & risks. TSO, London.

Serhan, C.N., Chiang, N. & Dyke, T.E.V. (2008). Resolving inflammation: Dual anti-inflammatory and pro-resolution lipid mediators. *Nat Rev Immunol*, Vol. 8, pp. 349-361

Shkoda, A., Werner, T., Daniel, H., Gunckel, M., Rogler, G. & Haller, D. (2007). Differential protein expression profile in the intestinal epithelium from patients with Inflammatory Bowel Disease. *Journal of Proteome Research*, Vol. 6, No. 3, pp. 1114-1125, ISSN: 1535-3893

Sidhu, K.S. (2003). Health benefits and potential risks related to consumption of fish or fish oil. *Regulatory Toxicology and Pharmacology*, Vol. 38, No. 3, pp. 336-344, ISSN: 0273-2300

Simopoulos, A.P. (1991). Omega-3-fatty-acids in health and disease and in growth and development. *American Journal of Clinical Nutrition*, Vol. 54, No. 3, pp. 438-463, ISSN: 0002-9165

Simopoulos, A.P. (2008). The importance of the omega-6/omega-3 fatty acid ratio in cardiovascular disease and other chronic diseases. *Exp Biol Med (Maywood)*, Vol. 233, No. 6, pp. 674-688, ISSN: 1535-3702

Stover, P.J. (2006). Influence of human genetic variation on nutritional requirements. *American Journal of Clinical Nutrition*, Vol. 83, No. 2, pp. 436S-442S, ISSN: 0002-9165

Stulnig, T.M., Huber, J., Leitinger, N., Imre, E.-M., Angelisová, P., Nowotny, P. & Waldhäusl, W. (2001). Polyunsaturated eicosapentaenoic acid displaces proteins from membrane rafts by altering raft lipid composition. *Journal of Biological Chemistry*, Vol. 276, No. 40, pp. 37335-37340

Subbiah, M.T.R. (2008). Understanding the nutrigenomic definitions and concepts at the food-genome junction. *Omics - a Journal of Integrative Biology*, Vol. 12, No. 4, pp. 229-235, ISSN: 1536-2310

Teitelbaum, J.E. & Allan Walker, W. (2001). Review: the role of omega 3 fatty acids in intestinal inflammation. *J Nutr Biochem*, Vol. 12, No. 1, pp. 21-32, ISSN: 1873-4847

Tirosh, O., Levy, E. & Reifen, R. (2007). High selenium diet protects against TNBS-induced acute inflammation, mitochondrial dysfunction, and secondary necrosis in rat colon. *Nutrition*, Vol. 23, No. 11-12, pp. 878-886, ISSN: 0899-9007

Trebble, T., Arden, N.K., Stroud, M.A., Wootton, S.A., Burdge, G.C., Miles, E.A., Ballinger, A.B., Thompson, R.L. & Calder, P.C. (2003). Inhibition of tumour necrosis factor-alpha and interleukin 6 production by mononuclear cells following dietary fish-oil supplementation in healthy men and response to antioxidant co-supplementation. *British Journal of Nutrition*, Vol. 90, No. 2, pp. 405-412, ISSN: 0007-1145

Triggs, C.M., Munday, K., Hu, R., Fraser, A.G., Gearry, R.B., Barclay, M.L. & Ferguson, L.R. (2010). Dietary factors in chronic inflammation: Food tolerances and intolerances of a New Zealand Caucasian Crohn's disease population. *Mutat Res*, pp. Fundam. Mol. Mech. Mutagen., ISSN: 0027-5107

Visioli, F., Rise, P., Barassi, M.C., Marangoni, F. & Galli, C. (2003). Dietary intake of fish vs. formulations leads to higher plasma concentrations of n-3 fatty acids. *Lipids*, Vol. 38, No. 4, pp. 415-418, ISSN: 0024-4201

Wahrburg, U. (2004). What are the health effects of fat? *Eur J Nurt*, Vol. 43, pp. I/6-I/11

Wall, R., Ross, R.P., Fitzgerald, G.F. & Stanton, C. (2010). Fatty acids from fish: The anti-inflammatory potential of long-chain omega-3 fatty acids. *Nutrition Reviews*, Vol. 68, No. 5, pp. 280-289, ISSN: 0029-6643

Weaver, K.L., Ivester, P., Seeds, M., Case, L.D., Arm, J.P. & Chilton, F.H. (2009). Effect of dietary fatty acids on inflammatory gene expression in healthy humans. *J Biol Chem*, Vol. 284, No. 23, pp. 15400-15407, ISSN: 0021-9258

Whelan, J. & Rust, C. (2006). Innovative dietary sources of n-3 fatty acids. *Annual Review of Nutrition*, Vol. 26, pp. 75-103, ISSN: 0199-9885

Whelan, J., Jahns, L. & Kavanagh, K. (2009). Docosahexaenoic acid: Measurements in food and dietary exposure. *Prostaglandins Leukotrienes and Essential Fatty Acids*, Vol. 81, No. 2-3, pp. 133-136, ISSN: 0952-3278

Yamamoto, T., Nakahigashi, M. & Saniabadi, A.R. (2009). Review article: diet and inflammatory bowel disease - epidemiology and treatment. *Alimentary Pharmacology & Therapeutics*, Vol. 30, No. 2, pp. 99-112, ISSN: 0269-2813

Ye, J. (2008). Regulation of PPARgamma function by TNF-alpha. *Biochemical and Biophysical Research Communications*, Vol. 374, No. 3, pp. 405-408, ISSN: 0006-291X

Zhao, X.M., Kang, B., Lu, C.L., Liu, S.Q., Wang, H.J., Yang, X.M., Chen, Y., Jiang, B., Zhang, J., Lu, Y.Y. & Zhi, F.C. (2011). Evaluation of P38 MAPK pathway as a molecular signature in Ulcerative Colitis. *Journal of Proteome Research*, Vol. 10, No. 5, pp. 2216-2225, ISSN: 1535-3893

Zhu, Y., Mahon, B.D., Froicu, M. & Cantorna, M.T. (2005). Calcium and 1α,25-dihydroxyvitamin D3 target the TNF-α pathway to suppress experimental inflammatory bowel disease. *European Journal of Immunology*, Vol. 35, No. 1, pp. 217-224, ISSN: 1521-4141